BIOPHYSICAL TECHNIQUES SERIES

Editor
R. A. DWEK

BIOPHYSICAL TECHNIQUES SERIES

1 S. W. HOMANS *A dictionary of concepts in NMR*

A Dictionary of Concepts in NMR

S. W. HOMANS
University Lecturer
Department of Biochemistry
University of Dundee

CLARENDON PRESS • OXFORD
1992

Oxford University Press, Walton Street, Oxford OX2 6DP

Oxford New York Toronto
Delhi Bombay Calcutta Madras Karachi
Petaling Jaya Singapore Hong Kong Tokyo
Nairobi Dar es Salaam Cape Town
Melbourne Auckland

and associated companies in
Berlin Ibadan

Oxford is a trade mark of Oxford University Press

Published in the United States
by Oxford University Press, New York

First published 1989
Reprinted 1991
Revised paperback edition published 1992

British Library Cataloguing in Publication Data

Homans, S. W.
A dictionary of concepts in NMR.
1. Nuclear magnetic resonance
I. Title II. Series
538'.362

ISBN 0–19–855274–2
ISBN 0–19–854765–X (Pbk)

Library of Congress Cataloging in Publication Data

Homans, S. W.
A dictionary of concepts in NMR/S. W. Homans.
(Biophysical techniques series)
Bibliography:
Includes index.
1. Nuclear magnetic resonance spectroscopy—Dictionaries.
I. Title II. Title: Dictionary of concepts in nuclear magnetic resonance. III. Series: Biophysical techniques series (Oxford, England)
QD96.N8H65 1989 543'.0877'03—dc20 89-3378 CIP
ISBN 0–19–855274–2
ISBN 0–19–854765–X (Pbk)

Printed in Great Britain by
Bookcraft (Bath) Ltd, Midsomer Norton, Avon

Preface

THE aim of this work is to aid chemists and biochemists familiar with the basic principles of NMR to understand the bewildering array of acronyms and technical jargon which is to be found in the literature. I have chosen a dictionary format since this work is intended to be used as a reference source rather than to be read from cover to cover. In common with present experimental trends, the text is biased heavily towards two-dimensional NMR methods in liquids. These have had a particularly significant impact in studies upon biological systems, and it is hoped that this book will be of particular value to biochemists interested in the inner workings of the experiments and techniques which they routinely use. To this end I have tried to describe the various experiments available to date in particular detail, with cross-reference to the various technical terms where necessary.

I emphasize that I claim no originality for the theoretical framework described here. I have drawn heavily upon the literature of recent years, but have attempted to describe some of the more difficult concepts in a manner which hopefully will be understandable to all who have a basic knowledge of NMR. Although the descriptions are often mathematical, the reader should not recoil from the apparent complexity associated with many of the entries. From personal experience this approach looks more difficult than it really is, and all that is required to understand it is a very rudimentary knowledge of mathematics. The advantage of a quantum mechanical treatment of concepts rather than a simple classical picture, is that one can gain an essentially complete understanding of a given experiment which helps enormously in optimizing it for a given application.

At the end of many entries will be found references for further reading. I have kept these to a minimum, since the purpose of this work is to obviate the need to plough through the original literature in search of a particular concept or technique. Explicit reference in the text is also avoided for the sake of clarity, with apologies to those whose work this approach fails to accredit.

Clearly a work of this size would not have been possible without the contributions of colleagues both past and present. Special thanks are due to Jonathan Boyd, who guided my early interests in NMR, to members of Ray Freeman's research group particularly Chris Bauer, Tom Frenkiel, James Keeler, and David Neuhaus who corrected many misconceptions, and to my colleagues Renzo Bazzo, Iain Campbell, Rino Esposito, Daryl

Fernandes, Robin Leatherbarrow, Annalise Pastore, Rod Porteous, Christina Redfield, Nick Soffe, Bob Williams, and Wrenn Wooten of the Oxford Enzyme Group for stimulating discussions and collaborations. I would also like to thank Steve Adams, Bill Haynes, Bill Hutton, Sean Nugent, and Ernie Jaworski of the Monsanto Co. USA for many useful discussions in both Oxford and St Louis. I wish to express my deep gratitude to Raymond Dwek, in whose laboratory my experience with NMR was gained, and without whom this work would not have been possible. Finally, this monograph could not have been written without the patience and support of my wife Felicia, who also carefully typed various versions of the manuscript.

Oxford
May 1988

S. W. H.

Contents

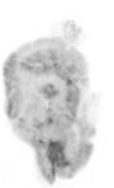

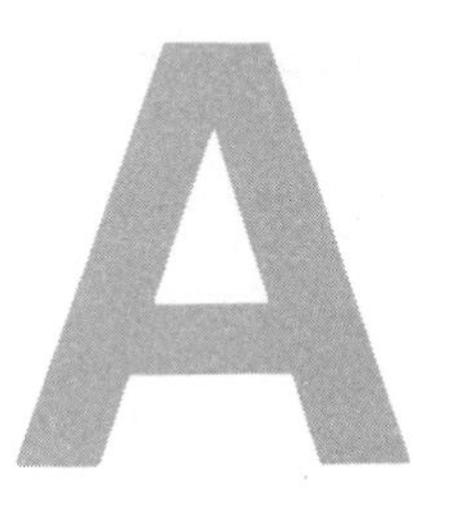

Absolute-value mode The absolute-value mode is defined as the square root of the power spectrum. Thus, if the absorption and dispersion mode components (see **lineshape**) are denoted by U and V respectively, then the absolute-value mode (A) is calculated from

$$A = (U^2 + V^2)^{\frac{1}{2}}. \tag{A1}$$

The absolute-value mode was important in two-dimensional NMR before the advent of **phase-sensitive experiments**. Earlier experiments relied upon echo selection to achieve quadrature detection in the ω_1 domain (see **antiecho**), resulting in the appearance of the undesirable (but unavoidable) phase-twist lineshape. This consists of an admixture of absorption mode and dispersion mode lineshapes. The resonance lines in the two-dimensional spectrum can therefore not be adjusted to pure absorption phase. To overcome this difficulty, it is convenient to calculate the absolute-value mode which by definition always has positive intensity. However, since the dispersion-mode component is still present, the ultimate resolution attainable in an absolute-value two-dimensional spectrum is lower than the equivalent phase-sensitive spectrum. In addition, the signal-to-noise ratio is degraded by $\sqrt{2}$. It should be noted that some peaks in spectra derived from certain two-dimensional experiments (e.g. **relayed correlation spectroscopy**) can only be plotted satisfactorily in the absolute-value mode.

Absorption-mode lineshape See **lineshape**.

Aliasing In the conversion of an analogue signal from the NMR receiver to its digital equivalent, the analogue signal is sampled periodically by the **analogue-to-digital converter** (ADC). The sampling theorem states that in order to reproduce faithfully an analogue signal of frequency f, the sampling rate of the ADC is required to be at least $2f$ (see Fig. A1). This is called the Nyquist frequency.

If a signal is present at the ADC input with a frequency which is greater than half the Nyquist frequency, then this signal will nevertheless be digitized but the frequency component of the output signal will apparently differ from that at the input (see Fig. A2). This is known as aliasing. It should be emphasized that this phenomenon differs from a

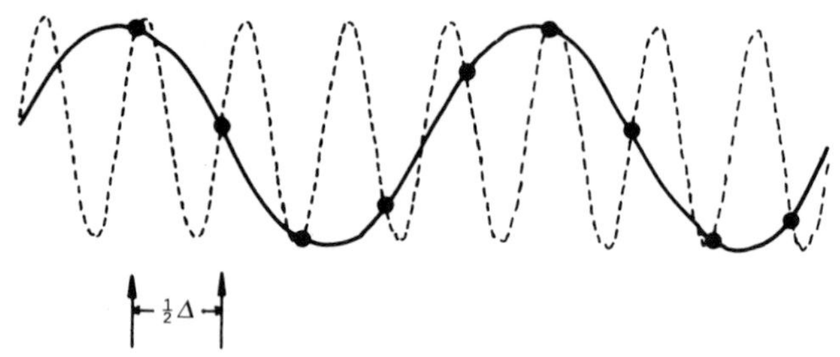

Fig. A1. A sampling rate of 1500 Hz obeys the sampling theorem with respect to the 300 Hz sine wave (solid line). However, the 1200 Hz sine wave (dotted line) is not sampled at an adequate rate and will generate an 'aliased' signal after Fourier transformation (see Fig. A2).

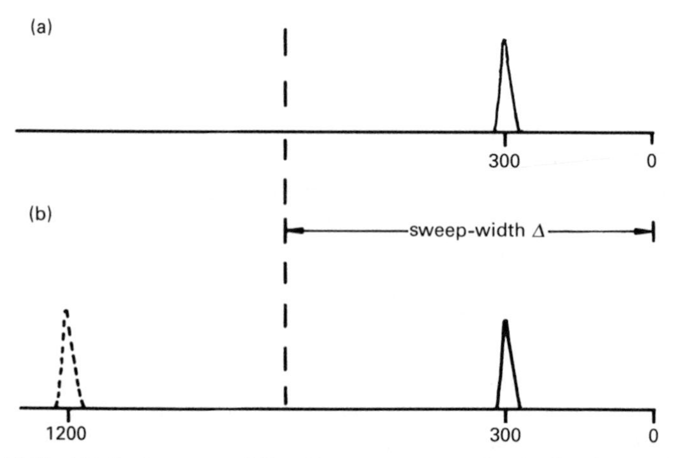

Fig. A2. (a) The 300 Hz sine wave of Fig. A1 generates an authentic signal at 300 Hz. (b) The 1200 Hz sine wave is aliased into the spectrometer sweep-width to generate a spurious signal at 300 Hz.

true frequency shift as generated by, for example, a **phase-sensitive detector**. The effect of aliasing in the NMR spectrum is to generate a resonance line with an anomalous chemical shift. The presence of aliasing is easily detected by altering the **sweep-width** of the spectrometer, when the aliased line will appear to shift. Moreover, aliased resonances often are difficult to phase since their true frequency is usually outside the bandwidth of the **audio-filter** which generally matches the sweep-width. A simple expedient to avoid aliasing is to record a trial spectrum with a large sweep-width such that the sampling frequency is always at least twice that of the largest frequency to be digitized.

Amplifier An amplifier is a device which increases the amplitude of a signal at its input to give a larger signal at its output. In NMR, it is crucial that the output signal is a faithful reproduction of the input signal, i.e. the amplifier should be distortionless. An ideal amplifer would be a piece of wire with gain. In practice, the devices used to provide amplification invariably introduce some distortion. However, under the correct conditions this can be kept to a very low level. Various types of amplifier can be found in a modern spectrometer, as defined by their operating frequency. Working from the probe inwards, the low-level e.m.f. generated in the receiver coils is amplified to a more tractable level by the spectrometer preamplifier. Since no frequency changing has yet taken place, this preamplifier works at the Larmor frequency (see **Larmor precession**) of the nuclei under investigation which is a radiofrequency (r.f.). For protons, this can be of the order of 600 MHz. In many respects the preamplifier is the most crucial device within the spectrometer, since its properties dictate the overall sensitivity and freedom from spurious effects within the NMR spectrum. In order to achieve the best possible performance, the preamplifier must be capable of amplifying signals with amplitudes of a fraction of a microvolt, i.e. almost on the **noise** level, without introducing any additional noise. Unfortunately, thermal noise within the components of the preamplifier will invariably introduce some additional noise (determined by the **noise figure**), but modern components allow this to be kept to an acceptable level. In addition, the preamplifier is sited as close as possible to the **probe**, in order to reduce signal loss along the connecting cables. Once the signal has been amplified, such stringent requirements can be relaxed in subsequent amplification without significant degradation of the overall signal-to-noise ratio of the spectrometer.

An additional requirement of the preamplifier is its ability to amplify large signals without overload, i.e. it should have a large dynamic range. Any shortcomings here will cause serious distortions in the NMR spectrum of a sample containing an intense resonance line, e.g. a solvent peak (see Hoult (1978)). Of course, this problem can be alleviated by attenuating the input signal to the preamplifier, but this merely degrades the noise figure and is no substitute for a well-designed device.

In most spectrometers, the r.f. signal from the preamplifier is converted to a lower, intermediate frequency (i.f.) by the **phase-sensitive detector**(s). It is then amplified further by the i.f. amplifier(s) which provide most of the overall gain of the spectrometer. The i.f. gain is usually under the control of the experimenter in order to match the output signal of the i.f. amplifier to within the dynamic range of the **analogue-to-digital-converter**. See also **linear amplifier**.

FURTHER READING

For an analysis of amplifier design, see Hoult, D. I. (1978). *Prog. NMR Spectr.* **12,** 41–77.

Amplitude modulation The mode of radio transmission known as amplitude modulation is familiar to many from the tuning dials on their radio receivers. In this mode, the amplitude of an r.f. carrier wave is modulated by the information (e.g. speech or music) which it is desired to transmit. Figure A3 illustrates this diagrammatically for a modulating sine wave.

In theoretical terms, the modulation process is represented by the product of the two waveforms. Thus, if the r.f. carrier is represented by $i_c = I_c \cos \omega_c t$ and the modulating cosine wave by $i_m = I_m \cos \omega_m t$ then the resulting signal is described by

A2 $$i = I_c(1 + K \cos \omega_m t) \cos \omega_c t,$$

where $K = I_m/I_c$ is called the modulation depth. By simple trigonometric identity, this can be re-expressed as

A3 $$i = I_c \cos \omega_c t + (KI_c/2) \cos(\omega_c + \omega_m)t + (KI_c/2) \cos(\omega_c - \omega_m)t.$$

In other words, two sidebands are produced which are equidistant by a frequency ω_m from the carrier. It is precisely this mechanism which gives rise to **spinning sidebands** in NMR spectra. A similar situation exists in certain NMR experiments where **density matrix** elements or spin operators are associated with simple sinusoidal or cosinusoidal oscillations in **chemical shifts** or **spin couplings**. As an example, the term $I_x \cos \omega_I t$ which represents x magnetization of spin I modulated by the **Larmor precession** frequency of spin I, can be thought of as an amplitude modulation. Using the identity $\cos x = \frac{1}{2}[\exp(ix) + \exp(-ix)]$, it is seen that an amplitude-modulated function can be decomposed into a sum of phase modulated signals (see **phase modulation**). On **Fourier transformation**, the frequency-domain signal $S(t) = \frac{1}{2}[\mathrm{Abs}(\omega_x) + \mathrm{i\,Dis}(\omega_x) + \mathrm{Abs}(-\omega_x) + \mathrm{i\,Dis}(-\omega_x)]$, where Abs and Dis represent the absorption-mode and dispersion-mode lineshapes (see **lineshape**). The real part of this function (the detected signal), $\frac{1}{2}[\mathrm{Abs}(\omega_x) + \mathrm{Abs}(-\omega_x)]$,

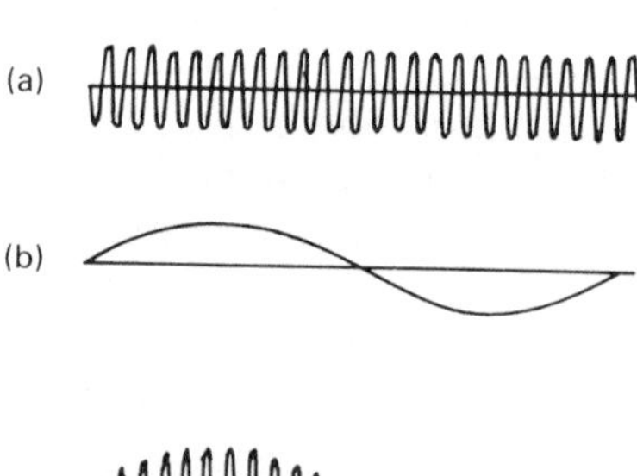

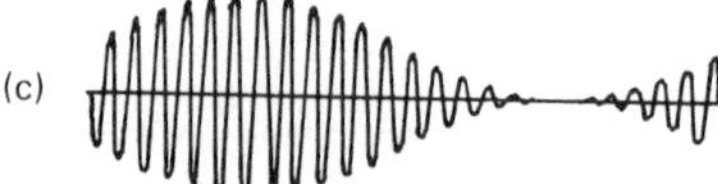

Fig. A3. (a) A sine wave. (b) A low-frequency modulating signal. (c) The sine wave (a) amplitude modulated by (b).

shows that there is no sign discrimination of the Larmor precession frequency, and two resonance lines will be found on either side of the transmitter reference frequency. In **two-dimensional NMR**, it is important to obtain sign discrimination in both dimensions, which can be achieved by either using phase modulation, or more usefully by so-called **phase-sensitive experiments**.

FURTHER READING

Keeler, J. and Neuhaus, D. (1985). *J. Magn. Reson.* **63,** 454.

Analogue-to-digital converter (ADC) In Fourier transform NMR, all post-acquisition data manipulation is performed using digital computers. The very low-level e.m.f. generated in the receiver coils by the sample is first amplified (see **amplifier**), and then converted to a lower frequency signal by a **phase-sensitive detector**. This low-frequency (**audio-frequency**) signal is of course an analogue signal, i.e. it varies continually with time. It must therefore be digitized before it can be handled by the computer. This is achieved by an **analogue-to-digital converter**, or ADC. Of particular importance in NMR of biological molecules is the dynamic range of the ADC. That is, the ability of the ADC to digitize weak signals faithfully in the presence of strong signals. This ability is dependent upon the wordlength of the ADC. We often refer to '12-bit ADCs' or '20-bit ADCs'. This simply means that the wordlength which characterizes the ADC is 12 or 20 bits. The largest integer that can be registered in a single computer word will therefore be $2^{12} - 1 = 4095$ or $2^{20} - 1 = 1\,048\,575$. If the ratio of the intensities of the strongest and weakest signals is greater than either 4095 or 1 048 575, then the input data will exceed the dynamic range of the ADC, and the small signal will not be digitized accurately. Bearing in mind that the concentration of protons in H_2O is 110 M, and that often NMR studies of macromolecules in 90% H_2O/10% D_2O are performed at concentrations of a few mM, it can be seen that a high-quality ADC is required. In practice the required fidelity is reduced by irradiation of the H_2O resonance (see **solvent suppression**). In other experiments in D_2O, the signal-to-noise ratio is often quite poor, and under these circumstances the precision of digitization can be much lower since the dynamic range is low. In some circumstances, the use of a lower ADC resolution is valuable, since a larger number of transients can be co-added without overflowing the available wordlength. Thus, an ADC resolution of 10 bits on a 20-bit wordlength computer allows 1024 experiments to be accommodated, but with an ADC resolution of 16 bits, only 16 experiments can be accommodated. Alternatively, double-precision arithmetic can be employed, whereby two computer words are used for one integer.

Angular momentum The studies of Bohr on the spectrum of the hydrogen atom introduced the postulate that the angular momentum of a system was quantized, i.e. it could only take values which were integer multiples of $h/2\pi$, where h is Planck's constant. Several years later it was suggested by Sommerfeld that the directions of orientation of the electronic angular momentum vector were restricted to certain orientations when the electron was in a closed orbit. In other words, the direction as well as the magnitude of the angular momentum vector was quantized.

In classical mechanics the angular momentum of a particle about a fixed point x is given by

A4 $$I = r \times P$$

where r is the position vector of a particle with respect to x, and P is the linear momentum.

In quantum mechanics the components of position and linear momentum of a particle obey the commutation relations (see **commutator**)

A5 $$[r_n, P_m] = \mathrm{i}\delta_{nm}$$

A6 $$[r_n, r_m] = 0$$

A7 $$[P_n, P_m] = 0$$

$$n, m = x, y, z$$

where $\delta_{nm} = 1$ if $n = m$ and is zero otherwise. We can apply these relations to find the commutation rules for the components of angular momentum I_x, I_y, I_z:

A8 $$I_x = (r_y P_z - r_z P_y)$$

A9 $$I_y = (r_z P_x - r_x P_z)$$

A10 $$I_z = (r_x P_y - r_y P_x).$$

Thus, for example,

A11 $$\begin{aligned}[I_x, I_y] &= (r_y P_z - r_z P_y)(r_z P_x - r_x P_z) - (r_z P_x - r_x P_z)(r_y P_z - r_z P_y) \\ &= \mathrm{r_y P_x (P_z r_z - r_z P_z) + r_x P_y (r_z P_z - P_z r_z)} \\ &= \mathrm{i}(r_x P_y - r_y P_x) \\ &= \mathrm{i}I_z.\end{aligned}$$

A similar procedure for the other combinations gives the full commutation relations:

A12 $$[I_x, I_y] = \mathrm{i}I_z$$

A13 $$[I_y, I_z] = \mathrm{i}I_x$$

A14 $$[I_z, I_x] = \mathrm{i}I_y.$$

The non-commutation of the components of angular momentum is a consequence of quantization. The **uncertainty principle** therefore makes it impossible to measure simultaneously the values of any two components of angular momentum. A further consequence of quantization is that the total angular momentum of a nucleus can take only discrete values, namely $[I(I+1)]^{\frac{1}{2}}\hbar$, where $\hbar = h/2\pi$ and I is the spin quantum number or 'spin', which has half-integral values. The observable magnitudes of a given component of the angular momentum are expressed in terms of the magnetic quantum number m, e.g. $I_z = m\hbar$, where $m = I$, $(I-1)$, $(I-2), \ldots -I$, giving $(2I+1)$ values. This expression for m is consistent with the selection rule that $\Delta m = \pm 1$. Thus if $I = \frac{1}{2}$ (as for protons) then there are two values of m, $\pm\frac{1}{2}$, and two possible values of I_z, $\pm\frac{1}{2}\hbar$.

The commutation relations in (A12)–(A14) define the components of spin angular momentum as a set of spin angular momentum **operators**. If we consider a spin $\frac{1}{2}$ system described by the **orthonormal** wave functions $|\alpha\rangle$ and $|\beta\rangle$ (expressed in the **bra-ket notation**), then the operators I_x, I_y, and I_z behave as follows:

$$\begin{aligned} I_x\,|\alpha\rangle &= \tfrac{1}{2}\,|\beta\rangle \\ I_x\,|\beta\rangle &= \tfrac{1}{2}\,|\alpha\rangle \\ I_y\,|\alpha\rangle &= \tfrac{1}{2}\mathrm{i}\,|\beta\rangle \\ I_y\,|\beta\rangle &= -\tfrac{1}{2}\mathrm{i}\,|\alpha\rangle \\ I_z\,|\alpha\rangle &= \tfrac{1}{2}\,|\alpha\rangle \\ I_z\,|\beta\rangle &= -\tfrac{1}{2}\,|\beta\rangle. \end{aligned} \qquad \text{A15}$$

Here, the **eigenvalues** of I_z, $\frac{1}{2}$ and $-\frac{1}{2}$, in units of $\hbar$ correspond exactly to the two values of m. In general, the various **Hamiltonians** under which spin systems evolve in NMR experiments can be formulated in terms of I_x, I_y, and I_z. These operators are therefore of fundamental importance for the quantum mechanical description of NMR and (A12)–(A15) form the basis of this description. The **matrix representations** of I_x, I_y, and I_z are the well-known **Pauli-spin matrices**.

FURTHER READING

The following texts describe the quantum mechanical principles of angular momentum in detail:

Edmonds, A. R. (1974). *Angular momentum in quantum mechanics*, (2nd edn). Princeton University Press, Princeton.

Rose, M. E. (1957). *Elementary theory of angular momentum*. Wiley, New York.

Angular momentum operators See **angular momentum**.

Anisotropic chemical shift relaxation The chemical shift of a nucleus is dependent upon the orientation of the molecule in a magnetic field.

Rapid molecular motions in liquid state result in an **averaging** of all possible values, resulting in an average chemical shift which is the trace (see Appendix 3) of the chemical shielding **tensor**:

A16 $$\sigma = \tfrac{1}{3}(\sigma_{xx} + \sigma_{yy} + \sigma_{zz}).$$

On a shorter time-scale the nucleus experiences fluctuations in the local magnetic field, and if the chemical shielding tensor is anisotropic (i.e. $\sigma_{xx} \neq \sigma_{yy} \neq \sigma_{zz}$), then this provides a relaxation mechanism. The relaxation rate is dependent upon the **Larmor precession** frequency ω, upon the molecular **correlation time** τ_c, and upon the magnitude of the static field B_0:

A17 $$\frac{1}{T_1} = \frac{1}{15}\gamma^2 B_0^2(\sigma_{\parallel} - \sigma_{\perp})^2 \cdot \frac{2\tau_c}{1+\omega^2\tau_c{}^2}$$

A18 $$\frac{1}{T_2} = \frac{1}{90}\gamma^2 B_0^2(\sigma_{\parallel} - \sigma_{\perp})^2\left[\frac{6\tau_c}{1+\omega^2\tau_c{}^2} + 8\tau_c\right]$$

where γ is the **magnetogyric ratio** and $\sigma_{\parallel}$ and $\sigma_{\perp}$ refer to shielding along and perpendicular to the symmetry axis, assuming axial symmetry. In the **extreme narrowing** limit, (A17) and (A18) reduce to

A19 $$\frac{1}{T_1} = \frac{2}{15}\gamma^2 B_0^2(\sigma_{\parallel} - \sigma_{\perp})^2\tau_c$$

A20 $$\frac{1}{T_2} = \frac{7}{45}\gamma^2 B_0^2(\sigma_{\parallel} - \sigma_{\perp})^2\tau_c$$

and T_1 does not equal T_2 under extreme narrowing conditions, in contrast to the situation under exclusive dipole–dipole **relaxation**.

FURTHER READING

Abragam, A. (1961). *The principles of nuclear magnetism*, Chapter 8. Clarendon Press, Oxford.

Anisotropic motion In **relaxation** theory, the **autocorrelation function** characterizes the type of molecular motion responsible for the relaxation. A particularly simple assumption is that the correlation function is an exponential with a time constant equal to the **correlation time** τ_c. This is a reasonable assumption for certain types of motion, for example rotation of a spherical molecule. In the case of other types of motion, for example relaxation caused by random translational diffusion, the correlation function cannot be represented adequately by a single exponential. Another complication which is of particular importance in biological NMR is the possibility of a distribution of correlation times caused by internal motion. In other words, motion within the macromolecule

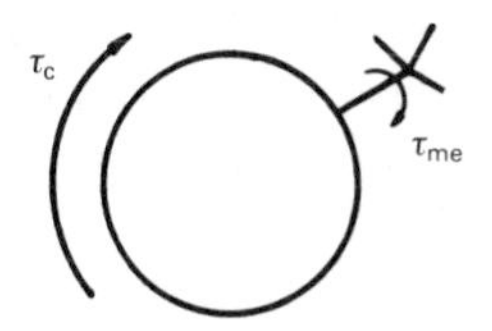

Fig. A4. Diagrammatic representation of a methyl group anisotropically rotating on a globular macromolecule. The correlation times are denoted by τ_{me} and τ_c respectively.

cannot be described by a single correlation time. In such cases the correlation function may again be non-exponential, and a suitable model for the anisotropic motion must be derived.

One example which has been studied in great detail is the rotation of a methyl group on the surface of a protein. The spectral density function (see **relaxation**) for the anisotropic rotation of the internuclear vector between two spins in the methyl group has been derived on the assumption that the methyl group rotates around a spinning axis on the globular protein (Fig. A4). Two correlation times must thus be considered: first, the correlation time characterizing the (fast) spinning of the methyl group about the spinning axis (τ_{me}), and secondly the isotropic reorientation of the spinning axis, which can be assumed to be identical to the rotational correlation time of the macromolecule (τ_c). Under these conditions the spectral densities have been calculated by Woessner:

A21 $$J(0) = \tfrac{1}{4} \cdot \tau_c + \tfrac{3}{4} \cdot \tau_r$$

A22 $$J(\omega) = \frac{1}{4} \cdot \frac{\tau_c}{1+\omega^2\tau_c^2} + \frac{3}{4} \cdot \frac{\tau_r}{1+\omega^2\tau_r^2}$$

A23 $$J(2\omega) = \frac{1}{4} \cdot \frac{\tau_c}{1+4\omega^2\tau_c^2} + \frac{3}{4} \frac{\tau_r}{1+4\omega^2\tau_r^2}$$

where ω is the Larmor frequency of the methyl protons, $1/\tau_r = 1/\tau_c + 1/\tau_{me}$ for a model involving jumping of the methyl group between three sites, and $1/\tau_r = 1/\tau_c + 4/\tau_{me}$ for a diffusional model. The correlation time τ_{me} is that characterizing the methyl group rotation. The magnitudes of the **spin–lattice relaxation** rate ($1/T_1$) and the **spin–spin relaxation** rate ($1/T_2$) can be computed in the usual way from these equations. Although the decay of both longitudinal and transverse magnetization is predicted to be a simple exponential, this is not always found to be the case experimentally. The discrepancy arises from the fact that cross-correlation of proton pairs has been neglected in the Woessner theory, i.e. the motion of each methyl proton is assumed to be uncorrelated with its neighbours. However, this assumption is not justified in certain cases and cross-correlation gives rise to deviations from simple exponential behaviour. A theoretical formalism which includes cross-correlation effects has been described by Werbelow and Marshall. This treatment predicts that the decay of longitudinal magnetization shows nearly exponential behaviour, whereas the decay of transverse magnetization is strongly non-exponential, and is in fact composed of a sum of three exponentials. This is reflected in the lineshapes of methyl groups anisotropically rotating on large proteins, which in general are composed of a broad component, and a narrow component which in turn is a superposition of two Lorentzians. The exact shape depends upon ω, τ_c, and τ_{me}.

FURTHER READING

Werbelow, L. G. and Marshall, A. G. (1973). *J. Magn. Reson.* **11,** 299.
Woessner, D. E. (1962). *J. Chem. Phys.* **36,** 1.
A detailed discussion of the effect of internal motion in proteins can be found in Kalk A. and Berendsen, H. J. C. (1976). *J. Magn. Reson.* **24,** 343.

Anisotropy Anisotropy is manifest in an NMR spectrum when certain components of the **Hamiltonian** of the system do not average to zero. In NMR of liquids, certain components average naturally due to random reorientation in ordinary coordinate space. In fact only scalar chemical shifts and scalar indirect spin–spin couplings survive. These are the interactions which cause the structures of high-resolution NMR spectra. Where molecules have restricted motion, i.e. in nematic liquids and solids, such averaging does not occur, and additional components of the Hamiltonian contribute to the spectrum (see **powder spectrum**). Examples are dipolar couplings and magnetic shielding. These have an orientation-dependence of the spins with respect to the applied field. In favourable circumstances such anisotropies can be averaged in ordinary coordinate space (see **magic-angle spinning**) or in **spin space**.

FURTHER READING

Haeberlen, U. (1976). High resolution NMR in solids. *Adv. Mag. Reson. suppl.* 1.

Antiecho In the absence of **phase cycling**, most **two-dimensional NMR** experiments are associated with **amplitude modulation** of **magnetization** during the t_1 period. An amplitude-modulated signal, given for example by $\cos(\omega_1 t)$ can be decomposed into a sum of phase-modulated signals, since $\cos(\omega_1 t) = \frac{1}{2}(\exp(i\omega_1 t) + \exp(-i\omega_1 t))$. After **two-dimensional Fourier transformation**, signals are found at $\pm\omega_1$ (see **amplitude modulation**). Therefore, unless the **carrier** is displaced to one side of the spectrum, signal overlap will result. In order to avoid this problem, the signs of the ω_1 frequencies must be discriminated. A common approach has been to convert the modulation of the signals during t_1 to one of phase (see **phase modulation**). This is achieved by phase cycling the receiver reference and all pulses preceding t_1 (transmitter phase shift) by $\pi/2$ radians (or $\pi/2n$ for n-quantum experiments). If the phase shifts are in the same sense, signals are detected with identical signs in ω_1 and ω_2, whereas if the phases are cycled in the opposite sense, signals are detected having apparent signs of precession frequencies in ω_1 opposite to those in ω_2. The former signals are known as antiecho or P-type peaks, while the latter are known as echo or N-type peaks. Each type of signal has the undesirable phase-twist lineshape, and ω_1 discrimination can be achieved in a more satisfactory manner using **phase-sensitive experiments**. The key principle to the mechanism of, for example echo selection, is the detection of a second amplitude-modulated component (see **amplitude modulation**) (resulting from the transmitter phase shift) which has sine rather than cosine modulation. Addition of the sine and cosine modulated signals, together with the receiver reference phase shift, results in the time-domain signal

$$\begin{aligned} S(t_1, t_2) &= \cos(\omega_1 t_1)\exp(\mathrm{i}\omega_2 t_2) \\ &\quad + \exp(\mathrm{i}\pi/2)\sin(\omega_1 t_1)\exp(\mathrm{i}\omega_2 t_2) \\ &= \exp(\mathrm{i}\omega_1 t_1)\exp(\mathrm{i}\omega_2 t_2). \end{aligned} \tag{A24}$$

Upon Fourier transformation in both dimensions, the real part (see **complex number**) of the spectrum is a single phase-twist line at $+\omega_1$, $+\omega_2$:

$$\mathrm{Re}[S(\omega_1, \omega_2)] = (\mathrm{Abs}\ \omega_1^+\ \mathrm{Abs}\ \omega_2^+ - \mathrm{Dis}\ \omega_1^+ \mathrm{Dis}\ \omega_2^+). \tag{A25}$$

FURTHER READING

Keeler, J. and Neuhaus, D. (1985). *J. Magn. Reson.* **63,** 454.

Apodization See **convolution**.

Audio-filter Before the **audio-frequency** signal derived from the final detector in an NMR **spectrometer** is digitized (see **analogue-to-digital converter**), it undergoes a stage of audio-filtration. The sampling theorem shows that in order to reproduce faithfully a waveform of frequency f, the sampling rate of the ADC must be $2f$, i.e. twice per cycle (see **aliasing**). If the offset of the most distant resonance line from the **carrier** is known, then it is a simple matter to ensure that the sampling rate is sufficiently high to allow each resonance to be recorded with its true **Larmor precession** frequency. This is in fact achieved automatically when the **sweep-width** of the spectrometer is adjusted. However, although there may be no signals present at greater than f, **noise** will certainly be present, and since the sampling rate is fixed at $2f$, this noise will be aliased into the spectrum. Degradation of the signal-to-noise ratio will therefore result. To prevent this, the signal is stripped of any significant noise above f by passing it through a low-pass audio-filter whose function is to attenuate any signals (i.e. noise) above *f*. In practice, no filter has a step-function cutoff. A filter of the four-pole Butterworth type, for example, has a typical rolloff of 24 dB per octave, which is sufficiently sharp to prevent degradation of the signal-to-noise ratio of the NMR spectrum.

Audio-frequency In some respects, the term audio-frequency implies that this class of signals can actually be heard. However, audio-frequencies are formally a part of the electromagnetic spectrum lying below radio frequencies, and the human ear is, of course, insensitive to electromagnetic radiation. However, if audio-frequency energy can be made to induce pressure changes in a medium (by employing a transducer) such signals will be 'audible'. In an NMR spectrometer, audio-frequency signals exist after the final detection stage, and these frequencies may range from d.c. (see **d.c. offset**) to several KHz. In a similar fashion to the reception of radio signals by a domestic radio receiver, such signals could be heard in an NMR spectrometer by adding a transducer to the output of the detector but this would be of dubious value to the experimenter. Rather, such signals, after filtration (see **audio-filter**) are presented to an **analogue-to-digital converter** (ADC) after which they are **Fourier transformed** within the host computer. The resulting frequency-domain signal (the NMR spectrum) shows the individual frequency components of the composite time-domain signal (see **free induction decay**).

Autocorrelaton function Autocorrelation is cross-correlation (see **cross-correlation function**) of a function with itself. Mathematically, it is described by the following integral:

A26 $$\rho(t) = \int_{-\infty}^{\infty} f^*(\tau) \, . \, f(t+\tau) \, \mathrm{d}\tau$$

where * represents the complex conjugate (see **complex number**) of the function. This is a measure of the correlation between the value of a function at times differing by τ. The magnitude of $\rho(t)$ will depend upon the degree of coherence of the function. A sinusoidal function, for example, will generate a finite value for $\rho(t)$, whereas if the function is simply random noise then $\rho(t)$ rapidly decays with time. An important property of $\rho(t)$ is that its **Fourier transform** is called the power spectrum of the original function. This has important consequences in **relaxation** theory, where the power spectrum of random molecule motion is required in order to determine the energy generated at the **Larmor precession** frequency. In this particular case the power spectrum is more properly referred to as the spectral density function (see **relaxation**).

FURTHER READING

Bracewell, R. M. (1965). *The Fourier transform and its applications*. McGraw-Hill, New York.

Average Hamiltonian theory When the **density matrix** (ρ) of a **spin system** evolves under a **Hamiltonian** ($\mathcal{H}$), the solution of the **Liouville–von Neumann equation** tells us that the state of the density matrix at time t [$\rho(t)$] is related to the initial density matrix [$\rho(0)$] by

A27 $$\rho(t) = T\exp\left(-\mathrm{i}\int_0^t \mathcal{H}(t')\,\mathrm{d}t'\right)\rho(0)\exp\left(+\mathrm{i}\int_0^t \mathcal{H}(t')\,\mathrm{d}t'\right)$$

where T is the Dyson time ordering operator (see **Dyson expression**). The Hamiltonian can often be made time-independent for finite periods of time by selecting a suitable **rotating frame**. Under these circumstances (A27) reduces to the form

A28 $$\rho(t) = \exp(-\mathrm{i}\mathcal{H}_1\tau_1)\rho(0)\exp(\mathrm{i}\mathcal{H}_1\tau_1).$$

The **exponential operators** in (A28) can easily be obtained in their **matrix representation**.

In those circumstances where the Hamiltonian varies continuously from, say, $t = 0$ to $t = t$, $\rho(t)$ can more easily be evaluated using average Hamiltonian theory. The framework necessary to develop this theory is rather complex, and readers primarily interested in the result should proceed to (A54).

Consider a system of like spins in a magnetic field. $I_z = \sum_i I_{zi}$, the z-component **angular momentum** operator, is the operator of infinitesimal rotations about the z-axis in **spin space**. In classical NMR, we are familiar with the rotating frame of coordinates which appears to cancel the precession of the bulk magnetization vector (see **classical formalism**) about B_0. The rotating frame is actually a geometric (i.e. 'visual') interpretation of an interaction representation, which removes single-spin Hamiltonians (in this case I_z) from the total Hamiltonian of the system. In this simple case, the appropriate interaction representation to remove I_z (the Zeeman term) can be described by

A29 $$U_z = \exp(-\mathrm{i}\mathcal{H}_z t),$$

where

A30 $$\mathcal{H}_z = \omega_i I_{zi}.$$

A less tractable but nevertheless more informative example can be given by considering a system with a total Hamiltonian:

A31 $$\mathcal{H}_{\mathrm{TOT}} = \mathcal{H}_{\mathrm{TD}}(t) + \mathcal{H}_i$$

where $\mathcal{H}_{\mathrm{TD}}$ is dependent upon time (for instance $\mathcal{H}_z$ in the laboratory frame) and the 'internal' Hamiltonian $\mathcal{H}_{\mathrm{i}}$ collects terms such as the scalar spin–spin Hamiltonian, $\mathcal{H}_J$. We can equate the state of the system represented by the density matrix $\rho(t)$ with its equivalent interaction representation $\tilde{\rho}(t)$,

A32 $$\rho(t) = U_{\mathrm{TD}}(t)\tilde{\rho}(t)U_{\mathrm{TD}}^{-1}(t)$$

where

A33 $$U_{\mathrm{TD}}(t) = T\exp\left[-\mathrm{i}\int_0^t \mathcal{H}_{\mathrm{TD}}(t')\,\mathrm{d}t'\right].$$

$\tilde{\rho}(t)$ evolves according to the **Liouville–von Neumann equation**:

A34 $$\dot{\tilde{\rho}}(t) = -\mathrm{i}[\tilde{\mathcal{H}}_{\mathrm{i}}(t), \tilde{\rho}(t)]$$

where

A35 $$\tilde{\mathcal{H}}_{\mathrm{i}}(t) = U_{\mathrm{TD}}^{-1}(t)\mathcal{H}_{\mathrm{i}}U_{\mathrm{TD}}(t).$$

In analogy to (A27), the formal solution of (A34) is

A36 $$\tilde{\rho}(t) = U_{\mathrm{i}}(t)\tilde{\rho}(0)U_{\mathrm{i}}^{-1}(t)$$

where

A37 $$U_{\mathrm{i}}(t) = T\exp\left[-\mathrm{i}\int_0^t \tilde{\mathcal{H}}_{\mathrm{i}}(t')\,\mathrm{d}t'\right].$$

Combining (A32) and (A36) gives

A38 $$\rho(t) = U(t)\tilde{\rho}(0)U^{-1}(t)$$

where

A39 $$U(t) = U_{\mathrm{TD}}(t)U_{\mathrm{i}}(t).$$

Equation (A38), which provides us with a solution for $\rho(t)$, is deceptively simple. $U(t)$ consists of a complex series of exponentials, and the overall aim of this treatment is to express $U(t)$ in the form of a single exponential. A particular important case for our purposes is where the interaction $\mathcal{H}_{\mathrm{TD}}(t)$ of the system is cyclic, i.e. if $\mathcal{H}_{\mathrm{TD}}$ is periodic:

A40 $$\mathcal{H}_{\mathrm{TD}}(t+\tau) = \mathcal{H}_{\mathrm{TD}}(t)$$

and in addition if $U_{\mathrm{TD}}(t)$ as defined by (A33) is periodic:

A41 $$U_{\mathrm{TD}}(t) = U_{\mathrm{TD}}(t+\tau_{\mathrm{c}}).$$

If (A40) and (A41) hold, then τ_{c} will be an integer multiple of τ.

Since $U_{\mathrm{i}}(0) = 1$, i.e. at $t = 0$ the system is unchanged, it follows from

(A41) that the value of U_i after $N\tau_c$ for N integer will be

A42 $$U_i(N\tau_c) = T\exp\left[-i\int_0^{N\tau_c} \mathscr{H}_{TD}(t')\,dt'\right] = 1$$

τ_c is called the cycle time. Returning to our simple example for the moment, we note that the Zeeman interaction of a system of equivalent spins is a cyclic interaction. The period of $\mathscr{H}_{TD} = \mathscr{H}_Z$ is infinitely small. The cycle time, τ_c is equal to the period of the **Larmor precession** of the spins.

The cyclic nature of $\mathscr{H}_{TD}(t)$ determines that $U_{TD}(t)$ transfers its periodicity to $\tilde{\mathscr{H}}_i(t)$. From (A35), it is clear that

A43 $$\tilde{\mathscr{H}}_i(t + N\tau_c) = \tilde{\mathscr{H}}_i(t) \quad \text{for } N \text{ integer.}$$

Using (A43), (A37) becomes

A44 $$U_i(N\tau_c) = T\exp\left[-i\int_0^{N\tau_c} \tilde{\mathscr{H}}_i(t')\,dt'\right]$$

A45 $$= \left[T\exp\left(-i\int_0^{\tau_c} \tilde{\mathscr{H}}_i(t')\,dt'\right)\right]^N$$

A46 $$= [U_i(\tau_c)]^N.$$

Using this result, together with the fact that $U_1(N\tau_c) = 1$ (A42), gives, from (A39),

A47 $$\rho(N\tau_c) = [U_i(\tau_c)]^N \rho(0)[U_i^{-1}(\tau_c)]^N.$$

In other words, in order to describe the state of the system at an integer multiple of τ_c, the single-cycle propagator is raised to the Nth power. To obtain $[U_i(\tau_c)]^N$ in the form of a single exponential, it is convenient to perform a Magnus expansion on $U_i(\tau_c)$:

A48 $$U_i(\tau_c) = T\exp\left[-i\int_0^{\tau_c} \tilde{\mathscr{H}}_i(t')\,dt'\right]$$
$$= \exp[-iF\tau_c],$$

where F is a time-independent operator

A49 $$= \exp[-i(\bar{\mathscr{H}}_0 + \bar{\mathscr{H}}_1 + \bar{\mathscr{H}}_2 + \ldots)\tau_c]$$

where

A50 $$\bar{\mathscr{H}}_0 = \frac{1}{\tau_c}\int_0^{\tau_c} \tilde{\mathscr{H}}_i(t)\,dt$$

A51 $$\bar{\mathcal{H}}_1 = \frac{-\mathrm{i}}{2\tau_c}\int_0^{\tau_c} \mathrm{d}t_2 \int_0^{t_2} \mathrm{d}t_1 [\tilde{\mathcal{H}}_i(t_2), \tilde{\mathcal{H}}_i(t_1)]$$

A52 $$\bar{\mathcal{H}}_2 = -\frac{1}{6\tau_c}\int_0^{\tau_c} \mathrm{d}t_3 \int_0^{t_3} \mathrm{d}t_2 \int_0^{t_2} \mathrm{d}t_1 \{[\tilde{\mathcal{H}}_i(t_3), [\tilde{\mathcal{H}}_i(t_2), \tilde{\mathcal{H}}_i(t_1)]] + [\tilde{\mathcal{H}}_i(t_1), [\tilde{\mathcal{H}}_i(t_2), \tilde{\mathcal{H}}_i(t_3)]]\}.$$

If (A47) and (A49) are now combined,

A53 $$\rho(N\tau_c) = \exp[-\mathrm{i}FN\tau_c]\rho(0)\exp[+\mathrm{i}FN\tau_c],$$

or if t is restricted to integer multiples of τ_c,

A54 $$\rho(t) = \exp[-\mathrm{i}Ft]\rho(0)\exp[\mathrm{i}Ft].$$

Equation (A54) is of central importance since it shows that a system subjected to cyclic interactions, the observation of which is restricted to $t = N\tau_c$, behaves as if it were developing according to a constant Hamiltonian F. The lowest-order approximation of F is $\bar{\mathcal{H}}_0$ which is the zero order or average Hamiltonian. The importance of $\bar{\mathcal{H}}_1$, $\bar{\mathcal{H}}_2, \ldots$ depends upon the properties of the cycle. The value of average Hamiltonian theory is that the effect of an arbitrarily complex pulse sequence can be evaluated, when the more exact **density matrix** treatment would be prohibitively cumbersome.

In order to demonstrate the use of average Hamiltonian theory we will consider two examples. Consider first the hypothetical case where $\mathcal{H}(t)$ jumps once in the interval $0 \rightarrow \tau_c$ (Fig. A5). Rewriting (A50)–(A52) in the following form:

A55 $$\bar{\mathcal{H}}_0 = (1/\tau_c)\{\mathcal{H}_1\tau_1 + \mathcal{H}_2\tau_2 + \ldots + \mathcal{H}_n\tau_n\}$$

A56 $$\bar{\mathcal{H}}_1 = -(\mathrm{i}/2\tau_c)([\mathcal{H}_2, \mathcal{H}_1]\tau_2\tau_1 + [\mathcal{H}_3, \mathcal{H}_1]\tau_3\tau_1 + [\mathcal{H}_3, \mathcal{H}_2]\tau_3\tau_2 + \ldots)$$

A57 $$\bar{\mathcal{H}}_2 = -(1/6\tau_c)(\{[\mathcal{H}_3, [\mathcal{H}_2, \mathcal{H}_1]] + [[\mathcal{H}_3, \mathcal{H}_2], \mathcal{H}_1]\}\tau_3\tau_2\tau_1 + \ldots + \tfrac{1}{2}\{[\mathcal{H}_2, [\mathcal{H}_2, \mathcal{H}_1]\tau_2^2\tau_1 + [[\mathcal{H}_2, \mathcal{H}_1], \mathcal{H}_1]\tau_2\tau_1^2 + \ldots\}).$$

If $\mathcal{H}_1\tau_1 = A$ and $\mathcal{H}_2\tau_2 = B$, we find

A58 $$\bar{\mathcal{H}}_0 = (1/\tau_c)(A + B), \qquad \bar{\mathcal{H}}_1 = -(\mathrm{i}/2)[B, A]$$
$$\bar{\mathcal{H}}_2 = -(1/12)\{[B, [B, A]] + [[B, A], A]\}.$$

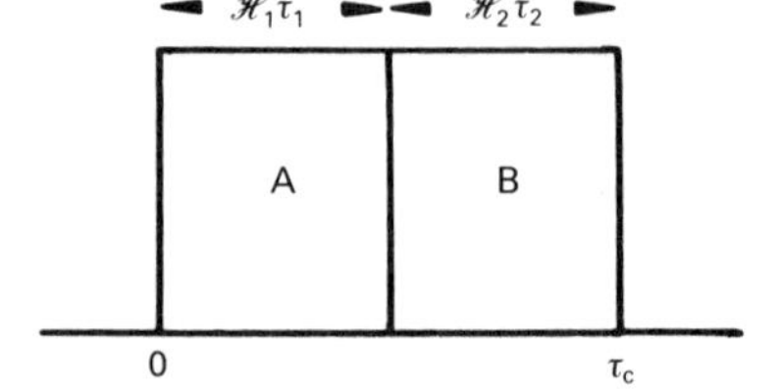

Fig. A5. Hypothetical case where the Hamiltonian $\mathcal{H}(t)$ jumps from A to B during the interval τ_c.

Incidentally, it follows that

A59 $$e^{-iB}e^{-iA} = \exp(-i(A+B) - \tfrac{1}{2}[B, A] + (i/12)\{[B, [B, A]] + [[B, A], A]\} + \ldots)$$

which is the Baker–Campbell–Hausdorff formula for the expression of two non-commuting operators (see **commutator**) in terms of a single exponential.

As a second example of the use of average Hamiltonian theory we will compute the average Hamiltonian corresponding to the WAHUHA pulse sequence and show its effect upon chemical shifts and dipolar couplings in solids. The WAHUHA pulse sequence is shown in Fig. (A6). In order to examine its effect upon dipolar couplings, it is necessary to examine the values of the internal Hamiltonian that are proportional to $\mathbf{I}\cdot\mathbf{S} - 3I_zS_z$, i.e. the dipolar Hamiltonian. Now since the r.f. pulses in Fig. A6 effect rotations of the spin operators, and the scalar product of two vectors is invariant to rotation (i.e. $\mathbf{I}\cdot\mathbf{S} = I_xS_x + I_yS_y + I_zS_z$ is invariant to the pulses of the sequence) then we need only consider the term I_zS_z. Its value in the interaction frame is shown in Fig. A6. These values can be verified using the rules for the transformation of product operators (see **product operator formalism**) under r.f. pulses. Now using (A55), we can derive an expression for the average Hamiltonian:

$$\bar{\mathcal{H}}_0 = \mathbf{I}\cdot\mathbf{S} - (3/\tau_c)\{I_zS_z\tau + I_yS_y\tau + 2I_xS_x\tau + I_yS_y\tau + I_zS_z\tau\}$$

and since $\tau_c = 6\tau$,

A60 $$\bar{\mathcal{H}}_0 = \mathbf{I}\cdot\mathbf{S} - (I_xS_x + I_yS_y + I_zS_z) = 0$$

and thus the system behaves as if dipolar couplings are zero.

Similarly, for a Hamiltonian proportional to I_z (such as the zeeman Hamiltonian responsible for chemical shifts) using the value of I_z in the

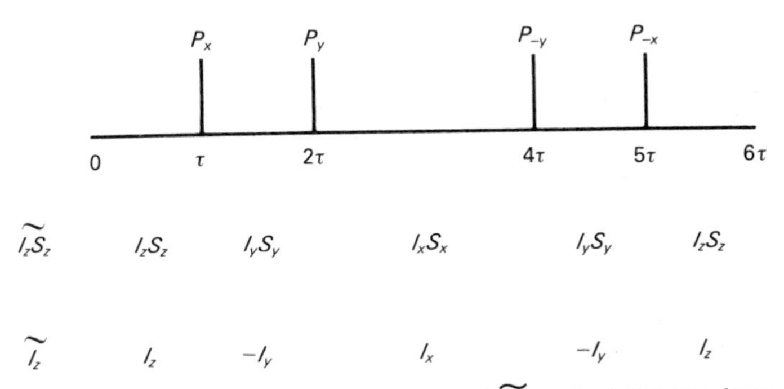

Fig. A6. The WAHUHA pulse sequence, and the value of $\widetilde{I_zS_z}$ in the interaction frame at each interval.

interaction frame (Fig. A6) we find for example:

$$\mathcal{H}_z = \omega_I I_z,$$

A61
$$\bar{\mathcal{H}}_0 = (1/3)\omega_I(I_x + I_y + I_z) = (1/\sqrt{3})\omega_I I_{111}$$

where

$$I_{111} = (I_x + I_y + I_z)/\sqrt{3}$$

and thus all shift interactions are scaled by $1/\sqrt{3}$. The WAHUHA sequence is an example of a cyclic sequence, and as such has the useful property that the first-order and all other odd-order correction terms to the average Hamiltonian vanish.

FURTHER READING

Haeberlen, U. (1976) High resolution NMR in solids. *Adv. Magn. Reson., Suppl* 1.
Haeberlen, U. and Waugh, J. S. (1968). *Phys. Rev.* **175,** 453.

Averaging The concept of averaging in NMR can be thought of as a 'visual' interpretation of the results of **average Hamiltonian theory**. In order to examine the processes which result in averaging, we must be aware of the distinction between ordinary (cartesian) coordinate space and **spin space**. It is quite easy to grasp the manifestations of averaging in ordinary coordinate space. A simple example is the averaging of **dipolar couplings** between nuclei in liquid samples. The random reorientational motions of molecules in the static magnetic field result in the averaging of the dipolar **Hamiltonian** part of the internal Hamiltonian to zero. In fact, the only parts of the internal Hamiltonian which survive in liquids are scalar **chemical shifts** and scalar spin–spin (J) couplings (see **spin coupling**). These are the interactions responsible for the morphology of the corresponding NMR spectra.

A second example of averaging in ordinary coordinate space is the spinning of a sample about an axis perpendicular to the applied field. The purpose of this practice is to reduce the inhomogeneity broadening of resonance lines. A further related example is **magic-angle spinning** about the applied field in order to suppress the dominant anisotropic interactions of spins in solids.

It should be obvious that the first example of averaging occurs naturally. The latter examples, however, are deliberately imposed upon the spin system by the experimenter. Further simplifications of NMR spectra can be obtained by creating averages in **spin space**. Although averaging in spin space does occur naturally (resulting in the **high-field approximation**), more generally the experimenter chooses to remove the effects of chosen parts of the internal Hamiltonian by engineering rotations in spin space using special sequences of r.f. pulses. See also **average Hamiltonian theory**.

FURTHER READING

Haeberlen, U. (1976). High resolution NMR in solids. *Adv. Magn. Reson. Suppl.* 1.

Axial peak An axial peak is a resonance line present in **two-dimensional NMR** spectra. It derives from relaxation during the interpulse delay(s). For example, consider a basic COSY experiment (see **correlated spectroscopy**). After the first pulse along the x' coordinate, the bulk magnetization vector (BMV) will lie along the y' direction in the x'–y' **rotating frame** as shown in Fig. A7. During the t_1 period, the BMV will possess a component in the z direction due to relaxation (Fig. A7). For convenience, precession of isochromats in the $x'y'$ plane is ignored here. After the second pulse along the x' direction, the z' magnetization will be converted into observable x'–y' magnetization, leading to axial peaks in the two-dimensional NMR spectrum. Since axial peaks do not undergo any modulation with respect to t_1, they appear at zero frequency in ω_1 after **two-dimensional Fourier transformation**. In general, axial peaks are undesirable in two-dimensional NMR spectra, and they are usually eliminated using **phase cycling** procedures.

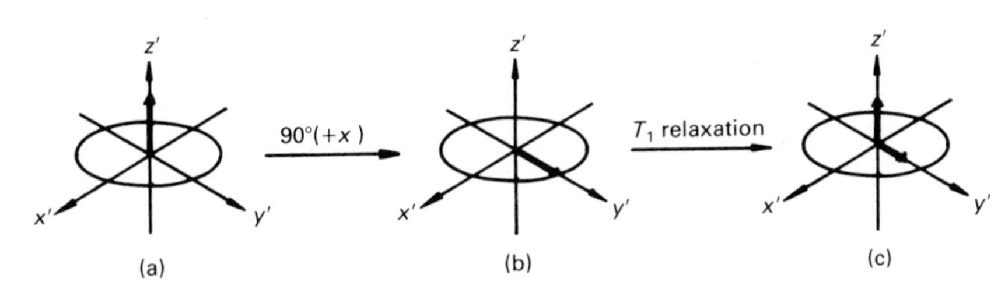

Fig. A7. (a) The bulk magnetization at equilibrium lies along the $+z'$ axis. (b) The first pulse in the COSY sequence creates transverse magnetization. (c) Longitudinal relaxation during t_1 results in the recreation of magnetization along the $+z'$ axis. After the second pulse (with arbitrary phase) in the COSY sequence, this magnetization will be tipped into the x'–y' plane, resulting in observable magnetization which gives rise to axial peaks.

B

Bandwidth An important parameter of any NMR receiver is its bandwidth, i.e. the range of frequencies to which the receiver is sensitive. Receivers designed for radio communication purposes have their bandwidths defined at their **intermediate frequency**. In contrast, the bandwidth of NMR receivers is generally defined at **audio-frequency**. This is achieved by the application of an **audio-filter**, whose purpose is to restrict signals at the input to the **analogue-to-digital converter** to within a given range. See also **sweep-width**.

Basis set See **basis state**.

Basis state The energy of a spin system in a magnetic field is quantized. Like the individual nuclei, the spin system as a whole exists in certain states, called stationary states. Each stationary state is characterized by a wave function or **eigenfunction**, ψ. For a given spin system, therefore, there exists a set of such wave functions, one for each state. Each wave function is sometimes referred to as a basis state, and the set is referred to as a basis set or simply basis. In order to calculate the energies or **eigenvalues** of the spin system, we insert each basis state into the **Schrödinger equation**.

As an example of the form of a basis set, consider two uncoupled protons A and B in a static magnetic field. Since each proton can exist in two possible orientations, that is aligned with or against the field, there are four possible states for the system (Fig. B1). If we now label a spin-up state with the symbol β, and a spin-down state with α, we can redraw Fig. B1 as shown in Fig. B2. The four states $\alpha\alpha$, $\alpha\beta$, $\beta\alpha$, and $\beta\beta$ are the basis-states of the two-spin system and are by definition **orthonormal**. These states are known as product-functions (or collectively **product basis**) since they are each composed of the product of the wavefunctions of each individual nucleus (see **Schrödinger equation**). The product basis is often represented in ket notation (see **bra-ket notation**);

$$\alpha\alpha \rightarrow |\alpha\alpha\rangle$$

$$\alpha\beta \rightarrow |\alpha\beta\rangle$$

$$\beta\alpha \rightarrow |\beta\alpha\rangle$$

$$\beta\beta \rightarrow |\beta\beta\rangle.$$

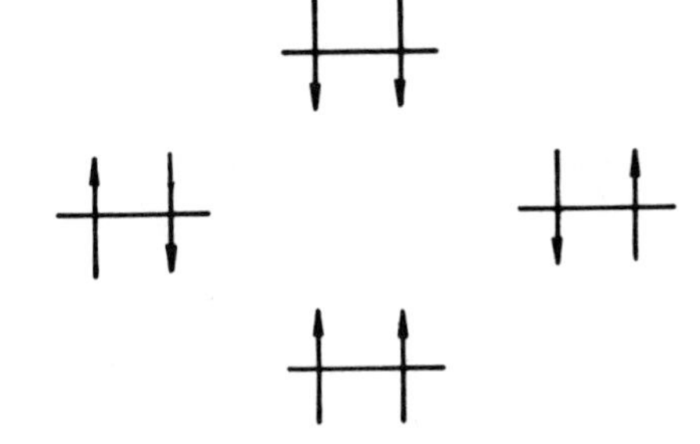

Fig. B1. The four energy levels of a loosely coupled two-spin system.

This clarifies the **matrix representation** of operators. If each basis state is an eigenstate of the system, the basis set is usually referred to as the **eigenbasis**. For the simple system above, the product basis is identical to the eigenbasis, as indeed it is for any loosely coupled spin system (see **spin coupling**). However, in strongly-coupled systems (see **strong coupling**), the product basis is not the eigenbasis. It is important to work in the eigenbasis for a spin system when performing calculations, since then the **Hamiltonian** representing evolution of the spin system under spin-coupling terms gives a particularly simple diagonal matrix representation.

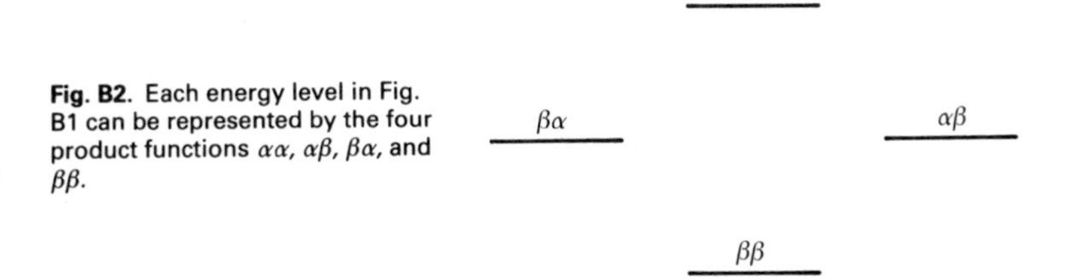

Fig. B2. Each energy level in Fig. B1 can be represented by the four product functions $\alpha\alpha$, $\alpha\beta$, $\beta\alpha$, and $\beta\beta$.

Bloch equations The phenomenologically formulated Bloch equations describe the magnetic resonance phenemonon in terms of a classical vector model (see **classical formalism**). An ensemble of nuclei in a magnetic field will generate a total magnetic moment per unit volume since an excess of nuclei align with the field (see **Boltzmann distribution**). At equilibrium, the state of the spin system can therefore be described in terms of cartesian coordinates in the laboratory frame (Fig. B3). M_0 can be resolved into three components, M_x, M_y, and M_z. In the absence of any exciting (B_1) field, M_z will not change with time:

B2 $$\frac{dM_x}{dt} = \gamma B_0 M_y$$

B3 $$\frac{dM_y}{dt} = -\gamma B_0 M_x.$$

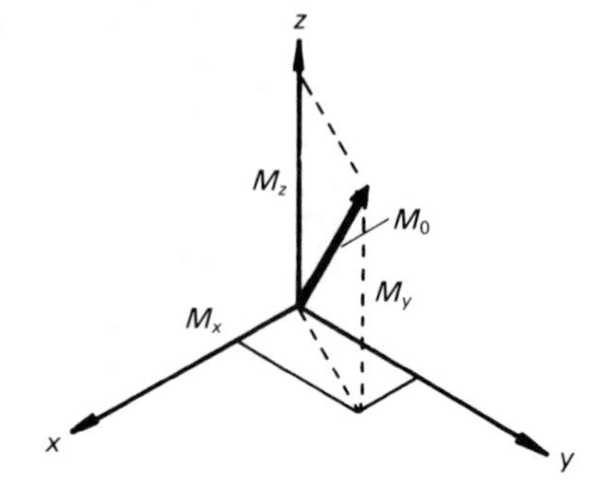

Fig. B3. A magnetization vector M_0 can be decomposed into three orthogonal components M_x, M_y, and M_z.

If an r.f. field of amplitude $2B_1$ is now applied, one of the components which rotates about the z axis in the same sense as the **Larmor precession** will stimulate transitions. The x and y components of this field of magnitude B_1 as it precesses about the z are given by

B4 $$B_{1x} = B_1 \cos(\omega t)$$

B5 $$B_{1y} = -B_1 \sin(\omega t).$$

The magnetization along the x axis will now contain not only a component of M_y rotating about B_0, but also a component M_z rotating about B_1. The time rate of change of M_x, M_y, and M_z therefore becomes

B6 $$\frac{\mathrm{d}M_x}{\mathrm{d}t} = \gamma[M_y B_0 - M_z B_{1y}]$$

B7 $$\frac{\mathrm{d}M_y}{\mathrm{d}t} = -\gamma[M_x B_0 + M_z B_{1x}]$$

B8 $$\frac{\mathrm{d}M_z}{\mathrm{d}t} = -\gamma[M_x B_{1y} - M_y B_{1x}].$$

In order to obtain the full Bloch equations, it is necessary to include terms which describe the relaxation in the longitudinal (z) and transverse (x, y) directions. These are described by time constants T_1 and T_2 respectively:

B9 $$\frac{\mathrm{d}M_x}{\mathrm{d}t} = \gamma[M_y B_0 + M_z B_1 \sin(\omega t)] - \frac{M_x}{T_2}$$

B10 $$\frac{\mathrm{d}M_y}{\mathrm{d}t} = -\gamma[M_x B_0 + M_z B_1 \cos(\omega t)] - \frac{M_y}{T_2}$$

B11 $$\frac{\mathrm{d}M_z}{\mathrm{d}t} = -\gamma[-M_x B_1 \sin(\omega t) - M_y B_1 \cos(\omega t)] - \frac{M_z - M_0}{T_1}.$$

Equations (B9)–(B11) are the Bloch equations in the laboratory frame. However, it is more convenient to examine NMR phenomena in the **rotating frame**. Under these conditions, and with excitation applied along the x' axis, the Bloch equations become

B12 $$\frac{dM_{x'}}{dt} = (\omega_0 - \omega)M_{y'} - \frac{M_{x'}}{T_2},$$

B13 $$\frac{dM_{y'}}{dt} = -(\omega_0 - \omega)M_{x'} - \frac{M_{y'}}{T_2} + \gamma B_1 M_z,$$

B14 $$\frac{dM_z}{dt} = -\gamma B_1 M_{y'} - \frac{(M_z - M_0)}{T_1},$$

where ω_0 is the on-resonance precession frequency. The steady state solution of these equations describes the observed magnetization. If we apply a simplification here, $\gamma B_1^2 T_1 T_2 \ll 1$, i.e. the r.f. power is sufficiently low to prevent saturation, then $M_{x'}$, $M_{y'}$, and $M_{z'}$ are described as follows:

B15 $$M_{x'} = M_0 \frac{\gamma B_1 T_2^2(\omega_0 - \omega)}{1 + 4\pi^2 T_2^2(\omega_0 - \omega)^2},$$

B16 $$M_{y'} = M_0 \frac{\gamma B_1 T_2}{1 + 4\pi^2 T_2^2(\omega_0 - \omega)^2},$$

B17 $$M_z = M_0 \frac{1 + 4\pi^2 T_2^2(\omega_0 - \omega)^2}{1 + 4\pi^2 T_2^2(\omega_0 - \omega)}.$$

The Bloch theory thus predicts that two components are detectable in the x'–y' plane. The signal observed along $M_{x'}$ has the form shown in Fig. B4 and is known as the dispersion mode signal. Conversely, the form of $M_{y'}$ shown in Fig. B4 is the absorption mode signal, and is the signal which is normally detected. The dispersion and absorption components are also known as the real and imaginary parts. The two components are related by the **Hilbert transform**. It should be noted that an admixture of the two components will be observed if the detector (see **phase-sensitive**

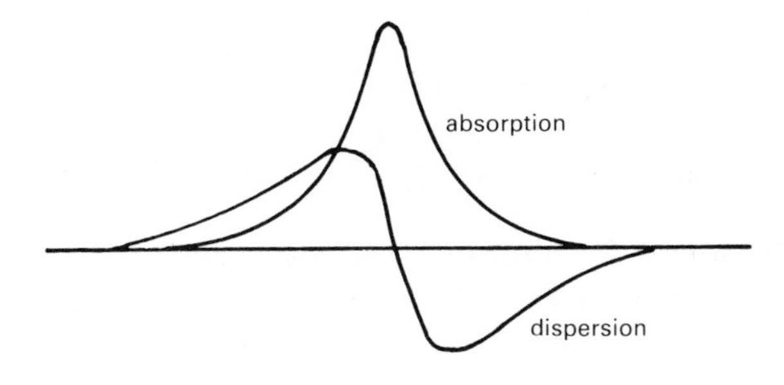

Fig. B4. The absorption and dispersion components of transverse magnetization.

detector) is not exactly aligned (in terms of **phase**) along the x' or y' *plane.*

FURTHER READING

Ernst, R. R., Bodenhausen, G. and Wokaun, A. A. (1987) *Principles of NMR in one and two dimensions.* p. 116ff. Clarendon Press, Oxford.

Bloch–Siegert shift In several NMR experiments, selective irradiation is applied at the resonance frequency of a given nucleus. For example, consider **spin decoupling** of an AX spin system, by irradiation with a B_2 field at the **carrier** frequency of A. It is generally assumed that irradiation at the resonance frequency of A has no effect upon the spectrum other than that resulting from perturbation of A. However, this assumption is only true when $\gamma B_2 < |\omega_A - \omega_X|$, where ω_A and ω_X are the resonance frequencies of spins A and X respectively. If this assumption is not valid, then a Bloch–Siegert shift may be observed. This arises from the presence of an additional field in the rotating frame due to B_2. In the above example, a small shift in frequency of the resonance corresponding to the X nucleus is observed during irradiation of A. The Bloch–Siegert shift can cause difficulties in spin decoupling difference spectroscopy if the decoupler is switched off to obtain an unperturbed spectrum. A poor difference spectrum will obviously result. For this reason the decoupler should remain on during the acquisition of the unperturbed spectrum, and its frequency adjusted to a region which is clear of resonances.

A quantitative measure of the Bloch–Siegert shift can be had by noting that with the appropriate rotating component of B_2, the spins experience an effective field which is the resultant of the resonance offset ΔB and B_2. This increases the precession frequency by an amount $\gamma(B_{\text{eff}} - \Delta B)/2\pi$. Usually it is the case that the resonance offset is very much greater than the strength of the B_2 field (measured in units of frequency), i.e. $\Delta B \gg B_2$. This gives a Bloch–Siegert shift which is of the order of

$$\Delta f = 1/2(\gamma B_2/2\pi)^2/(\gamma\,\Delta B/2\pi).$$

Since B_2 is usually intense in practical cases, and since ΔB may be much smaller than the Larmor precession frequency, the Bloch–Siegert shift can be quite large.

FURTHER READING

Bloch, F. and Siegert, A. (1940). *Phys. Rev.* **57,** 522.
Ramsey, N. F., (1955). *Phys. Rev.* **100,** 1191.

Boltzmann distribution The Boltzmann law allows us to calculate the relative populations of states with differing energies. For example, in a proton NMR experiment, an ensemble of equivalent spins will partition between

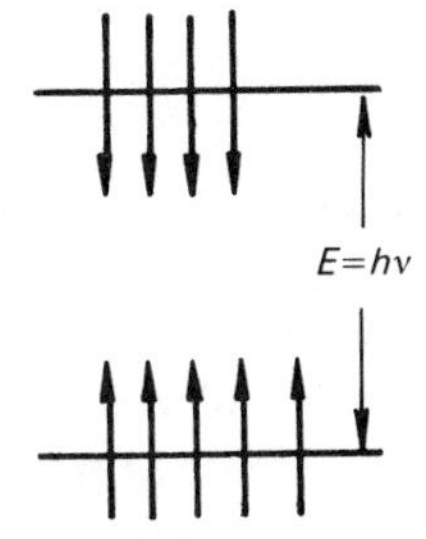

Fig. B5. At thermal equilibrium, a net excess of spins exists in the low spin state. At room temperature this excess is very small.

the lower and upper spin states (Fig. B5). From the Boltzmann law, the relative populations of the states is given by

B18 $$\frac{n_l}{n_u} = \exp\left[\frac{E}{KT}\right] = \exp\left[\frac{h\nu}{KT}\right]$$

where n_l is the number of nuclei in the low spin state, n_u is the number of nuclei in the upper spin state, E is the energy difference between the states, K is the Boltzmann constant, and T is the absolute temperature.

Since $h\nu$ is very much smaller than KT at normal temperature in an NMR experiment, and given that

B19 $$\exp(x) = 1 + x + \frac{x^2}{2!} + \frac{x^3}{3!} + \dots$$

the exponent can be expanded to give

B20 $$\exp\frac{h\nu}{KT} \simeq 1 + \frac{h\nu}{KT}.$$

In other words, there is an excess of $h\nu/KT$ spins in the low spin state. This can be calculated to be 1 part in 10^9 at normal temperatures. Since this excess is proportional to the signal inducible in the **probe**, NMR is a very insensitive technique compared to other forms of spectroscopy, where the energy difference is very much larger.

Bra-ket notation A central concept of quantum mechanics is the existence of a wavefunction ψ, which describes the state of a given system. In order to predict the result of a given experiment upon the system, we perform mathematical manipulations upon the wavefunction. As an example, the application of the **Hamiltonian** operator on the wavefunction yields the product of **eigenvalue** and wavefunction (**eigenfunction**), as described by the time-independent **Schrödinger equation**:

B21 $$\mathscr{H}\psi = E\psi.$$

In what might appear to be a trivial substitution, we can rewrite (B21) as follows:

B22 $$\mathcal{H}\,|\psi\rangle = E\,|\psi\rangle$$

where the $|\,\rangle$ is the 'ket' notation for the eigenfunction. This notation was introduced by Dirac as a shorthand notation for use in quantum mechanical calculations. Its value is more readily appreciated if we examine a more complex example. Consider a quantum system (e.g. an ensemble of coupled spins) with states represented by the wavefunctions $\psi_1, \psi_2, \ldots, \psi_n$. A fundamental concept of quantum mechanics dictates that these functions are normalized:

B23 $$\int \psi_n^* \psi_n \, \mathrm{d}v = 1,$$

and orthogonal:

B24 $$\int \psi_m^* \psi_n \, \mathrm{d}v = 0, \qquad n \neq m$$

where * represents the complex conjugate (see **complex number**). In Dirac's notation, the complex conjugate is represented in 'bra' notation by $\langle \psi|$. Hence, the integrals in (B23) and (B24) can be written as

B25 $$\begin{aligned} \langle \psi_n | \psi_n \rangle &= 1 \quad \text{or} \quad \langle n | n \rangle = 1 \\ \langle \psi_m | \psi_n \rangle &= 0 \quad \text{or} \quad \langle m | n \rangle = 0. \end{aligned}$$

The beauty of the bra-ket notation is that integrals can be related to matrix elements. If A is any operator corresponding to a physical quantity, the array of integrals

B26 $$A_{mn} = \int \psi_m^* A \psi_n \, \mathrm{d}v = \langle m|\, A \,|n\rangle$$

are known as the matrix elements of A and give a **matrix representation** of the operator. We always need to evaluate (B26) when predicting the results of NMR experiments using the **density matrix** formalism. For further information see **matrix representation**.

Broadband decoupling It is well known that two scalar coupled nuclei (A and X) can be decoupled by the application of an intense r.f. field at the Larmor frequency of one of the nuclei. This is known as **spin decoupling**. In this type of experiment the Fourier relationship (see **Fourier transform**) between a long pulse in the time domain and its transform in the frequency domain is exploited in the linear approximation to irradiate a given resonance selectivity. However, in certain experiments it is desirable to irradiate a group of nuclei over a large bandwidth. As an example, when observing resonances from C^{13} nuclei, it is desirable to suppress the couplings to bonded protons. In other words, effective irradiation across the whole proton bandwidth of the sample is desirable in order to achieve broadband decoupling. One way to achieve this would be to reduce the width of the irradiating r.f. pulse. However, a very large amount of power would be required to effect efficient decoupling across the whole bandwidth. A much more efficient method of achieving broadband decoupling depends upon the application of a train of **composite pulses** to the spin system. Such pulses are of central importance for efficient heteronuclear decoupling. They rely upon the fact that it is possible to refocus the effects of heteronuclear *IS* couplings (for weak *II* interactions) by an inversion pulse applied to the *I* spins. By use of a repetitive sequence of accurate inversion pulses, continuous refocusing is possible, i.e. spin decoupling. If inversion pulses are combined to give cyclic sequences, described by a **propagator** which is an approximate unity operator (see **identity operator**), then the highest possible degree of decoupling is obtained over a variety of offset conditions, flip angles, and coupling constants.

Composite inversion sequences are described under the heading composite pulses. In fact the first such sequence to be described (equation (C37)) is used in the MLEV decoupling sequence. Here the composite inversion pulse (abbreviated R) is combined into a cycle:

B27 $$C = RR\overline{RR}$$

where the bar indicates that all r.f. pulses are shifted in phase by π radians. To improve the cyclic nature of the sequence, it is possible to derive the permuted sequence:

B28 $$CP = \bar{R}RR\bar{R}$$

and CP itself can be phase-inverted to give the supercycle

B29 $$CP\overline{CP} = RR\overline{RR}\;\bar{R}RR\bar{R}\;\overline{RR}RR\;R\overline{RR}R$$

which is called the MLEV-16 supercycle. Such sequences can be rationalized by examining magnetization trajectories, or more elegantly using **average Hamiltonian theory**. A second generation of sequences termed WALTZ are based upon the inversion sequence

B30 $$R = (\beta)_0(2\beta)_\pi(3\beta)_0,$$

with $\beta \approx \pi/2$, which has better offset compensation than the MLEV inversion element, and is less sensitive to errors in r.f. phase shifts. The WALTZ-4 sequence is obtained by the following permutations of R:

B31 $$\text{WALTZ-4} = RR\overline{RR}$$

which can be written in obvious notation

B32
$$RR\overline{RR} = 1\bar{2}3\ 1\bar{2}3\ \bar{1}2\bar{3}\ \bar{1}2\bar{3}$$
$$= 1\bar{2}4\bar{2}3\ \bar{1}2\bar{4}2\bar{3}, \qquad \text{(B32)}$$

since pulses of width β and equal phase can be combined. If a $(\pi/2)_0$ pulse is now permuted cyclically from beginning to end of $RR\overline{RR}$, we find

B33
$$K\bar{K} = \bar{2}4\bar{2}3\bar{1}2\bar{4}2\bar{3}1$$

which can be combined with its phase-alternated counterpart to give WALTZ-8:

B34
$$K\overline{KK}K = \bar{2}4\bar{2}3\bar{1}\ 2\bar{4}2\bar{3}1\ 2\bar{4}2\bar{3}1\ \bar{2}4\bar{2}3\bar{1}$$

and finally a $(\pi/2)_\pi$ pulse is permuted from end to beginning of $K\overline{KK}K$, and a phase-inverted sequence is appended to give WALTZ-16:

B35
$$Q\overline{QQ}Q = \bar{3}4\bar{2}3\bar{1}2\bar{4}2\bar{3}\ 3\bar{4}2\bar{3}1\bar{2}4\bar{2}3\ 3\bar{4}2\bar{3}1\bar{2}4\bar{2}3\ \bar{3}4\bar{2}3\bar{1}2\bar{4}2\bar{3}$$

which is one of the most efficient broadband decoupling sequences discovered to date.

FURTHER READING

The following references describe the derivation of MLEV and WALTZ:

Levitt, M. H. and Freeman, R. (1981) *J. Magn. Reson.* **43,** 502.
Levitt, M. H., Freeman, R., and Frenkiel, T. (1982) *J. Magn. Reson.* **47,** 328.
Levitt, M. H., Freeman, R., and Frenkiel, T. (1982) *J. Magn. Reson.* **50,** 157.
Levitt, M. H., Freeman, R., and Frenkiel, T. (1988). *Adv. Magn. Reson.* **11,** 47.
Shaka, A. J., Keeler, J., Frenkiel, T. and Freeman, R. (1983) *J. Magn. Reson.* **52,** 335.

An evaluation of the relative merits of these sequences is given in:

Shaka, A. J., Keeler, J., and Freeman, R. (1983) *J. Magn. Reson.* **53,** 313.

Broadening probe See **paramagnetic centre**.

Bulk magnetization vector See **classical formalism**.

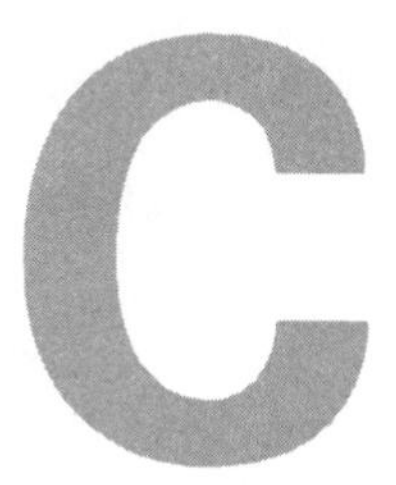

Camelspin See **rotating frame Overhauser effect spectroscopy**.

Carrier In radio communication, the carrier is the r.f. wave which is modulated by the relevant information to be transmitted. Depending upon the mode of transmission, the carrier itself may or may not be transmitted. In the case of **amplitude modulation** (AM) the carrier and both sidebands are transmitted. In contrast, double sideband transmission uses both sidebands but no carrier, whereas single sideband transmission requires one sideband only. In NMR, the carrier normally refers to the transmitter reference frequency, although this is often identical to the receiver reference frequency. The concept of a carrier in NMR is actually not very different from that inferred from radio-frequency communication, since an r.f. pulse is a carrier wave modulated by a d.c. pulse. Although the concept of sidebands is not easy to grasp in this case, we can introduce these by amplitude modulation of a continuous wave carrier. In this manner it is possible to selectively irradiate at more than one frequency in a NMR spectrum without using multiple signal generators.

Carr–Purcell–Meiboom–Gill (CPMG) sequence The discovery of spin echoes by Hahn demonstrated that the effect of magnetic field inhomogeneity upon linewidth could be removed. In order to reduce the diffusion term which is manifest in the **spin echo** sequence, Carr and Purcell proposed an alternative pulse sequence involving $\pi/2$ (90°) and π (180°) r.f. pulses. It can be understood using the simple **classical formalism**. Suppose that at $t = 0$ a $\pi/2$ pulse is applied at resonance along the $+x'$ axis of the **rotating frame**. The magnetization, which before the pulse is presumed to be along the $+z'$ axis (i.e. at equilibrium), will be along the $+y'$ axis after the pulse (Fig. C1). Due to magnetic field inhomogeneity, the magnetization vectors dephase in the $x' - y'$ plane for a time τ (Fig. C1), at which time a π pulse is applied along the $+x$ axis. This pulse flips the magnetization into the $-y$ axis. The effect of the 180° pulse, as shown in the diagram, is to cause a refocusing, or 'echo' of magnetization at $t = 2\tau$. The complete **pulse sequence** is therefore $90°_x - \tau - 180°_x - \tau -$ acquisition. If the $(\tau - 180° - \tau)$ part of the sequence is repeated, a train of echoes is formed. If there is no diffusion, a spin dephases during τ following each echo and rephases during the

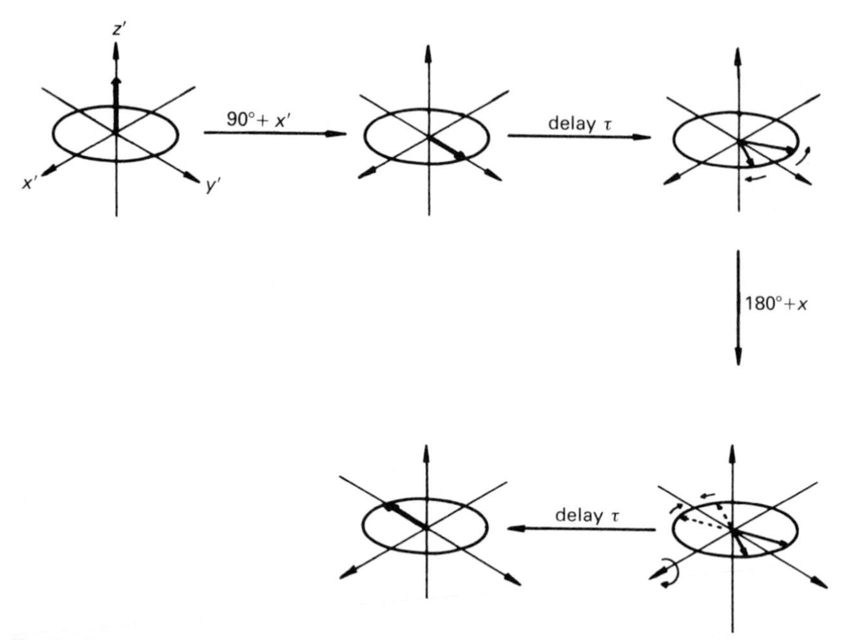

Fig. C1. Classical description of the Carr–Purcell sequence. A 90° pulse applied along the x' axis of the rotating frame creates precessing transverse magnetization which is initially aligned along the y' axis. After a delay τ the isochromats have dephased, and are refocused by a 180° pulse applied along the x' axis to produce an echo at a time 2τ.

interval after the π pulse. Any diffusion makes rephasing imperfect and reduces the intensity of the next echo. Of course T_2 relaxation (see **relaxation, spin–spin relaxation**) causes the echo amplitude to decrease also, but the reduction in echo amplitude caused by T_2 will only depend upon on the total time elapsed. In contrast, the diffusion term will be dependent upon τ. This, if τ is changed, but $n2\tau$ is held constant, it is possible to vary the contribution due to diffusion but not T_2. Thus the effect of the diffusion term can be made negligible.

The Carr–Purcell sequence can contain many pulses. Until now it has been assumed tacitly that these are perfect pulses, i.e. containing no timing or phase errors. If the pulse rotations for the π pulses deviate slightly, there are cumulative effects which become large and serious. For example, if the pulse is actually less than π refocusing will not occur exactly in the xy plane. In fact, these errors will always arise since an r.f. pulse is never uniform across a sample due to r.f. field inhomogeneity. Meiboom and Gill showed a simple solution to this problem. They introduced a 90° phase shift between the initial $\pi/2$ pulse and subsequent π pulses. Thus, for a $\pi/2$ pulse along the $+x$ axis, subsequent π pulses are applied along the $+y$ axis. All echoes then form along the $+y$ axis, and furthermore r.f. pulse imperfections cancel with each π pulse and the error is not cumulative. The CPMG sequence is therefore

$$90°_x - \tau - 180°_y - 2\tau - 180°_y - 2\tau - 180°_y - 2\tau \ldots \quad \text{acquisition.}$$

In practice, the CPMG sequence is of value in the measurement of spin–spin relaxation.

FURTHER READING

Carr, H. Y. and Purcell, E. M. (1954). *Phys. Rev.* **94,** 630.
See also
Schlichter, C. P. (1978). *Principles of magnetic resonance* (2nd edn). Springer-Verlag, Berlin.

Cartesian operators See **product operator formalism**.

Chemical exchange From the theory of the **chemical shift**, it is clear that the resonance frequency of a given nucleus will depend upon its environment. This in turn will give rise to an absorption line at a certain discrete chemical shift which can often be used to characterize the environment qualitatively. However, it is sometimes not possible to describe 'the environment' of the nucleus since in certain dynamic systems it may exist in more than one environment. This is known as chemical exchange. An example is the equilibrium between a ligand molecule bound to its receptor and the same molecule free in solution. It might be thought that this system would give rise to two resonance lines for a given nucleus within the ligand, reflecting the presence of free and bound ligand. Although this is certainly a possibility, it is equally possible that a single resonance line would be observed, despite the fact that the nucleus in question exists in two quite different environments. These different effects upon the NMR spectrum can be understood with reference to the time-scale of the exchange phenomenon. If the exchange rate is slow in comparison with the chemical shift difference (in radians per second) between the resonant frequencies of the resonances which characterize each state (e.g. free or bound), then we speak of slow exchange. In this case two discrete resonances would indeed be observed for a given nucleus. However, if the exchange rate is fast in comparison with the chemical shift difference, we call this fast exchange. A single resonance would now be observed, with a chemical shift which is the average of the chemical shifts observed in the slow exchange case, but weighted by the relative populations of the two states. A further situation arises when the exchange rate is similar to the chemical shift difference. This is known as intermediate exchange, which is characterized by line broadening. These qualitative aspects can be understood in a more formal manner by consideration of a simple example. Consider two species A and B. In the absence of chemical exchange these will produce two resonance lines at the characteristic **Larmor precession** frequencies ω_A and ω_B. If the concentrations are equal, we can equate the rate constants for chemical exchange between these species:

$$A \underset{K_{BA}}{\overset{K_{AB}}{\rightleftharpoons}} B$$

C1 $$K_{AB} = K_{BA} = K.$$

The appearance of the spectrum for various values of K is shown in Fig. C2. When exchange is slow between the two species ($[\omega_A - \omega_B] \gg K$) the resonances are resolved but are broadened by an amount $\Delta\omega = K/\pi$. This is rationalized by noting that each species exists in a given state for $1/K$ s, and from the **uncertainty principle** the resonances will be 'lifetime broadened' by an amount proportional to K; there is an uncertainty K/π in the resonance frequencies.

In fast exchange ($[\omega_A - \omega_B] \ll K$) the nuclei visit each site many times on the time-scale of the measurement, and so a single signal is obtained at the average frequency, $(\omega_A - \omega_B)/2$. In those cases where the concentration in each site is not equal, then the average frequency is weighted linearly with respect to the two concentrations. The width of the resonance line in fast exchange decreases as the exchange rate

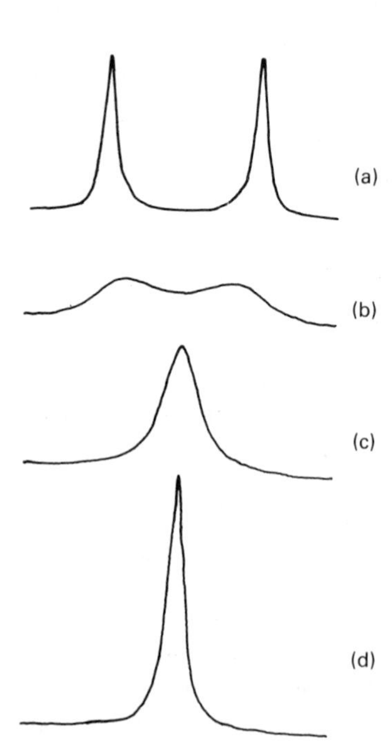

Fig. C2. Lineshapes during chemical exchange between two sites A and B (see text). The values of K are (a) 0.1π $(\omega_A - \omega_B)$; (b) 0.5π $(\omega_A - \omega_B)$; (c) 2π $(\omega_A - \omega_B)$; (d) 4π $(\omega_A - \omega_B)$.

increases since the averaging becomes more complete; $\Delta\omega = \pi(\omega_A - \omega_B)^2/2K$. In intermediate exchange ($[\omega_A - \omega_B] \approx K$), the lineshape is rather complex, and is best quantified by fitting to the **Bloch equations** modified by inclusion of chemical exchange.

The separation of the lines in slow and intermediate exchange is given by

C2 $$\Delta\omega = [(\omega_A - \omega_B)^2 - 2K^2/\pi^2]^{\frac{1}{2}}$$

which shows that the lines slowly merge as K increases.

In many situations of interest in biological NMR, the concentrations of nuclei in each site are dissimilar. For example, the concentration of ligand bound to an enzyme is very much smaller than free ligand. In these circumstances it is often possible only to observe the lineshape and shift of the free ligand. Under these conditions, the relaxation times of the bound ligand will usually be much shorter than free ligand, since the former is dominated by the slow rotational **correlation time** of the macromolecule. In such cases with unequal populations and relaxation times, Swift and Connick have derived expressions for the observed shifts and relaxation times. The chemical shift of the ligand in the bulk environment measured with respect to the shift of the 'pure' ligand is given by

C3 $$\Delta\omega = \frac{P_b(\omega_A - \omega_B)}{(1/T_2' + K)^2 + (\omega_A - \omega_B)^2/K^2}$$

where P_b is the fraction of bound ligand and T_2' is the spin–spin relaxation time in the bound environment. In the limit of fast exchange, (C3) reduces to

C4 $$\Delta\omega = P_b(\omega_A - \omega_B)$$

which is effectively the weighted average described qualitatively above.

The observed relaxation rates of the ligand in bulk solution are given by

C5 $$\frac{1}{T_{1,\,obs}} = \frac{1}{T_{1,\,A}} + \frac{P_b}{T_{1,\,B} + K^{-1}}$$

C6 $$\frac{1}{T_{2,\,obs}} = \frac{1}{T_{2,\,A}} + \frac{P_b}{K^{-1}}\left[\frac{\frac{1}{T_{2,\,B}}\left(\frac{1}{T_{2,\,B}} + K\right) + (\omega_A - \omega_B)^2}{\left(\frac{1}{T_{2,B}} + K\right)^2 + (\omega_A - \omega_B)^2}\right]$$

where the subscripts are in obvious notation. The linewidth is easily determined from (C6).

FURTHER READING

For a detailed description of chemical exchange in a variety of systems, see
Dwek, R. A. (1973). *NMR in biochemistry*, Clarendon Press, Oxford.
Swift, T. J. and Connick, R. E. (1962). *J. Chem. Phys.* **37,** 307.

Chemical shift The fundamental equation of NMR, $\omega = \gamma B_0$, tells us that if every nucleus in a sample was subject to the same magnetic field B_0, then the NMR spectrum of the sample would be composed of a multitude of resonance lines of identical frequency. This is of course not the case, and each nucleus (or group of magnetically equivalent nuclei) resonates with a characteristic frequency, or chemical shift. Perhaps the most often used example to illustrate chemical shifts is ethanol. The ^{1}H NMR spectrum of ethanol (Fig. C3) consists of three lines, whose intensities are in the ratio 3:2:1. Each line is further split due to **spin coupling**.

The three lines are clearly due to the three 'types' of nucleus. Furthermore, the relative intensity ratios suggest that the CH_3 protons are equivalent, as are the CH_2 protons, with the OH proton forming a third 'group'. Obviously the nuclei experience local fields due to their molecular surroundings which are different from B_0. In addition, if we were to measure the difference in chemical shift *vs.* B_0, we would find that the following relationship holds:

C7 $$\omega = \gamma(B_0 - \sigma B_0)$$

where σ is called the screening constant. In comparing chemical shifts, therefore, we are measuring the differences in σ associated with different molecular environments. An important property of molecular screening is that it is anisotropic, i.e. it differs along various axes within the molecule with respect to B_0. Therefore σ is a **tensor** (see **chemical shift**

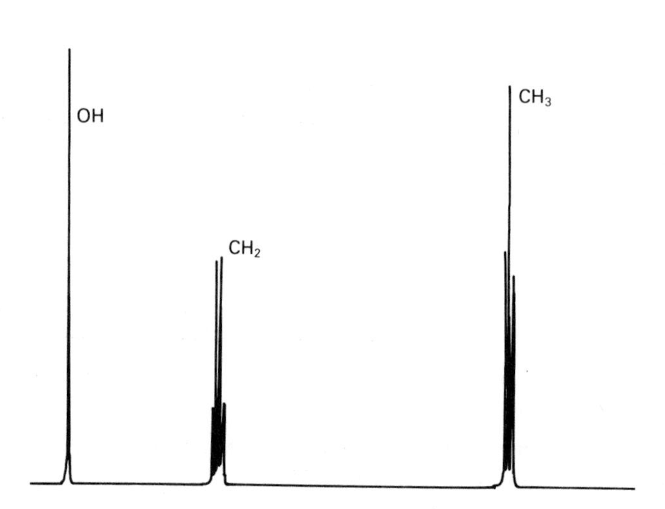

Fig. C3. ^{1}H NMR spectrum of ethanol.

anisotropy). However, in the gas or liquid phase, due to rapid molecular motion, a nucleus is subjected to an average value of σ, represented by the trace of the tensor (see Appendix 3).

Chemical shifts arise from the simultaneous interaction of a nucleus with an electron and of the electron with the applied static field B_0. It is practically impossible to calculate a value for the screening constant due to the complexity of the mechanisms which give rise to it. However, chemical shifts can be understood empirically with regard to several types of effect, as discussed below.

1. PARAMAGNETIC TERM

The contribution of the paramagnetic term to σ cannot readily be described classically. It can be loosely described as the generation of electronic asymmetry by the electric fields of nearby nuclei. In the case of protons, the paramagnetic term does not contribute to σ since s electrons have no orbital angular momentum. For other nuclei it is the dominant effect and is usually much larger than the diamagnetic term. For this reason the range of chemical shifts for the proton are small in comparison with other nuclei.

2. DIAMAGNETIC TERM

This originates in the electronic shielding of the nucleus. The presence of a group in the molecule which donates or withdraws electrons will therefore affect the chemical shift of a nearby nucleus. An example is the low-field (deshielded) resonance position of the C1 proton of glucose (and many other carbohydrates) due to the electron-withdrawing properties of the ring oxygen. Diamagnetic effects are important contributors to proton magnetic resonance spectra.

3. MAGNETIC ANISOTROPY

Local magnetic fields can be generated at a given nucleus due to anisotropy in neighbouring groups. A particularly important example in biological NMR is the so called **ring current shift** due to the aromatic rings of histidine, phenylalanine, tyrosine, and tryptophan residues in proteins. These act as natural probes of structure. A further example of anisotropy effects is the extreme low-field shifts found for aldehyde protons due to anisotropy of the carbonyl group.

4. ELECTRIC FIELDS

If a strongly polar group is present in a molecule, the molecular electron distribution will be influenced. This, in turn, affects σ. The effect is composed of two terms. The first describes electron drift in the polar bond against the inherent electric field. The second term describes the asymmetry induced by this shift, resulting in paramagnetic deshielding. Electric field effects are significant in ^{19}F shifts.

5. UNPAIRED ELECTRON SHIFTS

The very large magnetic moment of an unpaired electron can have a dramatic effect on the NMR spectrum. The hyperfine coupling observed in ESR spectra will of course be observed in the NMR spectrum. In addition, dipolar coupling between the electron and the nucleus may broaden the NMR resonance line very significantly. Alternatively, if the magnitude of the hyperfine coupling is very much less than the electron relaxation rate, then sharp lines are observed in the NMR spectrum which show large shifts. This is the famous Knight shift which is a characteristic of the NMR spectra of metals. The explanation of the Knight shift involves considering the field experienced by the nucleus as a result of the interaction with conduction electrons through the hyperfine coupling. Since the electrons in a metal are delocalized, a given nucleus is magnetically coupled to many electrons. Therefore the coupling is averaged over the electron spin orientations of many electrons. However, the electron spins are polarized in the B_0 field, and thus there is a non-vanishing coupling. Since the interaction corresponds to the nucleus experiencing a magnetic field parallel to the electron magnetic moment, and since the electron moment is preferentially parallel to B_0, the effective field at the nucleus is increased.

6. SOLVENT EFFECTS

Solvents can induce shifts by three general mechanisms:

(a) Magnetic anisotropy

Effects similar to ring current shifts can exist in certain solvents, e.g. benzene. Due to molecular reorientation an average of this contribution to σ is seen by the solute. If the solvent molecule is asymmetric, a non-zero average will result in a 'solvent shift'.

(b) Orientation effects

These effects may occur when a polar solute is dissolved in a polar solvent. Ordering of solvent molecules around the solute can occur, which enhances the diamagnetic shielding caused by the electric dipole with the solute.

(c) Solvent–solute interactions

A common example of this type of interaction is hydrogen bonding. For example, the NH protons of *N*-acetylglucosamine are shifted in their hydrogen-bonded state with respect to their unbonded shifts. This has been used to investigate the solution conformations of polysaccharides. The basis for shifts induced by hydrogen bonds is not well understood, however, and the shifts can therefore only be characterized qualitatively.

In view of the difficulty of quantifying chemical shifts, their application in biological NMR is generally qualitative. A possible exception to this has been the use of ring current shifts to correlate crystallographic data with those obtained in solution. In all other respects, the chemical shift is interpreted qualitatively in terms of the type of group or groups which resonate at characteristic positions in the NMR spectrum with respect to an internal standard.

Chemical shift anisotropy (CSA) In discussing **chemical shift**, the concept of the screening or shielding constant was introduced, which was described as a **tensor**. A tensor, which in the present case is actually a 3×3 matrix, is a representation of the value of a particular function in terms of a set of coordinates relative to a particular coordinate system. In this case the latter is defined by the magnetic field direction. From a somewhat idealized viewpoint, the values of the function can be represented pictorially by the length of a line parallel to one of the axes of the coordinate system (the magnetic field) through the centre of an ellipsoid of revolution (Fig. C4). It should be clear from Fig. C4 that different orientations of the magnetic field relative to the molecular coordinates will result in different resonance positions for the same chemical species. This is known as chemical shift anisotropy. The absolute magnitudes of the lengths of each axis in Fig. C4 are known as the principal values. In liquids, all orientations are assumed by a molecule in a time short compared to the inverse of the chemical shift anisotropy. This time average (see **averaging**) over orientations results in a resonance line only at the average chemical shift, which is sometimes called the isotropic value of σ. It is equal to the trace (see Appendix 3) of the tensor:

$$\bar{\sigma} = \tfrac{1}{3}(\sigma_{xx} + \sigma_{yy} + \sigma_{zz}). \qquad \text{C8}$$

In contrast, the NMR spectra of powders (see **powder spectrum**), solids (see **solid state NMR**) and liquid crystalline samples show chemical shift anisotropy with characteristic lineshapes.

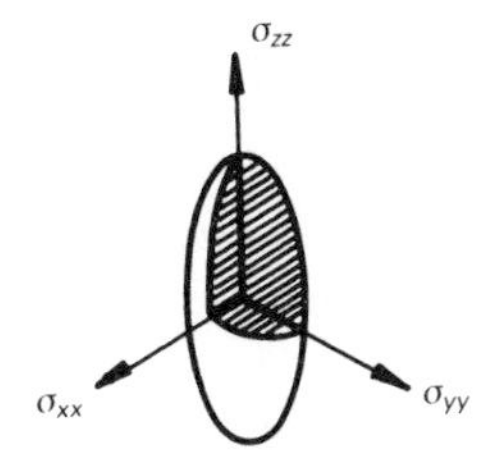

Fig. C4. Representation of chemical shift anisotropy as an ellipsoid of revolution.

In isotropic liquids, although chemical-shift anisotropy does not affect the **lineshape** as such, under certain circumstances it can act as an efficient **relaxation** mechanism (T_1 and T_2) and will therefore contribute to the linewidth. See **anisotropic chemical shift relaxation**.

Chemically induced dynamic nuclear polarization (CIDNP) CIDNP arises from a spin-sorting process acting during recombination of radical pairs, which leads to greatly perturbed populations of nuclear spin state levels. This in turn results in large intensity enhancements (see **Boltzmann distribution**) of NMR lines. Of course, free radicals are few and far between in biological systems, and therefore the experimenter is required to take certain steps to create them. A suitable method is known as photochemically induced dynamic nuclear polarization (photo-CIDNP), and can be described as follows.

A solution of the compound (usually a protein) is irradiated in the presence of a dye with an argon laser, which is aimed down the bore of the NMR probe. The dye becomes photoexcited and reacts reversibly with aromatic amino acid (tyrosine, histidine, tryptophan) sidechains on the surface of the protein to generate dye–protein radical pairs. The dissociation of the radical pairs generates nuclear spin polarization in the sidechains. If 'light' and 'dark' NMR spectra are recorded in alternative scans, a difference spectrum will give lines derived from the polarized residues. In this manner individual residues on the surface of the protein can be identified.

In biological systems, the radical pair mechanism of photo-CIDNP appears to be dominant. An encounter of two reactive radicals in solution may lead to a recombination reaction:

$$\boxed{R_1\cdot + R_2\cdot} \rightarrow R_1 - R_2. \qquad \text{C9}$$

This leads to **emission lines** in the spectrum.

Alternatively, an escape reaction may occur:

$$\boxed{R_1\cdot + R_2\cdot} \rightarrow R_1\cdot + R_2\cdot \qquad \text{C10}$$

leading to enhanced absorption signals.

The actual path followed depends partly on the spin states of the nuclei present in the radicals. This is a consequence of two assumptions of the radical pair theory. First, the reaction probability of a radical pair depends on the electronic spin state of the pair. Second, there are nuclear spin-dependent interactions involved in interconverting singlet and triplet radical pair states.

A schematic diagram showing typical photo-CIDNP difference spectra of the amino acids histidine, tyrosine, and tryptophan is shown in Fig. C5. The presence of a strong emission line in the aromatic region of tyrosine is very useful in the assignment of this residue. Histidine and

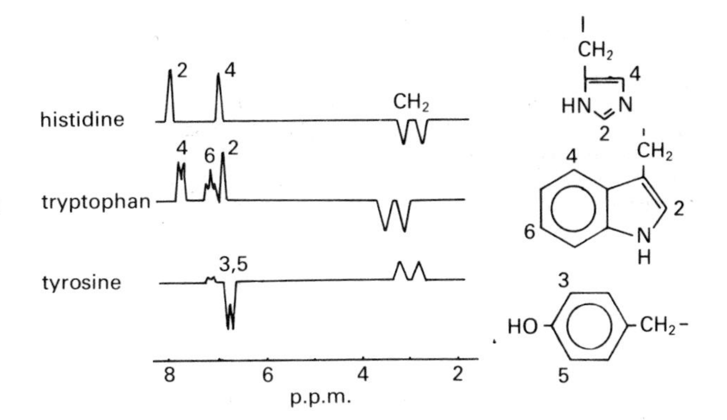

Fig. C5. Typical photo-CIDNP spectra of histidine, tyrosine, and tryptophan. Reproduced from Kaptein (1982), with permission.

tryptophan, on the other hand, can be distinguished by the pH dependence of the former.

The accessibility of a tyrosine, histidine, or tryptophan residue may be modified by the presence of ligands interacting with the protein. This is manifested by a change in CIDNP intensity, which therefore characterizes the residue at or near the binding site. This constitutes one of the major applications of the method.

FURTHER READING

For a review of photo-CIDNP as applied to proteins, see
Kaptein, R. (1982). *Biol. Magn. Reson.* **4,** 145–91.

CIDNP See **chemically induced dynamic nuclear polarization**.

Classical formalism In order to understand the workings of an NMR experiment, and thus to predict the result, we require a formalism with which to 'visualize' the evolution in time of the **spin system**. If we were to consider a single spin, a quantum mechanical formalism would be required. This is because atomic phenomena do not behave classically, i.e. they do not obey Newtonian mechanics. For example, if we were to attempt to measure the x or y components of the magnetization of a single proton, we would get one of two answers, $+\frac{1}{2}$ or $-\frac{1}{2}$ (in units of $\hbar$). However, if we repeated the measurement, the result would not always be the same. In other words, a single nucleus does not behave classically. Nevertheless, the phenomenologically formulated **Bloch equations** are perfectly consistent in describing simple NMR experiments in terms of classical mechanics. We resolve this apparent paradox by noting that the **expectation values** of the x and y components of the magnetization do behave classically. The signal observed in an NMR experiment derives from a large ensemble of spins, so the detected signal (expectation value

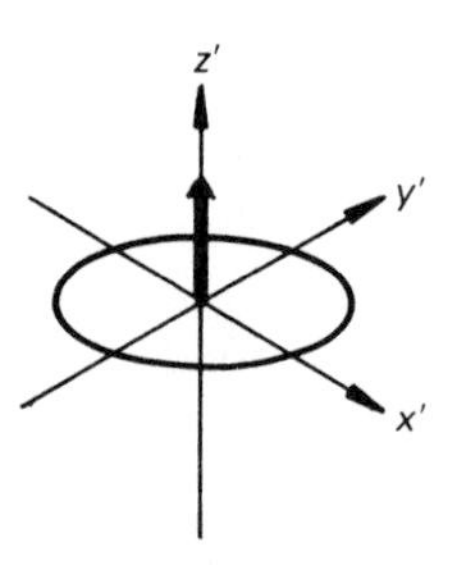

Fig. C6. The classical 'bulk magnetization vector', representing an excess of spins aligned along the static magnetic field B_0. The latter lies by convention along the $+z'$ axis.

of the x or y component of the magnetization) behaves in a classical manner. In some respects this must be intuitively obvious, since the NMR sample (as opposed to a single nucleus) is a classical object, and we therefore expect it to behave classically, in much the same way as a billiard ball.

The value of the classical formalism is that the bulk 'magnetization' from all of the spins in the sample can be represented by a vector. For example, at thermal equilibrium, this bulk magnetization vector lies by convention along the positive z' axis (so-called 'longitudinal magnetization') in a cartesian coordinate system in the **rotating frame** (Fig. C6). This represents a net excess of spins aligned along the static field, B_0. The effects of r.f. pulses are now represented by simple rotations of the bulk magnetization vector. For example, a 90° pulse along the $+x'$ axis will rotate the magnetization through 90° so that it is aligned along the $+y'$ axis (so-called 'transverse' magnetization). Using this formalism, complex pulse sequences such as the **Carr–Purcell–Meiboom–Gill sequence** are easily understood. Conversely, non-linear effects such as those giving rise to **multiple quantum coherence** cannot be represented by this simple formalism.

FURTHER READING

For a gentle introduction to NMR using the classical formalism see

Farrar, T. C. and Becker, E. D. (1971). *Pulse and Fourier transform NMR*. Academic Press, New York.

Coherence See **phase coherence**, **double-quantum coherence**, **multiple-quantum coherence**, **zero-quantum coherence**.

Coherence transfer Many **two-dimensional NMR** experiments depend upon the transfer of part of a coherence or the total coherence present between levels j and k to coherence between levels l and m. If both coherences are single-quantum coherences, we speak of magnetization transfer between transitions. More generally we use the term coherence transfer. Theoretically, coherence transfer is described by the action of **rotation operators**

upon the **density matrix**, or, equivalently, the transformation properties of product operators under **Hamiltonians** corresponding to r.f. pulses. Coherence transfer is responsible for the presence of crosspeaks in many two-dimensional spectra. Often, no net magnetization is transferred from one nucleus to the other, and the net integrated intensity of the crosspeak is then zero, i.e. the multiplet components are in antiphase. In other experiments which employ a different coherence transfer mechanism (see for example, **homonuclear Hartmann–Hahn spectroscopy**), net coherence transfer can be achieved, leading to in-phase multiplet structure in crosspeaks.

FURTHER READING

For a discussion of coherence transfer in a variety of systems, see

Ernst, R. R., Bodenhausen, G., and Wokaun, A. A. (1987). *Principles of NMR in one and two dimensions.* Chapter 8. Clarendon Press, Oxford.

Coherence transfer echo In all **two-dimensional NMR** experiments in inhomogeneous magnetic fields where the amplitude of a detected coherence is modulated as a function of t_1, coherence transfer echoes may be observed. The detected magnetization can be written as

$$M(t_1, t_2) = K \cos(\omega_{jk} t_1) \exp(\mathrm{i}\omega_{im} t_2) \tag{C11}$$

where the amplitude modulating function is $\cos(\omega_{jk} t_1)$ and K is a constant. Using the identity $\cos\theta = \frac{1}{2}(\mathrm{e}^{i\theta} + \mathrm{e}^{-i\theta})$, (C11) can be written as

$$M(t_1, t_2) = \tfrac{1}{2}K[\exp(-\mathrm{i}\omega_{jk} t_1 + \mathrm{i}\omega_{im} t_2) + \exp(\mathrm{i}\omega_{jk} t_1 + \mathrm{i}\omega_{im} t_2)]. \tag{C12}$$

Thus the detected signal is composed of two components modulated in opposite sense with respect to t_1. In the presence of magnetic field inhomogeneity, the first term on the right-hand side of (C12) will give rise to a so-called coherence transfer echo. This is because, during t_1, the **phase modulation** is opposite in sense to that in t_2, giving rise to a refocusing effect in an inhomogeneous magnetic field at a time dependent upon the order of the coherences and/or the nuclei involved in the coherence transfer. Since the phase modulation is in the same sense for the second term on the right-hand side of (C12), this aggravates the loss of **phase coherence** due to the magnetic field inhomogeneity, and this term is thus often referred to as the **antiecho**. The selective detection of the coherence transfer echo is implicit in two-dimensional experiments employing phase modulation during t_1. This is achieved by using either **phase-cycling** or **field gradient** procedures. The presence of the coherence transfer echo can often be observed in the **free induction decay** during the course of a two-dimensional NMR experiment. A practical example is illustrated in Fig. C7.

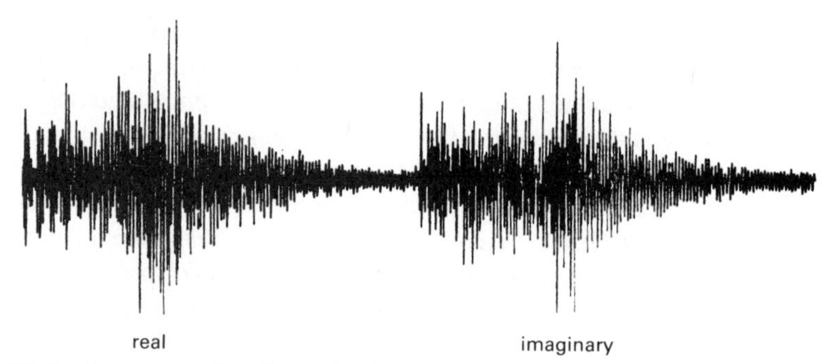

Fig. C7. A coherence transfer echo can be observed in these free induction decays derived from a conventional COSY experiment.

FURTHER READING

Maudsley, A. A., Wokaun, A., and Ernst, R. R. (1978). *Chem. Phys. Lett.* **55,** 9.

Coherence transfer pathways Many two-dimensional NMR experiments rely upon the same effective pulse sequence. Examples are **double-quantum filtered correlated spectroscopy** and **nuclear Overhauser effect spectroscopy**. The difference between these experiments lies in the exact **phase cycling** procedure used to select the desired coherence transfer pathway. The concept of a coherence transfer pathway is quite straightforward. From it stems a useful formalism due to Bodenhausen *et al.* (see Further reading) with which phase cycling procedures can be determined without explicit calculation.

To illustrate the principles of pathway selection, consider the pulse sequence appropriate for **correlated spectroscopy** (COSY). We assume that the spin system is at thermal equilibrium before the first pulse, and thus the 'coherence order' $p = 0$ (since only longitudinal magnetization exists). The first pulse can only create single-quantum coherences. These are described by $P = \pm 1$, since a given transition between eigenstates is associated with two coherences. Each coherence in this simple case corresponds with a classical magnetization vector (see **classical formalism**) which precesses in the rotating frame at $\pm\omega$, depending upon the respective sign of p. During the t_1 period, no change in coherence order can occur. The coherence transfer pathway ends with detection after the second pulse, at which stage single-quantum coherence $p = \pm 1$ must be available in order to induce an e.m.f. in the receiver coils. The complete procedure is shown in Fig. C8. The solid line shows the coherence transfer pathway $0 \rightarrow +1 \rightarrow -1$, which represents signals with precession frequencies of opposite sign in ω_1, ω_2 and thus corresponds to 'echo' peaks in the resulting spectrum. The dotted line represents **antiecho** peaks, where the precession frequencies are of the same sign in ω_1, ω_2. Let us assume for the moment that we wish to select echo-type

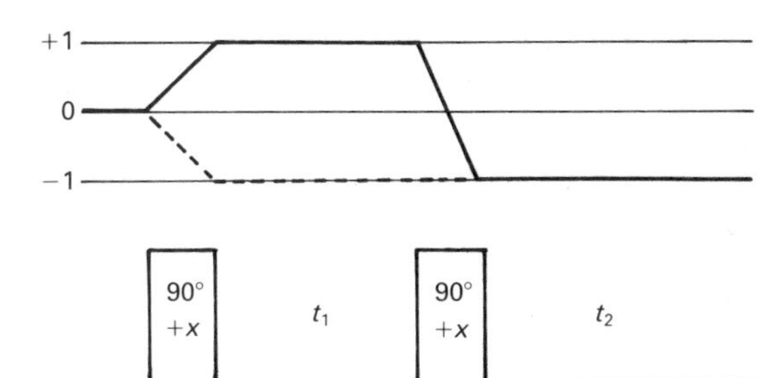

Fig. C8. Diagrammatic illustration of coherence transfer pathways in a conventional COSY experiment.

peaks. How is this achieved without explicit calculation (e.g. using the **density matrix** or **product operator formalisms**)? In order to answer this question it is necessary to examine the effect of a **phase** shift upon a coherence of order p. If we represent the phase shift by a rotation about the z axis, the properties of p-quantum coherence can be described by the following transformation:

C13 $$\exp(-\mathrm{i}\phi F_z)\sigma^p \exp(\mathrm{i}\phi F_z) = \sigma^p \exp(-\mathrm{i}p\phi)$$

where $F_z = \sum_{k=1}^{N} I_{K_z}$, and the density operator σ is represented by a sum of terms according to the coherence order p:

C14 $$\sigma(t) = \sum_p \sigma^p(t).$$

In the case of spins $\frac{1}{2}$, p extends over the total number of spins N; $p = \pm N$. Equation (C13) essentially tells us that a coherence of order p has a p-fold sensitivity to a phase-shift ϕ about the z-axis. Now in a two-dimensional experiment, n coherence transfer processes will generally be operative, and each can be represented by a **propagator** U:

C15 $$\sigma_{(0)} \xrightarrow{U_1} \xrightarrow{U_2} \xrightarrow{U_3} \ldots \xrightarrow{U_n} \sigma(t).$$

Each propagator causes coherence transfer from a particular order to numerous different orders (for example, note the effect of the pulses in Fig. C8).

After n coherence transfer steps, each pathway is represented by a set of n values representing the change in coherence at each step:

C16 $$\Delta p_i = p_{(+)} - p_{(-)}$$

where $p_{(+)}$ and $p_{(-)}$ are the coherence orders just after and just before the coherence transfer step. The complete pathway can thus be represented by a vector

C17 $$\mathbf{\Delta p} = [\Delta p_1, \Delta p_2, \ldots, \Delta p_n]$$

where the sum of the components is fixed since all pathways begin with $p=0$ and end with $p=-1$ (assuming **quadrature detection** to select signals precessing at $-\omega$ in t_2).

To restrict coherence transfer under a particular U (equation C15) to a particular change Δp_i in coherence order, it is necessary to perform N_i experiments where the phase ϕ_i of the propagator is incremented sequentially:

C18 $$\phi_i = K_i 2\pi/N_i, \qquad K_i = 0, 1, 2, \ldots, N_i - 1.$$

The N_i signals observed in the detection period are then combined according to a Fourier analysis (see **Fourier transform**) with respect to ϕ_i:

C19 $$S(\Delta p_i, t) = \frac{1}{N_i} \sum_{K_i=0}^{N_i-1} S(\phi_i, t) \exp(\mathrm{i}\Delta p_i \phi_i).$$

Thus, all coherence transfer pathways are selected which undergo a change in coherence order Δp_i under the propagator U_i. However, as a consequence of the sampling theorem (see **aliasing**), it is not possible to select a unique Δp_i, but rather a series of values:

C20 $$\Delta p_i \pm nN_i, \qquad n = 0, 1, 2, \ldots$$

and thus if a unique Δp_i value is to be chosen from a range of r consecutive values, N_i must be at least equal to r.

Using (C18) and (C20), it is now possible to design a suitable phase cycle for the detection of the $p=0 \rightarrow +1 \rightarrow -1$ coherence in Fig. C8 (solid line). Clearly, we specify the pathway uniquely if we select the change in coherence order due to the mixing pulse (second coherence transfer step) $\Delta p_2 = -2$. Following the formalism of Bodenhausen *et al.*, it is useful to create a list of changes in coherence order for a given coherence transfer step, and to emphasize the desired value in boldtype, while expressing the values which should be blocked in parentheses. Thus for coherence transfer step 2, we can write

C21 $$\Delta p_2 = \ldots -3, \mathbf{-2}, (-1), (0), 1, 2, 3, \ldots$$

since according to Fig. C8, **−2** is the desired change in coherence order, and -1 and 0 are changes which must be blocked. Therefore the number of consecutive values r from which the desired value must be extracted is 3, and this must be the minimum value of N_i. We can therefore choose a phase cycle such that (equation C18):

C22 $$\phi_2 = K_2(2\pi/3), \qquad K_2 = 0, 1, 2$$

i.e. ϕ_2 (the phase of the mixing pulse) is cycled through 0, 120°, 240°. This leads to the selection

C23 $$\Delta p_2 = \ldots (-3), \mathbf{-2}, (-1), (0), \mathbf{1}, (2), (3), \ldots$$

where the value +1 is also selected due to aliasing (equation C20). The above result indicates that a COSY experiment with echo selection (see **phase modulation**) can be performed with a three-step phase cycle, rather than the conventional four-step cycle. In fact the four-step cycle results in the non-essential (equation C21) suppression of the value +1:

C24 $$\Delta p_2 = (-3), \mathbf{-2}, (-1), (0), (1), \mathbf{2}, (3), \ldots.$$

To achieve the selection required in (C21), the signals must be combined according to (C19). This is achieved conveniently by phase shifting the receiver reference by

C25 $$\phi_{\text{ref}} = -\sum_i \Delta p_i \phi_i$$

and thus for the above three-step cycle,

C26 $$\phi_{\text{ref}} = -\Delta p_2 \phi_2 = +2\phi_2$$

which gives the complete procedure for the three-step cycle:

ϕ_1	ϕ_2	ref
0	0	0
0	$\frac{1}{3}(2\pi)$	$\frac{1}{3}(4\pi)$
0	$\frac{1}{3}(4\pi)$	$(8\pi/3) \equiv \frac{1}{3}(2\pi)$

or, for the four-step cycle;

ϕ_1	ϕ_2	ref
0	0	0
0	$\frac{1}{2}\pi$	π
0	π	$(2\pi) \equiv 0$
0	$\frac{1}{2}(3\pi)$	$\frac{1}{2}(6\pi) \equiv \pi$

The latter is recognized as the **phase cycling** procedure required for phase modulated (see **phase modulation**) COSY. Using the above formalism, a shorter, more efficient phase cycle has been discovered. If sensitivity is not limiting, then the number of scans per t_1 increment may thus be reduced.

If phase-sensitive experiments are required, then it is necessary to retain the 'mirror image' pathway in t_1 (dotted line in Fig. C8). We must therefore recast (C21) to give

C27 $$\Delta p_2 = -3, \mathbf{-2}, (-1), \mathbf{0}, 1, 2, 3, \ldots.$$

N_2 is now equal to 2 (selection from two consecutive values), and a two-step phase cycle is sufficient:

ϕ_1	ϕ_2	ref
0	0	0
0	π	$(2\pi) \equiv 0$

In many experiments more stringent pathway selection is required than can be obtained by cycling the phase of a single propagator U_i. In these cases, the desired pathway may be retained by cycling the phases of each propagator separately. The phase of U_{i-1} is cycled through all N_i steps before incrementing the phase of U_i. The total number of experiments thus equals $N_1 \,.\, N_2 \,.\, N_3 \,.\, \ldots \,.\, N_n$. The signals must then be combined according to the sum in (C25).

FURTHER READING

Bodenhausen, G., Kogler, H., and Ernst, R. R. (1984). *J. Magn. Reson.* **58,** 370.

Coherent averaging theory See **average Hamiltonian theory**.

Combination lines Combination lines arise from 'forbidden' transitions in multiple-spin systems. They cannot generally be observed in a conventional NMR experiment. To illustrate which transitions give rise to combination lines, consider the spin states and their transitions for a three-spin system with finite mutual spin couplings (Fig. C9). If **weak coupling** is assumed, the eight eigenstates of this system can be represented by the following product functions (see **product basis**):

$$
\begin{aligned}
(8) &= |\alpha\alpha\alpha\rangle \qquad & (4) &= |\alpha\alpha\beta\rangle \\
(7) &= |\alpha\beta\alpha\rangle & (3) &= |\alpha\beta\beta\rangle \\
(6) &= |\beta\alpha\alpha\rangle & (2) &= |\beta\alpha\beta\rangle \\
(5) &= |\beta\beta\alpha\rangle & (1) &= |\beta\beta\beta\rangle .
\end{aligned}
$$

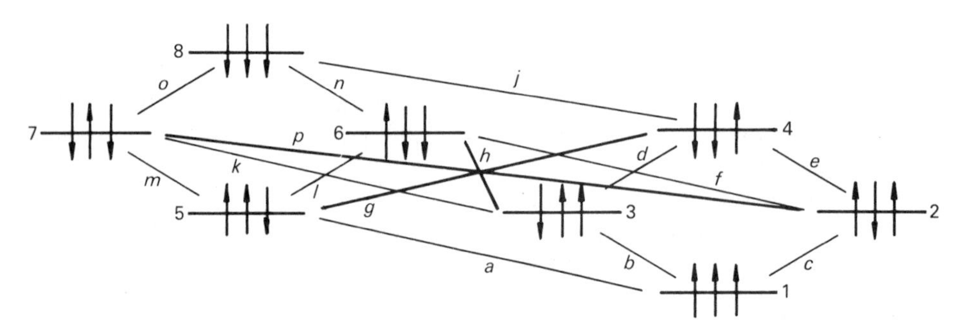

Fig. C9. The eight spin states of a weakly coupled three-spin system. Single-quantum transitions are shown by fine lines, whereas transitions leading to combination lines are shown in bold.

Each eigenstate is characterized by a value for the total spin, F. According to a selection rule, observable magnetization will only be obtained from those transitions where $\Delta F = \pm 1$. These are known as single-quantum transitions (see **multiple-quantum coherence**). There are fifteen in the three-spin system of Fig. C9, labelled a–p. Each transition is in general characterized by the flipping of a single spin. For example, transition b is derived from state $1 = |\beta\beta\beta\rangle$ under going a single spin-flip to state $3 = |\alpha\beta\beta\rangle$. However, three transitions, g, h, and p are seen to correspond to a more complex situation where two spins flip in one direction as a third flips in the other direction, e.g. states $2 = |\beta\alpha\beta\rangle$ and $7 = |\alpha\beta\alpha\rangle$. These transitions give rise to combination lines in the NMR spectrum. Since they are not of true 'single-quantum' character (despite the fact that they obey the 'selection rule') such lines are either absent or strongly inhibited in conventional NMR spectra.

Commutator In the world of classical mechanics we are familiar with algebraic expressions such as $A \,.\, B \,.\, C = D$. The equivalent operation, $B \,.\, A \,.\, C = D$, is equally valid. If we consider A and B to be **operators**, we could interpret the first equation in terms of B operating on C, (the operation being multiplication) followed by A operating on the result to give D. The second equation is the same except that A is the first operator. A simple physical interpretation of this can be obtained if A and B are operators corresponding to **observables**. If we make two measurements upon a classical object, we naturally get two results, and D would represent their product. It matters not which measurement we make first; the result is still D. However, in the world of quantum mechanics, we might get two different results depending upon which measurement we had made first. In terms of the algebraic expressions, therefore, $A \,.\, B \,.\, C = D$, but $B \,.\, A \,.\, C$ would not necessarily also equal D. The uncertainty depends upon whether the two operators commute, i.e. if $A \,.\, B = B \,.\, A$. We use a shorthand notation to test whether this is true:

$$[A, B] = AB - BA. \quad \text{(C28)}$$

If the value of $[A, B]$ is zero, the two operators are said to commute. If it is not zero, the result is called the commutator of A and B. The latter possibility is reminiscent of the fact that the product of two matrices is usually dependent upon the order of multiplication (see Appendix 3). Since quantum mechanical operators can be expressed in matrix form (see e.g. **Pauli-spin matrices**), it follows that the commutator of two non-commuting operators can also be represented by a matrix. This matrix is often another operator.

The presence of a commutator between two operators is fundamental to the workings of quantum mechanics. This can be seen with reference to the commutation rules of **angular momentum** operators. These are the fundamental equations governing the behaviour of cartesian product operators (see **product operator formalism**) under various rotations. Due to their importance, it is very worthwhile committing the commutation relations for angular momentum operators to memory.

Complex conjugate See **complex number**.

Complex number Complex numbers play an extremely useful role in NMR since they provide a particularly elegant means for the theoretical description of waveforms. A complex number comprises a real part (often abbreviated Re) and an imaginary part (Im):

$$x = a + \mathrm{i}b = \mathrm{Re} + \mathrm{Im} \tag{C29}$$

where $\mathrm{i} = \sqrt{-1}$. The imaginary part has no physical meaning as such, but can be represented together with the real part using an Argand diagram to obtain a vector representing x (Fig. C10). If x is multiplied by i, the product is $\mathrm{i}a - b$, which can be plotted as a second vector on the Argand diagram with the same magnitude as the first, but rotated by 90°. Thus multiplication by i results in a **phase** shift of 90°.

A function which is often found in theoretical NMR is the exponential function $\exp(\mathrm{i}\phi)$. This can be expanded into the well-known series;

$$\exp(\mathrm{i}\phi) = 1 + \mathrm{i}\phi + \mathrm{i}^2\phi^2/2! + \mathrm{i}^3\phi^3/3! + \mathrm{i}^4\phi^4/4! + \ldots. \tag{C30}$$

Now

$$\cos\phi = 1 - \phi^2/2! + \phi^4/4! + \ldots \tag{C31}$$

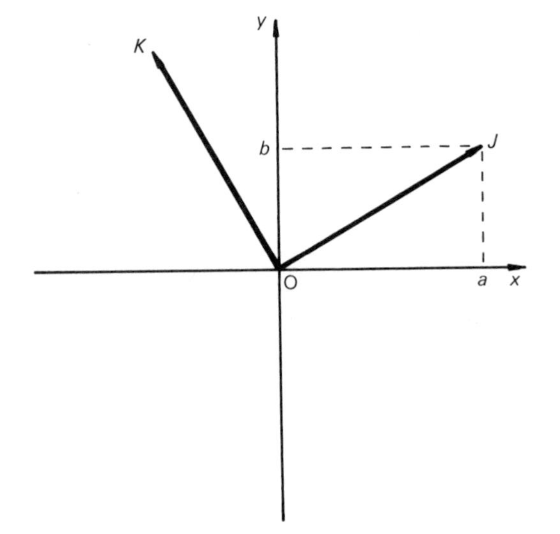

Fig. C10. A complex number can be represented by an Argand diagram where the real part is represented by the x coordinate and the imaginary part by the y coordinate. The complex number $a + ib$ is defined by the vector **OJ**, and multiplication by i results in the vector **OK**, which is phase shifted by 90° with respect to **OJ**.

and

C32 $$\sin\phi = \phi - \phi^3/3! + \ldots.$$

Therefore

C33 $$\exp(i\phi) = \cos\phi + i\sin\phi,$$

which is again a complex number. Often we require the complex conjugate of $\exp(i\phi)$ (denoted by $\exp(i\phi)^*$) which is simply given by

C34 $$\exp(i\phi)^* = \cos\phi - i\sin\phi.$$

Expressions of the form $A\exp(i\phi)$ are valuable since they contain information on amplitude (A) and phase (ϕ).

Composite pulses In many situations the response of the spin system to the effect of a single r.f. pulse is unsatisfactory. This is primarily due to the effects of r.f. field inhomogeneity and to off-resonance effects. In both cases these undesirable effects can be compensated by the application of a train of r.f. pulses which compensate for their own imperfections. This ensemble of pulses is known collectively as a composite pulse. A very large number of composite pulses has now been described in the literature. Two important applications are illustrated below.

Perhaps the simplest pulse which requires compensation is a $\pi/2$ (90°) pulse. Although a 90° pulse may be calibrated in principle to achieve accurate 'tipping' of the magnetization vector (see **classical formalism**) into the x–y plane for a given resonance, in practice a small error in the timing of the pulse width is likely. Although this does not cause a serious problem in 'pulse and collect' experiments, it can lead to systematic errors in others. If **off-resonance effects** can be neglected, the composite pulse

C35 $$P = (\beta)_0(\beta)_{\pi/2}$$

gives a more accurate β pulse. This can be understood by a simple geometrical argument for $\beta \approx \pi/2$. If the actual value of β is slightly less than $\pi/2$, the magnetization vector after the first pulse will lie just above the x–y plane, with a resulting small residual z-component. The second phase-shifted '$\pi/2$' pulse, which is again smaller than $\pi/2$ by the same amount, will rotate most of the residual z-magnetization into the x–y plane, and the transverse magnetization which is already in the x–y plane is unaffected (Fig. C11). A more efficient sequence which is rather more difficult to visualize graphically is the four-pulse sequence:

C36 $$P = (\beta)_{3\pi/2}(2\beta)_0(2\beta)_{\pi/2}(\beta)_0$$

where the flip-angle β is nominally $\pi/4$. Here again off-resonance effects are assumed to be small.

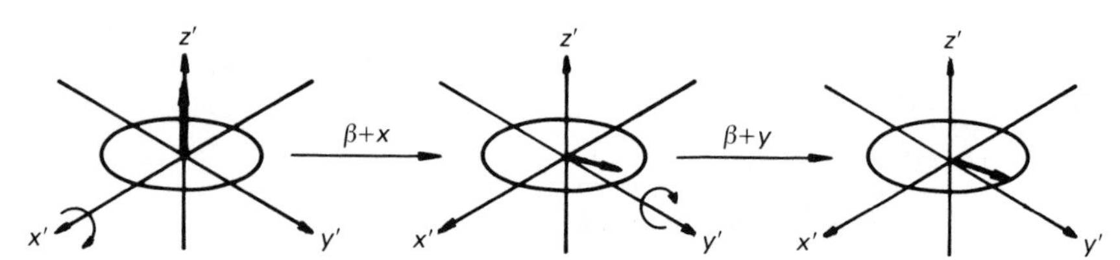

Fig. C11. Diagram illustrating the effect of a composite 90° pulse. See text for details.

A second, rather more important situation where composite pulse are of value is in the accurate inversion of magnetization, i.e. a perfect π (180°) pulse. This is highly sensitive to offset effects and pulse timing errors. Since accurate inversion is a very common requirement in both one-dimensional NMR (e.g. inversion recovery) and in **two-dimensional NMR** (refocusing of chemical shifts), a compensated inversion sequence is most useful. The first such sequence to be proposed is

C37 $$P = (\beta)_0(\beta')_{\pi/2}(\beta)_0$$

with rotation angles $\beta = \pi/2$ and $\beta' = \pi$. This again can be understood by a simple geometric argument. If $\beta < \pi/2$, the first pulse flips the magnetization vector to a position above the x–y plane, after which it is nutated to an approximately symmetrical position below the x–y plane. The third pulse then achieves very accurate inversion, since it rotates the vector by an angle less than 90°, in a similar fashion to the first pulse. The complete procedure is illustrated in Fig. C12. If $\beta > \pi/2$, the compensation can be understood by a similar argument.

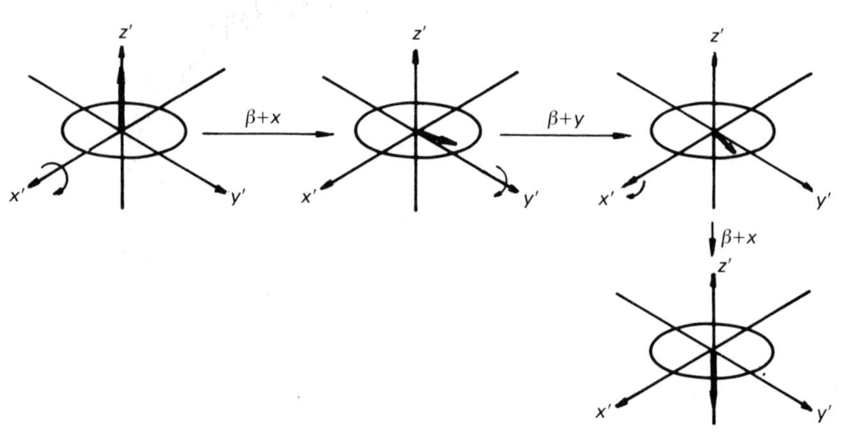

Fig. C12. Diagrammatic representation of the effect of a composite 180° pulse. See text for details.

The compensation of off-resonance effects in composite pulse sequences such as (C36) and (C37) cannot be understood geometrically, and it is necessary to integrate the **Bloch equations** numerically to examine offset dependence. In many cases this leads to more efficient 'pulse sandwiches'. For example, offset compensation considerations applied to sequence (C37) leads to the following modified sequence:

C38 $$P = (\beta)_0(\beta')_{\pi/2}(\beta'')_{3\pi/2}(\beta')_{\pi/2}(\beta)_0$$

where $\beta \approx \pi/2$, $\beta' \approx 1.12\pi$ and $\beta'' \approx 0.44\pi$. For further examples of composite pulses, see **Z-pulse** and **broadband decoupling**.

FURTHER READING

Composite pulses were first described by
Levitt, M. H. and Freeman, R. (1979). *J. Magn. Reson.* **33,** 473.

The following references describe the original derivations of the above pulses:
Composite 90° pulse:
Levitt, M. H. (1982). *J. Magn. Reson.* **48,** 234.
Levitt, M. H. and Ernst, R. R. (1983). *J. Magn. Reson.* **55,** 247.
Composite 180° pulse:
The above references, plus Levitt, M. H. (1982). *J. Magn. Reson.* **50,** 95.
Offset compensation:
Freeman, R., Kempsell, S., and Levitt, M. H. (1980). *J. Magn. Reson.* **38,** 453.

Connectivity networks Peak amplitudes and signs in two-dimensional correlation spectroscopy depend upon the connectivities in the energy level diagram of the **spin system**. Such connectivities can be classified by reference to the energy level diagram of a loosely coupled three-spin system *ISM* (Fig. C13). The connectivity of a pair of transitions can be determined most easily in terms of **shift operators** and **polarization operators**. For example, consider the connectivity between transitions 1–2 and 2–5. In terms of the above operators, we can represent these

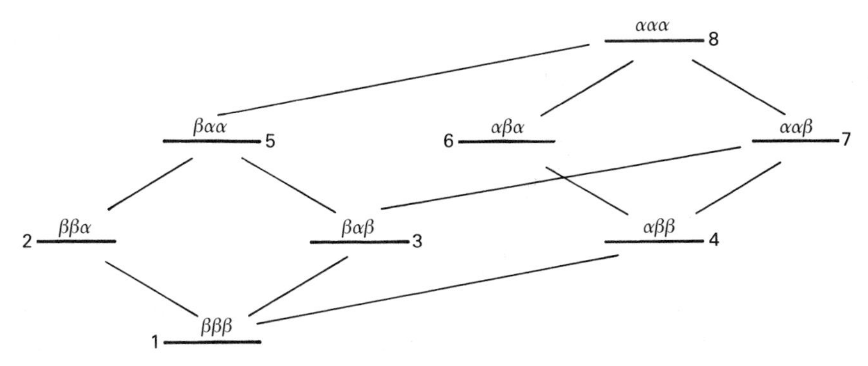

Fig. C13. Eight spin states of a three-spin system *ISM*.

transitions by

C39 $$1\text{–}2 = I^{\beta}S^{\beta}M^{+}, \qquad 2\text{–}5 = I^{\beta}S^{+}M^{\alpha}.$$

Since the 'active' spins (S and M) have opposite polarizations between transitions (S^{β}, M^{α}), this is known as a 'progressive' connectivity. The 'order' of this connectivity is zero, since the passive spin (I) has the same polarization. As another example consider the connectivity between transitions 2–5 and 7–8. In operator notation, these states are

C40 $$2\text{–}5 = I^{\beta}S^{+}M^{\alpha}, \qquad 7\text{–}8 = I^{\alpha}S^{\alpha}M^{+}.$$

Here again the 'active' spins are S and M, but the connectivity is 'regressive' since the polarizations are equal (M^{α}, S^{α}). Furthermore, the 'order' of the connectivity is 1, since the polarization of the passive spin is inverted. Now consider the operator notation for transitions 2–5 and 4–7:

C41 $$2\text{–}5 = I^{\beta}S^{+}M^{\alpha}, \qquad 4\text{–}7 = I^{\alpha}S^{+}M^{\beta}.$$

Both transitions only involve spin S, and the connectivity is thus described as 'parallel'. The order is 2, since two passive spins (I and M) have opposite polarizations.

Finally, both progressive and regressive connectivities can be categorized according to whether they share an energy level (direct connectivity) or not (remote connectivity).

The amplitudes and signs of peaks in correlation spectra (e.g. COSY) corresponding to transitions tu and rs depend upon the type of connectivity described above. According to Ernst, Bodenhausen, and Wokaun, the observed signal is given by

C42 $$S(\omega_1, \omega_2) = +Aa_{tu}(\omega_1)a_{rs}(\omega_2) - Bd_{tu}(\omega_1)d_{rs}(\omega_2)$$

where $a \equiv$ absorption, $d \equiv$ dispersion, and

C43 $$A = \pm(1/16)\sin^2\beta(\sin(\beta/2))^{2q}(\cos(\beta/2))^{2(N-2-q)}$$
$$B = 0$$

for progressive (+) and regressive connectivity of order q and flip angle β, and

C44 $$A = (1/8)\cos\beta(\sin(\beta/2))^{2q}(\cos(\beta/2))^{2(N-1-q)}$$

C45 $$B = -(1/8)(\sin(\beta/2))^{2q}(\cos(\beta/2))^{2(N-1-q)}$$

for parallel connectivity of order q.

For arbitrary β, the lineshapes are absorption-mode for the crosspeaks, but diagonal peaks are only pure dispersion for $\beta = 90°$. The coefficients A and B derive from the superposition of signals derived from **coherence transfer pathways** with symmetrical frequencies (i.e. echo and **antiecho** components). See also **flip-angle effects**.

FURTHER READING

Ernst, R. R., Bodenhausen, G., and Wokaun, A. A. (1987). *Principles of NMR in one and two dimensions*, pp. 414–22. Clarendon Press, Oxford.

Constant-time experiments Most two-dimensional NMR experiments may usefully be modified by the application of so-called constant-time evolution. The purpose of such modifications is generally to prevent the evolution of the spin system under spin couplings such that scalar decoupling of spins is achieved in the ω_1 dimension. The 'ω_1-decoupled COSY' experiment is a good example. Essentially the conventional COSY experiment (see **correlated spectroscopy**) is modified by the insertion of a 180° pulse in the t_1 period. Unlike conventional COSY, the time period τ_e between pulses remains fixed, and the normal, sequential incrementation of t_1 ensures that the 180° pulse is shifted sequentially across the τ_e period (Fig. C14). To analyse the inner workings of the experiment, the pulse sequence in Fig. C14 can be analysed for a weakly coupled two-spin system IS using the **product operator formalism.** Starting with the spin system at thermal equilibrium $(I_z + S_z)$, evolution within the time period $\frac{1}{2}(\tau_e + t_1)$, followed by the 180° pulse, and then by the time period $\frac{1}{2}(\tau_e - t_1)$ can be considered explicitly using the normal rules of the product operator formalism. The state of the spin system just before the final pulse is given by

$$\begin{aligned}\sigma_4 = &-I_y \cos \pi J_{IS}\tau_e \cos \omega_I t_1 \\ &+ I_x \cos \pi J_{IS}\tau_e \sin \omega_I t_1 \\ &+ 2I_x S_z \sin \pi J_{IS}\tau_e \cos \omega_I t_1 \\ &+ 2I_y S_z \sin \pi J_{IS}\tau_e \sin \omega_I t_1 + \text{terms in } S\end{aligned} \qquad \text{C46}$$

where for simplicity we only consider terms in spin I. The final pulse with $\beta = 90°$ of phase $+x$ then gives

$$\begin{aligned}\sigma_5 = &-I_z \cos \pi J_{IS}\tau_e \cos \omega_I t_1 \\ &+ I_x \cos \pi J_{IS}\tau_e \sin \omega_I t_1 \\ &- 2I_x S_y \sin \pi J_{IS}\tau_e \cos \omega_I t_1 \\ &- 2I_z S_y \sin \pi J_{IS}\tau_e \sin \omega_I t_1 + \text{terms in } S.\end{aligned} \qquad \text{C47}$$

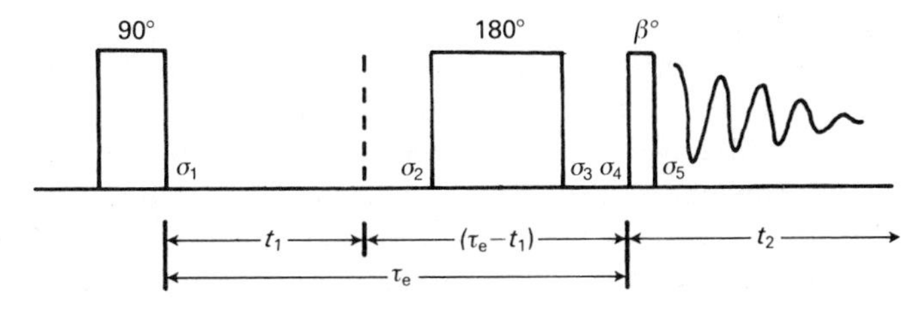

Fig. C14. Pulse sequence for constant time (ω_1 decoupled) COSY. See text for details.

The second term on the right-hand side of (C47) will give rise to a diagonal peak after evolution during t_2 and double **Fourier transformation**, whereas the fourth term will give rise to a crosspeak. These peak types have a cosinusoidal or sinusoidal dependence upon $\pi J_{IS}\tau_e$ respectively. Since τ_e is fixed, then there is effectively no evolution under spin coupling terms, and the COSY spectrum is decoupled in ω_1. However, the oscillatory dependence upon τ_e determines the crosspeak and diagonal peak intensities, and for a given value of τ_e, crosspeaks between spins with a particular value of J_{IS} may vanish. For a final pulse angle of 90°, the maximum crosspeak amplitude is clearly given by (C47) as $\tau_e = (2J_{IS})^{-1}$, which is also the condition for minimum diagonal peak amplitude. In larger spin networks a more complex transfer function results, and in general there is no optimum value of τ_e. While under some circumstances, the selection of crosspeak amplitudes based upon J may be advantageous, in many cases the low intensity of certain crosspeaks for a given value of τ_e is a severe disadvantage. This can actually be overcome to some extent by the use of a rotation angle $<\pi/2$ for the final pulse, but this prevents the generation of pure-phase (see **phase-sensitive experiments**) lineshapes. For these reasons, ω_1-decoupled COSY has only found use in a few specialized applications, where the collapse of multiplet structure in the ω_1 domain allows overlapping crosspeaks to be separated.

FURTHER READING

An early description of constant time experiments is given in Bax, A., and Freeman, R. (1981). *J. Magn. Reson.* **44,** 542.

For a practical application of ω_1-decoupled COSY see

Rance, M., Wagner, G., Sorensen, O. W., Wuthrich, K., and Ernst, R. R. (1984). *J. Magn. Reson.* **59,** 250.

Contact time See **Hartmann–Hahn condition**.

Convolution Convolution is a special transformation which can be used to describe a variety of physical processes. In the case of NMR, the most important of these is filtration, whereby the required signal is stripped of its noise components. The convolution $f(t)$ of two functions $x(t)$ and $h(t)$ can be thought of as a 'broadening' of one function by the other. In the case of NMR, we are often interested in stripping the spectrum of its noise components in order to improve the signal-to-noise ratio. In this case, if $x(t)$ represents the raw ('noisy') function, and $h(t)$ represents the weighting function (i.e. the function which causes the broadening), the output, or weighted function $f(t)$ is given by

$$f(t) = h(t) * x(t)$$

$$= \int_{-\infty}^{\infty} h(\tau) \,.\, x(t-\tau)\, \mathrm{d}\tau \tag{C48}$$

where $*$ denotes convolution.

These equations give little practical insight as to how convolution is achieved. Actually, the process is simplified somewhat by application of the convolution theorem. This states that the **Fourier transform** of the convolution of two functions is proportional to the products of the individual Fourier transforms. Conversely, the Fourier transform of a product of two functions is proportional to the convolution of their individual Fourier transforms. Thus, if

$$h(t) \xrightarrow{\mathscr{F}} H(\nu) \tag{C49}$$

$$f(t) \xrightarrow{\mathscr{F}} F(\nu) \tag{C50}$$

then

$$h(t) \,.\, f(t) \xrightarrow{\mathscr{F}} H(\nu) * F(\nu) \tag{C51}$$

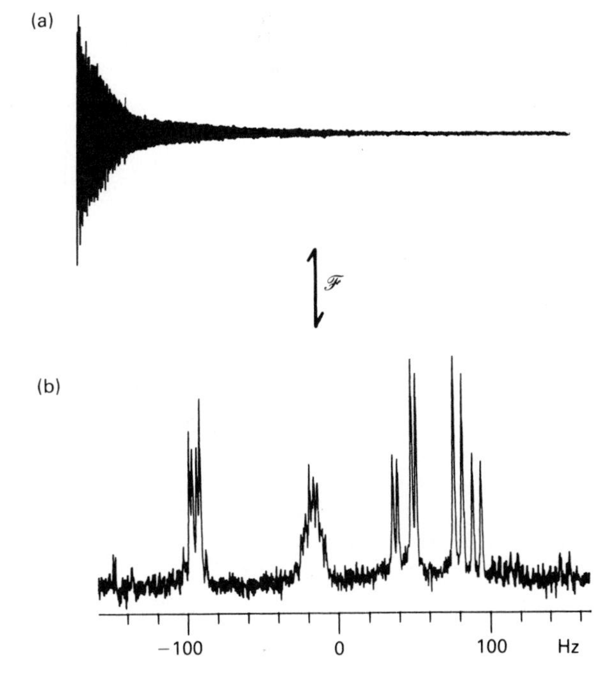

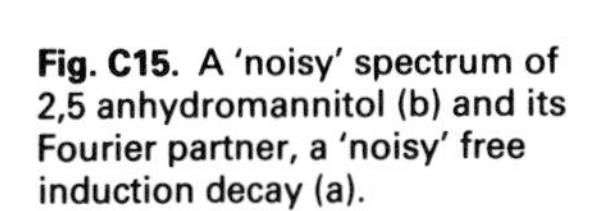
Fig. C15. A 'noisy' spectrum of 2,5 anhydromannitol (b) and its Fourier partner, a 'noisy' free induction decay (a).

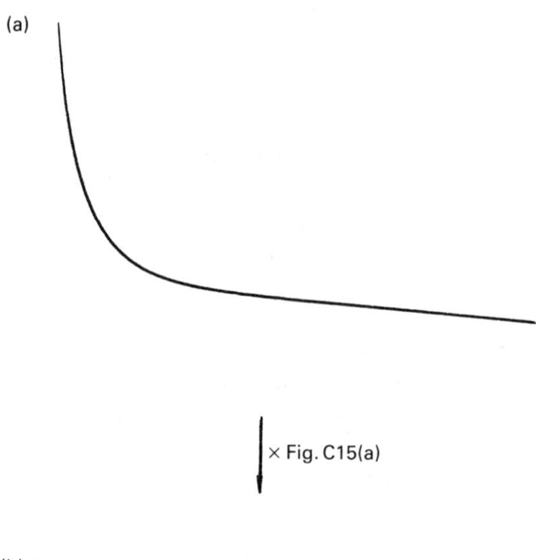

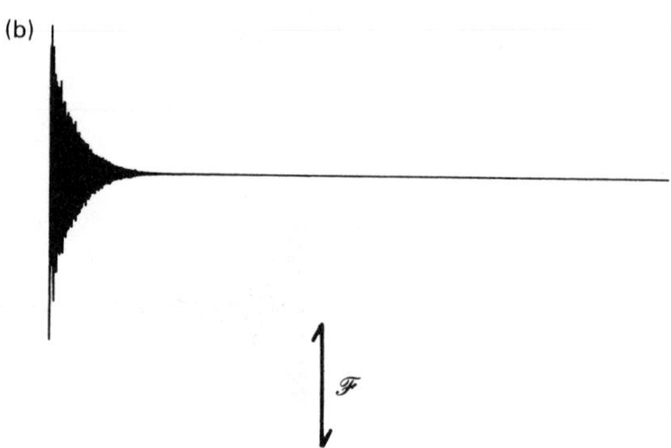

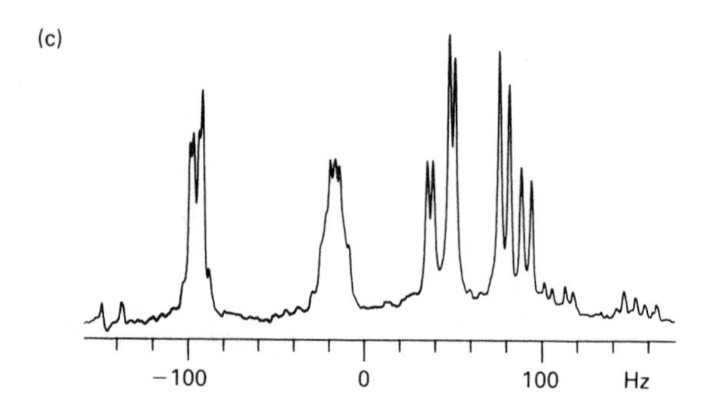

Fig. C16. Multiplication of the noisy free induction decay of Fig. C15 by a decaying exponential function (a) gives rise to a free induction decay (b) with fewer noise components. The corresponding spectrum (c) has decreased noise but broader lines.

where a Fourier transform is denoted by $\mathscr{F}$. It is perhaps now more obvious how convolution can be implemented in a NMR experiment. Remembering that the **free induction decay** is the time-domain Fourier partner of the NMR spectrum, then multiplication of the free induction decay by the Fourier transform of the desired function will generate a convoluted NMR spectrum on subsequent Fourier transformation. If we

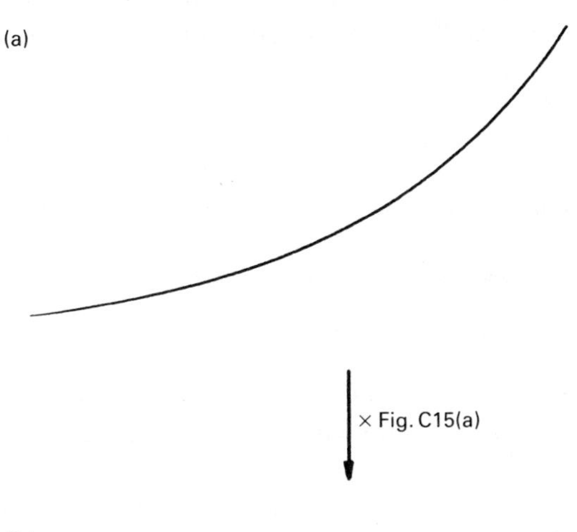

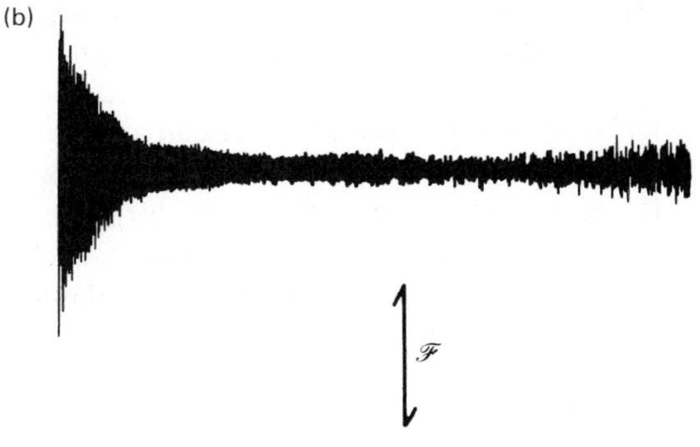

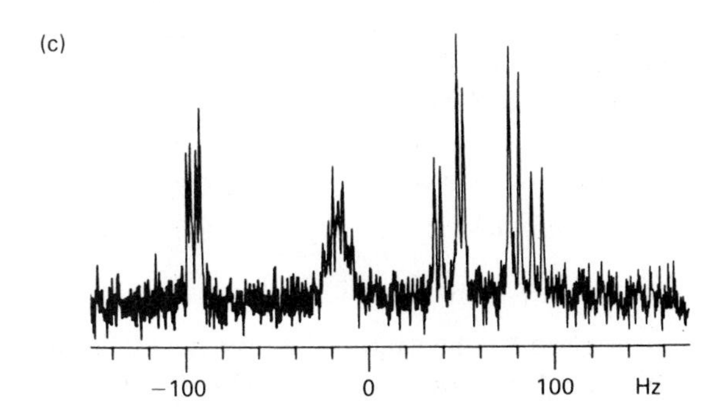

Fig. C17. Multiplication of the free induction decay in Fig. C15 by an increasing exponential (a), amplifies the noise components (b), giving rise to a noisy spectrum (c). The resolution is improved, however.

take the case of a noisy spectrum, its equivalent noisy free induction decay will be similar to that shown in Fig. C15. The Fourier transform of this free induction decay gives of course the noisy spectrum. If now the free induction decay is multiplied by a decaying exponential, of the form shown in Fig. C16, subsequent Fourier transformation shows a decrease in spectral noise. Note, however, that the linewidths are greater. The spectrum has been broadened by the weighting function $h(t)$. We have succeeded in filtering the noise from the spectrum at the expense of resolution. Theoretically, it can be shown that a matched filter, i.e. one which has the same bandshape as the signal to be recovered, gives optimal results, resulting in a twofold increase in linewidth. It perhaps comes as no surprise that in this case the time domain weighting function mimics the decay of the resonance line of interest. Since the free induction decay of the Lorentzian line is an exponential, the mathematical form of the weighting function is, correspondingly,

C52 $$h(t) = \exp(-t/T_c)$$

where T_c is a time constant representing the filter bandwidth. The use of a decaying exponential as described above is sometimes referred to as apodization.

It is possible to apply a variety of weighting functions to a free induction decay. If, instead of applying a decreasing exponential, an increasing exponential $h(t) = \exp(t/T_c)$ is applied, the effect is to improve resolution, but with severe degradation of the signal-to-noise ratio (Fig. C17). This is an example of deconvolution.

Since an increase in resolution is a desirable entity for the biological NMR spectroscopist, it is not surprising that much effort has been extended to find weighting functions which achieve increased resolution without severe signal-to-noise degradation. Three such functions are commonly employed:

1. LORENTZIAN TO GAUSSIAN TRANSFORMATION

In this procedure (Fig. C18), the free induction decay is multiplied by the Fourier transform of a Gaussian **lineshape** (which, incidentally is also Gaussian). In this manner, the lineshapes of the NMR resonances are converted to Gaussian, which has a sharper decay at the wings.

2. DOUBLE EXPONENTIAL MULTIPLICATION

As the name suggests, a double exponential function,

C53 $$h(j) = \exp\{(A_j - B_j^2)\}$$

is applied to the free induction decay, where j is the point index in an N-point free induction decay (Fig. C19).

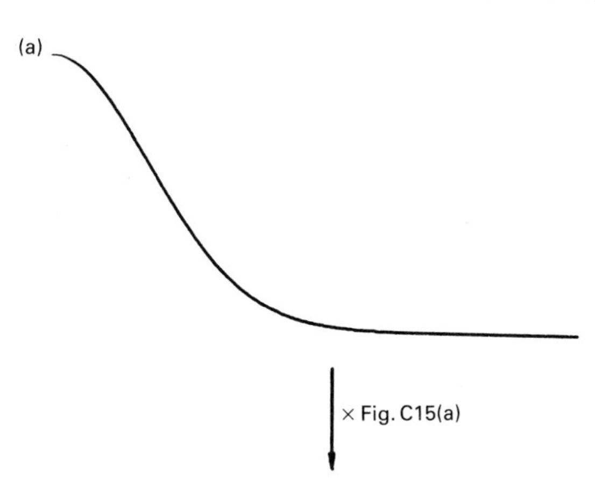

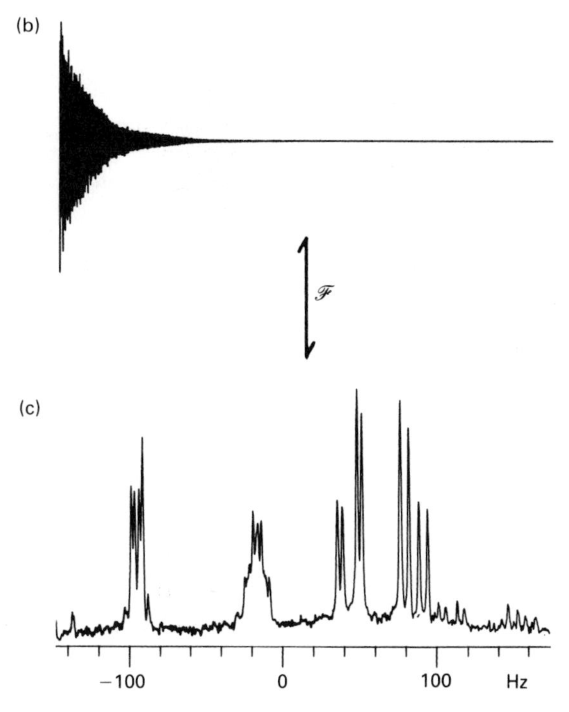

Fig. C18. Multiplication of the free induction decay of Fig. C15 by a Gaussian function (a) results in a free induction decay (b) which gives a spectrum whose lineshapes are Gaussian rather than Lorentzian (c).

3. SINE–BELL MULTIPLICATION

In this method the free induction decay is multiplied by a sine function (Fig. C20) which starts at zero, and has a value of $\pi/2$ at the middle of the free induction decay.

This is a rather severe weighting function which, although giving increased resolution, significantly degrades the signal-to-noise ratio. In addition, deep troughs are found on either side of the resonance lines.

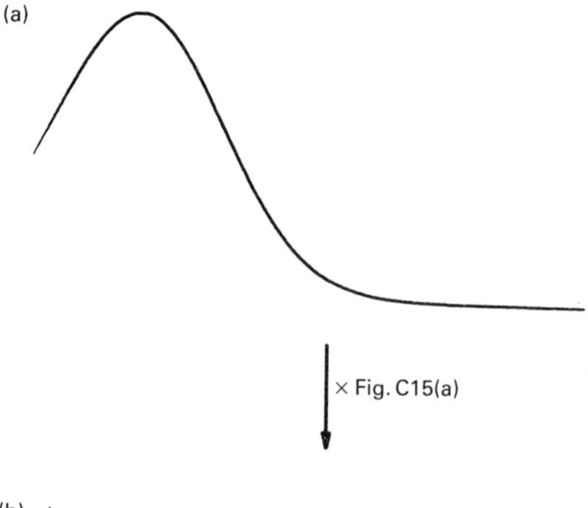

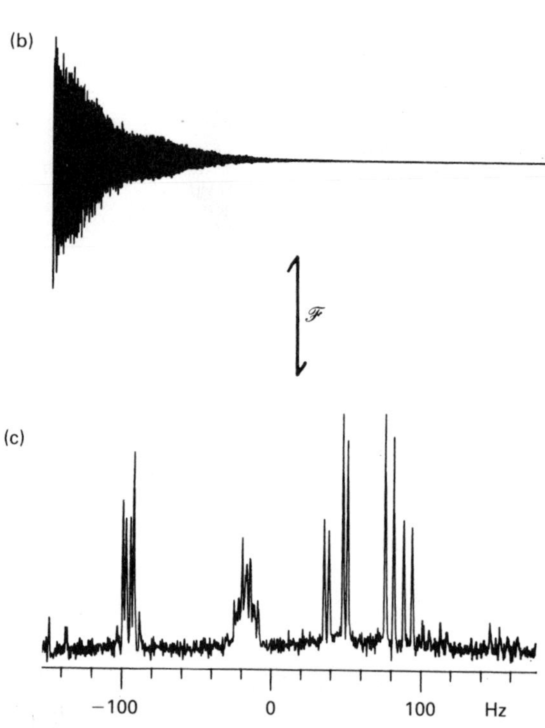

Fig. C19. Multiplication of the free induction decay of Fig. C15 by a double exponential function (a) gives a free induction decay (b) whose spectrum is resolution enhanced without severe degradation of the signal-to-noise ratio (c).

Despite these disadvantages, the sine–bell function has enjoyed popularity in improving the resolution of older phase-modulated two-dimensional NMR experiments where the familiar phase-twist lineshape gives poor resolution due to long dispersion 'tails' (see **antiecho**, **phase modulation**). An alternative strategy is to employ a phase-shifted sine-bell function, which does not have a value of zero at $t = 0$, resulting in rather better signal-to-noise ratios in convoluted spectra.

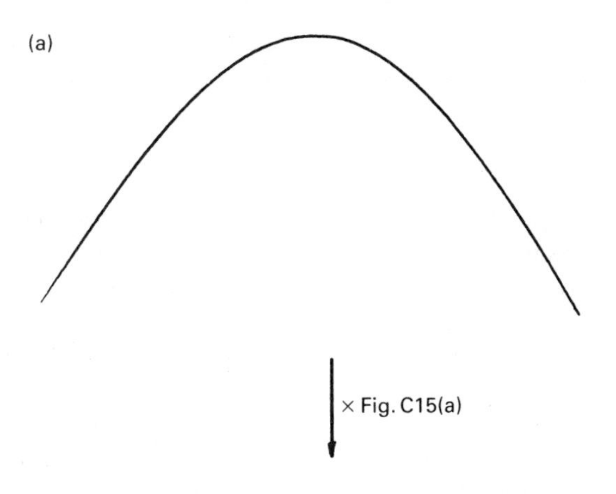

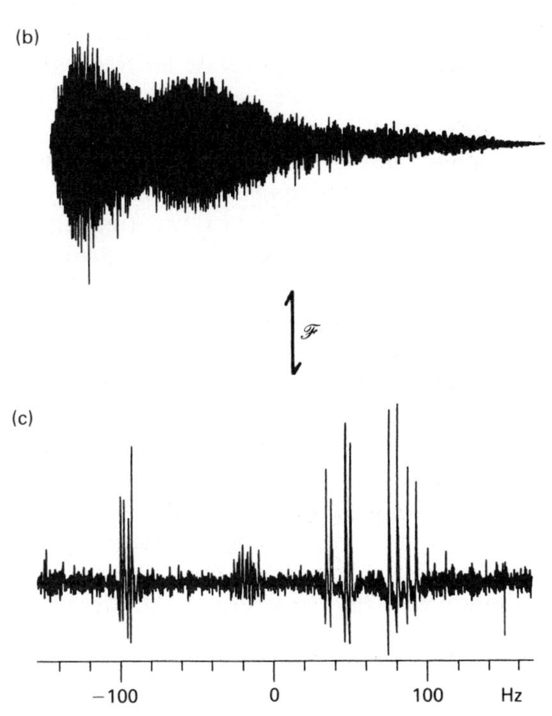

Fig. C20. Multiplication of the free induction decay of Fig. C15 by the sine–bell function (a) gives a free induction decay (b) whose spectrum (c) has a degraded signal-to-noise ratio and distorted lineshapes. However, there is a large improvement in resolution.

FURTHER READING

Bracewell, R. M. (1965). *The Fourier transform and its applications*. McGraw-Hill, New York.

Correlated spectroscopy (COSY) The COSY experiment is one of the simplest, and yet most useful, of the various **two-dimensional NMR** (2D NMR) experiments devised to date. In fact COSY was the first 2D NMR

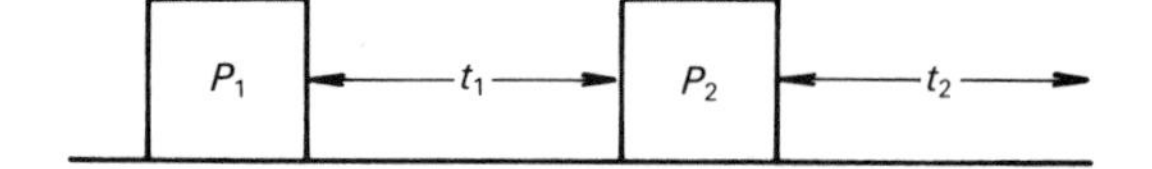

Fig. C21. The two-pulse sequence used in homonuclear correlated spectroscopy (COSY).

experiment to be described. In its homonuclear application, the experiment consists simply of two non-selective r.f. pulses, between which there is a variable delay t_1. Data are acquired after the second pulse, during a further period t_2 (Fig. C21). Before describing the theoretical and practical aspects of this important experiment in detail, it is worthwhile demonstrating in a purely classical manner how a two-dimensional spectrum can result from this sequence. This will involve several caveats which will be described in a more formal manner below.

Consider two protons, A and B, which are scalar coupled. The result of a simple pulse and collect sequence, followed by **Fourier transformation**, will generate an NMR spectrum as shown diagrammatically in Fig. C22. We use the terms ω_A, ω_B, J_{AB}, in obvious notation to denote the Larmor frequencies of spins A and B and their scalar (J) coupling. In essence, spin A has precessed with a Larmor frequency of ω_A during t_1, and spin B has precessed with a Larmor frequency of ω_B during t_1, although in fact two frequencies are involved for each spin ($\omega_A \pm \frac{1}{2}J_{AB}$ and $\omega_B \pm \frac{1}{2}J_{AB}$) due to the spin–spin coupling. Now consider what would happen if we were to use the pulse sequence of Fig. C21. Let us postulate that we could record data during both the t_1 and t_2 intervals. After pulse P_1 and the delay t_1, the situation is analogous to that of Fig. C22, i.e. each proton resonates with its characteristic Larmor frequency during t_1. After the pulse P_2, the situation becomes more complicated. In the first place, P_2 may appear to have no effect on the spins, i.e. they continue to resonate at ω_A and ω_B during t_2 just as they did in t_1. Alternatively, a portion of the magnetization associated with spin A during t_1 may 'jump' to spin B during t_2. In other words, a proportion of the magnetization which precessed at ω_A during t_1 now precesses at ω_B during t_2. This surprising result derives from a quantum mechanical

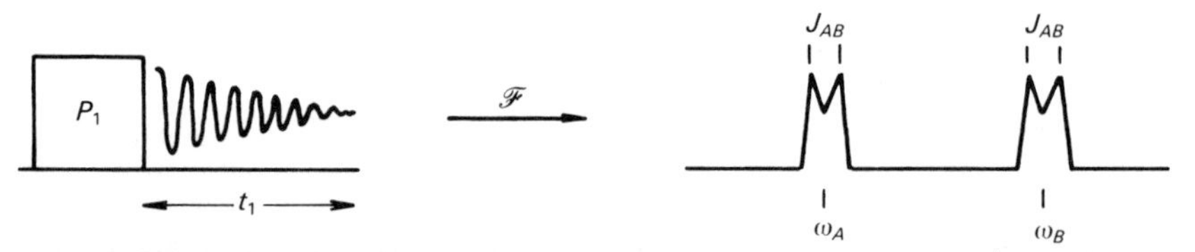

Fig. C22. Fourier transformation of the free induction decay resulting from the application of an r.f. pulse to a two-spin system results in the NMR spectrum.

process known as **coherence transfer** which will be shown formally below. In an analogous manner, a proportion of the magnetization which precessed at ω_B during t_1 now precesses at ω_A during t_2. Now, since we are observing the NMR spectrum with respect to two time periods it follows that we must employ a **two-dimensional Fourier transform** to observe the frequency components described above. This in turn suggests that we must display the spectrum in two orthogonal dimensions on paper. Such a display is shown in Fig. C23 for the two-spin case described above. The two-dimensional spectrum in Fig. C23 is displayed as a so-called contour plot i.e. we are observing the peaks from above, just as contour levels display mountain ranges in a two-dimensional map. The two-dimensional spectrum is a surface in three-dimensional space. The

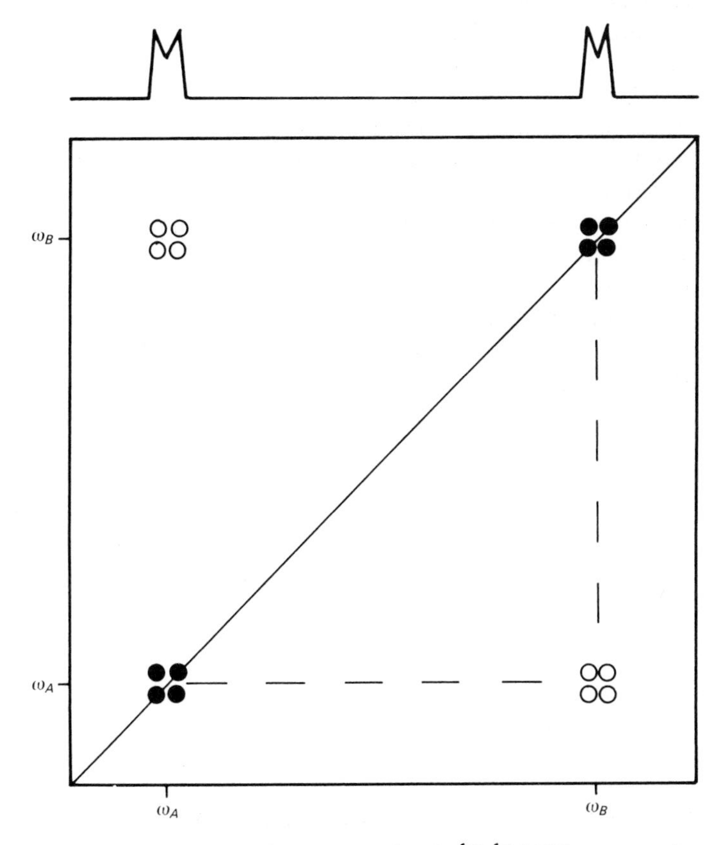

Fig. C23. Diagrammatic illustration of the contour plot of a ^1H–^1H COSY spectrum of two coupled spins. The filled circles represent diagonal peaks, whereas the open circles represent off-diagonal peaks or crosspeaks. The dotted line illustrates how crosspeaks correlate diagonal peaks derived from scalar coupled spins.

third dimension is of course intensity. We can now relate the four peaks in the spectrum with our classical description. Magnetization which remained with its parent spin during both t_1 and t_2 periods, i.e. was apparently unaffected by the P_2 pulse, will of course appear at the same coordinate in both ω_1 and ω_2 dimensions. For obvious reasons these are the so called diagonal peaks in two-dimensional spectra. Conversely, magnetization which 'jumped' as a result of the P_2 pulse will appear with different co-ordinates in the ω_1 and ω_2 dimensions. According to the above description they should be found at ($\omega_1 = \omega_A$, $\omega_2 = \omega_B$), and ($\omega_1 = \omega_B$, $\omega_2 = \omega_A$). These are the so-called crosspeaks in two-dimensional spectra. From Fig. C23 it should be clear that these crosspeaks effectively correlate the resonances of spin A with spin B. Now in this particular experiment, since the frequency 'jumping' or **coherence transfer** can only occur between spin-coupled nuclei, then the contour plot of Fig. C23 is a convenient means by which chemically bonded nuclei can be identified. This is particularly useful if only one of the resonances is assigned. Of course, the case of two coupled spins is a trivial example, but consider the case of a sample containing a large number of overlapping resonances. As an example, consider the 500 MHz ^{1}H NMR spectrum of the disaccharide galactose-α1-2-methyl-α-mannoside (Fig. C24). The two resonances at 5.15 p.p.m. and 5.09 p.p.m. are the H1 resonances of galactose and the mannoside respectively. These are shifted to low field due to the electron-withdrawing properties of the ring oxygens. Obviously we could determine the H2 resonance assignments from H1 by **spin decoupling**. However, due to severe resonance overlap, this method is unlikely to succeed in obtaining full resonance assignments. Now consider the

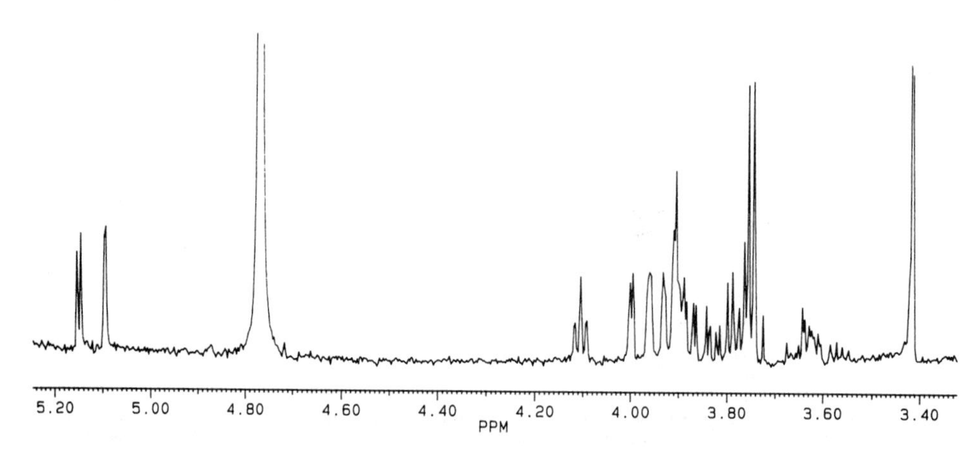

Fig. C24. One-dimensional ^{1}H NMR spectrum of the disaccharide galactose-α1-2-methyl-α-mannoside.

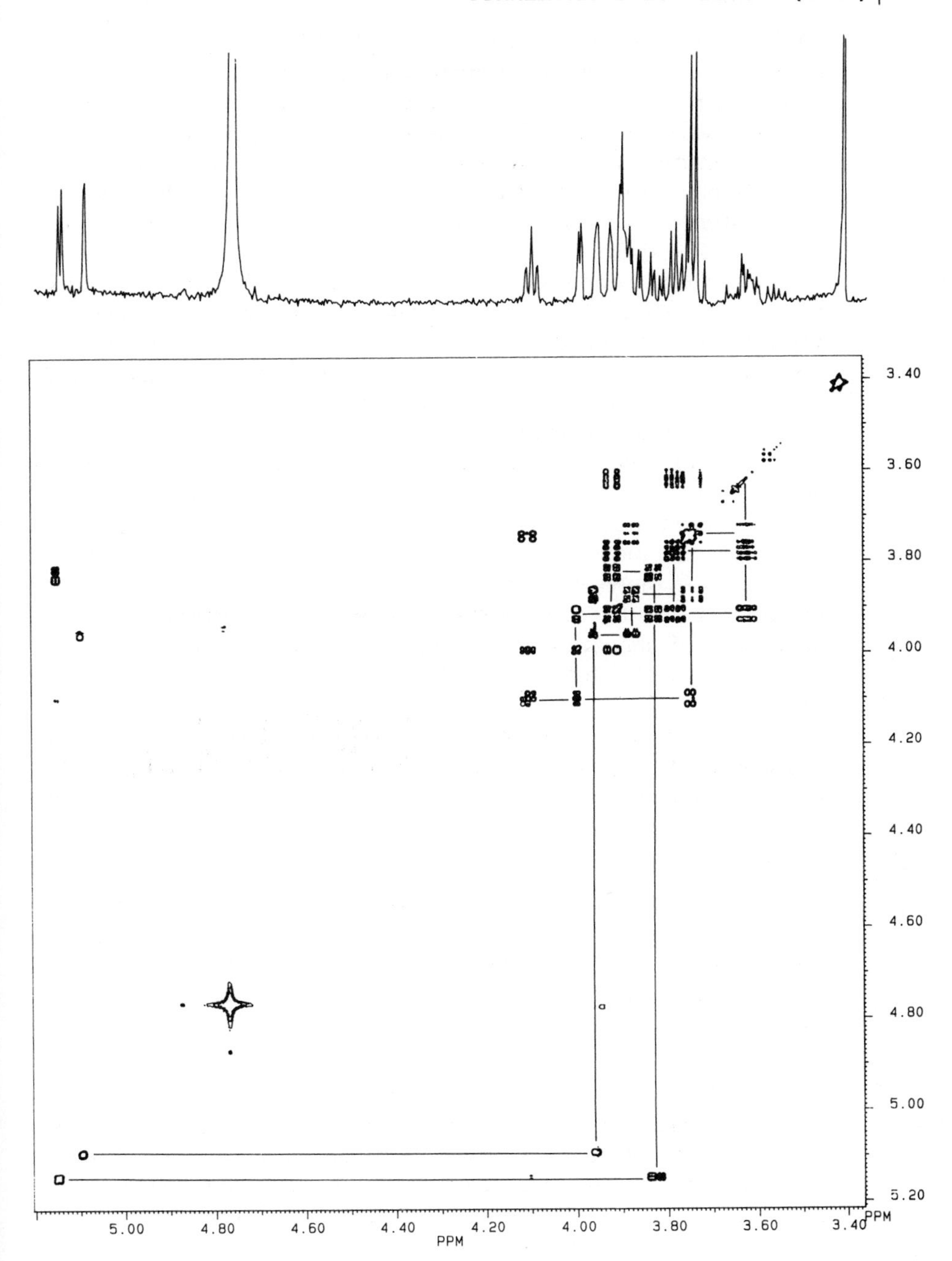

Fig. C25. $^1H-^1H$ COSY spectrum of galactose-α1-2-methyl-α-mannoside. In analogy to Fig. C23, scalar coupled protons can be identified as shown, using the resolved H1 protons of each monosaccharide ring as a starting point.

^1H–^1H COSY spectrum of the same sample (Fig. C25). We immediately observe that since the one-dimensional spectrum is effectively 'spread' into two-dimensions, the crosspeaks are resolved even in the region of the unresolved envelope. It is now a simple matter to make complete assignments using the H1 protons as a basis as shown. Furthermore, since the two-dimensional spectrum is a three-dimensional surface, we can project it on to any convenient axis to reconstruct the one-dimensional spectrum. It is shown in Fig. C25.

Having given a simplified description of the COSY experiment, and a typical application, it is now worthwhile examining the experiment in more detail. The precise mechanisms by which data are collected during the t_1 and t_2 dimensions are common to almost all **two-dimensional NMR** experiments, and the relevant details are described under this heading. It is the actual pulse sequence which distinguishes the various experiments. In order to examine the effects of the r.f. pulses in these experiments, it is necessary to employ a quantum mechanical formalism. The most complete formalism for such analyses relies upon the **density matrix**. However, the cumbersome complexity of this approach does not lend itself easily to physical insight into the workings of the experiment. We therefore employ the alternative **product operator formalism** for the sake of conceptual simplicity. As usual, we ignore relaxation during this treatment. In the limit of **weak coupling** the two formalisms are equivalent.

Consider a weakly coupled (see **weak coupling**) homonuclear two-**spin** $\frac{1}{2}$ **system** IS at thermal equilibrium. The initial density matrix expressed in the product operator formalism is composed simply of the terms I_z and S_z:

C54
$$\sigma(0) = I_z + S_z$$

If a 90° r.f. pulse is applied to the spin system, the evolution of the density matrix under the influence of the **Hamiltonian** corresponding to the r.f. pulse can be evaluated according to the rules described in Appendix 1. Assuming that the pulse **phase** is along the $+X$ axis, $\sigma(0)$ evolves as follows:

C55
$$I_z + S_z \xrightarrow{\pi/2(I_x+S_x)} -I_y - S_y = \sigma(1).$$

This corresponds to a classical magnetization vector initially collinear with the z axis, which is then tilted along the $-y$ axis by the r.f. pulse. The resulting transverse magnetization then evolves under a Hamiltonian composed of Zeeman and spin-coupling terms, to generate $\sigma(2)$:

C56
$$\begin{aligned}\sigma(1) \xrightarrow{\omega_I t_1 I_z + \omega_S t_1 S_z + \pi J_{IS} t_1 2I_z S_z} & [-I_y \cos \omega_I t_1 + I_x \sin \omega_I t_1 - S_y \cos \omega_S t_1 \\ & + S_x \sin \omega_S t_1] \cos \pi J_{IS} t_1 + [+2I_x S_z \cos \omega_I t_1 + 2I_y S_z \sin \omega_I t_1 \\ & + 2I_z S_x \cos \omega_S t_1 + 2I_z S_y \sin \omega_S t_1] \sin \pi J_{IS} t_1 = \sigma(2).\end{aligned}$$

$\sigma(2)$ is composed of terms corresponding to in phase and antiphase magnetization (see **product operator formalism**). The density operator after the second pulse is obtained from $\sigma(2)$ by following its evolution under the corresponding Hamiltonian:

C57

$$\sigma(2) \xrightarrow{(\pi/2)(I_x+S_x)} [-I_z \cos \omega_I t_1 + I_x \sin \omega_I t_1 - S_z \cos \omega_S t_1 + S_x \sin \omega_S t_1] \cos \pi J_{IS} t_1 - [2I_x S_y \cos \omega_I t_1 + 2I_y S_x \cos \omega_S t_1 + 2I_z S_y \sin \omega_I t_1 + 2I_y S_z \sin \omega_S t_1] \sin \pi J_{IS} t_1 = \sigma(3).$$

Note that the second pulse achieves transformations of the following type:

C58

$$2I_y S_z \sin \omega_I t_1 \rightarrow 2I_z S_y \sin \omega_I t_1$$

and

$$2I_z S_y \sin \omega_S t_1 \rightarrow 2I_y S_z \sin \omega_S t_1.$$

This first equation shows us that antiphase y magnetization of spin I with a Larmor frequency ω_I is transformed by the second pulse into antiphase y magnetization of spin S with a Larmor frequency ω_I. The second equation tells a similar story. This is the **coherence transfer** mechanism described earlier and will be seen to be responsible for the formation of crosspeaks in the COSY spectrum. Since coherence transfer can be thought of as a mixing of states, the second pulse is sometimes called a mixing pulse.

Each of the terms in $\sigma(3)$ now evolves during the t_2 period under the same Hamiltonian which was operative during t_1. This results in a very large number of terms, but only a few of them correspond to **observables**, and only these are of concern in the present context:

C59

$$\sigma(3) \xrightarrow{\omega_I t_1 I_z + \omega_S t_1 S_z + \pi J_{IS} t_1 2 I_z S_z} \left.\begin{aligned} & I_x \sin \pi J_{IS} t_1 \sin \pi J_{IS} t_2 \cos \omega_I t_2 \sin \omega_S t_1 \\ & + I_x \cos \pi J_{IS} t_1 \cos \pi J_{IS} t_2 \sin \omega_I t_1 \cos \omega_I t_2 \\ & + I_y \sin \pi J_{IS} t_1 \sin \pi J_{IS} t_2 \sin \omega_I t_2 \sin \omega_S t_1 \\ & + I_y \cos \pi J_{IS} t_1 \cos \pi J_{IS} t_2 \sin \omega_I t_1 \sin \omega_I t_2 \\ & + S_x \sin \pi J_{IS} t_1 \sin \pi J_{IS} t_2 \sin \omega_I t_1 \cos \omega_S t_2 \\ & + S_x \cos \pi J_{IS} t_1 \cos \pi J_{IS} t_2 \sin \omega_S t_1 \cos \omega_S t_2 \\ & + S_y \sin \pi J_{IS} t_1 \sin \pi J_{IS} t_2 \sin \omega_I t_1 \sin \omega_S t_2 \\ & + S_y \cos \pi J_{IS} t_1 \cos \pi J_{IS} t_2 \sin \omega_S t_1 \sin \omega_S t_2 \end{aligned}\right\} \text{observables only.}$$

In accordance with the rules for the form of observables in the product operator formalism, only terms in I_x, I_y, S_x, S_y have been retained in (C59). Nevertheless, this list of terms appears formidable at first sight. However, the situation begins to clarify after the application of some trigonometry. For the sake of argument, let us assume that the receiver phase is along the y axis of the rotating frame. We are then concerned only with terms in I_y and S_y. Strictly, if a comparison with the **density matrix** formalism is to be made, we should decompose the sine and cosine terms in (C59), which represent **amplitude modulation**, into two counter-rotating components. In this manner we would obtain a theoretical two-dimensional spectrum containing the **coherence transfer echo** and **antiecho** components. This is an unnecessary complication, however, since the modulating functions in the form shown in (C59) will be seen to generate a theoretical two-dimensional spectrum in a single quadrant which is identical to an experimental phase-sensitive COSY experiment. To see how this is achieved we take as an example the third term on the right-hand side of (C59):

C60 $$I_y \sin \pi J_{IS} t_1 \sin \pi J_{IS} t_2 \sin \omega_I t_2 \sin \omega_S t_1.$$

The four sine functions following I_y can be grouped into two pairs depending upon whether the dependence is upon t_1 or t_2:

C61 $$I_y \,.\, \sin \pi J_{IS} t_1 \sin \omega_S t_1 \,.\, \sin \pi J_{IS} t_2 \sin \omega_I t_2.$$

Using the trigonometric identity $\sin A \sin B = \frac{1}{2}[\cos(A - B) - \cos(A + B)]$, (C61) is conveniently expressed as

C62 $$I_y \,.\, \tfrac{1}{2}[\cos(\omega_S - \pi J_{IS})t_1 - \cos(\omega_S + \pi J_{IS})t_1] \\ .\, \tfrac{1}{2}[\cos(\omega_I - \pi J_{IS})t_2 - \cos(\omega_I + \pi J_{IS})t_2].$$

Using a similar trigonometric identity (see Appendix 2), the fourth term in (C59) can be expressed as

C63 $$I_y \,.\, \tfrac{1}{2}[\sin(\omega_I + \pi J_{IS})t_1 + \sin(\omega_I - \pi J_{IS})t_1] \\ .\, \tfrac{1}{2}[\sin(\omega_I + \pi J_{IS})t_2 + \sin(\omega_I - \pi J_{IS})t_2].$$

We are now in a position to interpret (C62) and (C63) in terms of the spectra to which they give rise. Each trigonometric function gives rise to a single line. The relative phases (positive or negative) of the lines is determined by their sign. The lineshape after real (cosine) **Fourier transformation** depends upon whether a cosine modulation (absorption) or a sine modulation (dispersion) is involved. Thus, from (C62) after Fourier transformation, we predict that four lines will be observed which are in antiphase absorption at $\omega_S \pm \pi J_{IS}$ in the t_1 dimension, and in antiphase absorption at $\omega_I \pm \pi J_{IS}$ in t_2. In other words, (C62) describes a crosspeak. In contrast, (C63) describes four lines which are in-phase dispersion at $\omega_I \pm \pi J_{IS}$ in t_1 and in-phase dispersion at $\omega_I \pm \pi J_{IS}$ in t_2.

Equation (C63) therefore describes a diagonal peak. Analogous expression can be derived for the terms in S_y in (C59). These results allow us to draw a theoretical plot for the experiment (Fig. C26). This corresponds exactly with an experimental phase-sensitive COSY experiment for an AX spin system.

We can draw some important practical conclusions from Fig. C26. Obviously, it is important that both crosspeaks and diagonal peaks are of sufficient **intensity** that they are not buried in the noise. The phase characteristics of diagonal peaks *vs.* crosspeaks have important implications in this regard. Since the crosspeak multiplets are composed of both positive and negative intensity, then it is important that these contributions should never be superimposed, or mutual cancellation will result. An obvious situation where this would occur is when J_{IS} is zero. Also, if J_{IS} is small, the multiplets may be sufficiently close to strongly inhibit crosspeak intensity. If we return to one of the terms responsible for crosspeak formation in (C59), e.g. the third term, we note that the function $\sin \pi J_{IS} t_1 \sin \pi J_{IS} t_2$ is responsible for the multiplicity of the

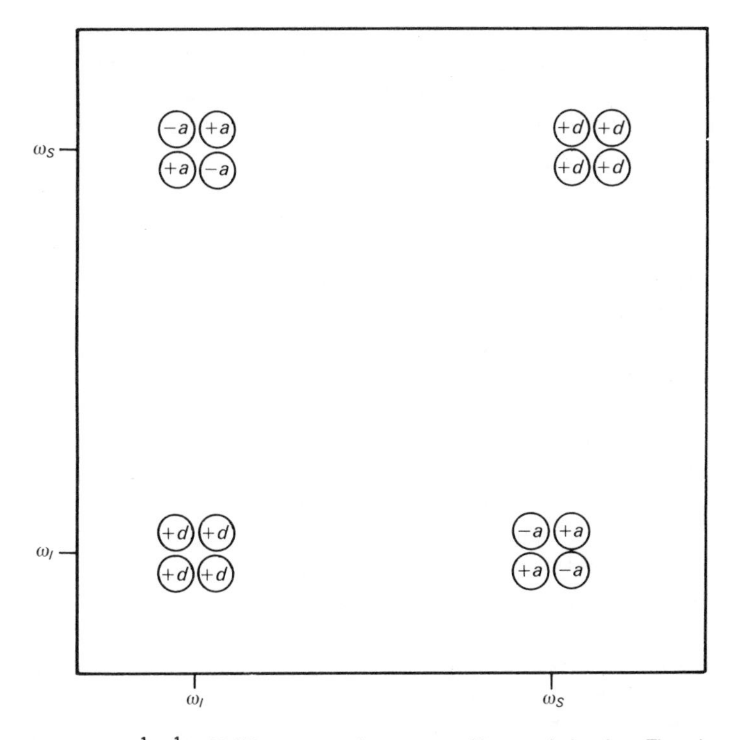

Fig. C26. Theoretical ^1H–^1H COSY spectrum for two weakly coupled spins. The phases are illustrated by + or −, while the lineshapes are designated as d or a, which are dispersion-mode and absorption-mode Lorentzian lines respectively.

crosspeak. One way of visualizing this is by considering two antiphase vectors in the receiver coil, which gradually move together during t_1 and t_2. In fact the third term in (C59) derives from an 'antiphase' operator product (see **product operator formalism**) of the form $2I_yS_z$ in $\sigma(3)$, so this mental picture should not be totally alien to us. The net result is that for maximum crosspeak intensity, the function $\sin \pi J_{IS} t_1 \sin \pi J_{IS} t_2$ should correspondingly be maximal. This occurs when both t_1 and t_2 extend for a time equal to $\frac{1}{2}J_{IS}$, and this constraint should obviously be observed if practically possible. Another consideration which is closely linked to the above is the question of **digital resolution**. Since the crosspeak multiplets are separated by J_{IS}, it is obviously necessary to digitize the data with a resolution of at least J_{IS} Hz/point. But of course for a given **sweep-width** and a given acquisition time as dictated by $\frac{1}{2}J_{IS}$ the number of data points will be fixed, and so this latter constraint is really just a reformulation of the former.

Turning now to the multiplicity of the diagonal peaks, we encounter the question of available resolution. Since the diagonal peaks are of in-phase dispersive nature, they possess inherently broad wings (see **lineshape**). Although there is no overriding requirement to remove these wings, they are undesirable, particularly when crosspeaks close to the diagonal are being observed, which happens all too often in biological 2D NMR. In early phase-modulated COSY experiments (see **phase modulation**) use was made of **flip-angle effects** to 'clean-up' the diagonal, but these cannot generally be applied to **phase-sensitive experiments**. An elegant alternative to remove the dispersive tails is to convert the in-phase dispersive lineshape to antiphase-absorption by employing a double-quantum filter (see **double-quantum filtered correlated spectroscopy**). In systems with more than two coupled spins, antiphase-dispersion components exist, but mutual cancellation of dispersive tails occurs to a large extent. If this method is not employed, then the only suitable alternative is to employ weighting functions in the time domain to improve the resolution. Here again the theoretical treatment allows us to suggest a suitable function. Unlike the magnetization responsible for the generation of crosspeaks which has zero integrated intensity at t_1, $t_2 = 0$, the magnetization responsible for the diagonal peaks is maximal at t_1, $t_2 = 0$. If, therefore, we apply a weighting function which decreases the magnitude of the free induction decay at t_1, $t_2 = 0$, we should find that the intensity of the diagonal peaks is reduced relative to the crosspeaks. In practice, it is found that a sine–bell function achieves this objective, while at the same time giving improved resolution. However, there is often significant decrease in the overall signal-to-noise ratio of the spectrum. The use of a sine–bell function in this application is an example of so-called **pseudo-echo transformation**.

To complete the analysis of the COSY experiment, we show the data routing and phase cycling required to perform a standard phase-sensitive COSY experiment using a complex **Fourier transform** in both dimensions. Since this is a simple experiment, we only require superficial phase cycling to remove **axial peaks**. The sequence below is normally repeated fourfold with implementation of **CYCLOPS**, giving a minimum of 16 scans per t_1 increment:

Scan	P1	P2	Receiver	
1	X	X	+	Location 1
2	X	$-X$	+	
3	Y	X	+	Location 2
4	Y	$-X$	+	

For a description of subsequent data processing, see **phase-sensitive experiments**. See also **double-quantum correlated spectroscopy, double-quantum filtered correlated spectroscopy**.

FURTHER READING

2D NMR was originally proposed by Jeener: see

Jeener, J. (1971). *Ampère International Summer School,* Basko Polje, Yugoslavia.

For a detailed theoretical analysis of COSY, see

Aue, W. P., Bartholdi, E., and Ernst, R. R. (1975). *J. Chem. Phys.* **64,** 2229.

For practical guidelines, see

Bax, A. and Freeman, R. (1981). *J. Magn. Reson.* **44,** 542.

Correlated spectroscopy (ω_1 decoupled) See **constant-time experiments**.

Correlation spectroscopy (rapid scan cross-correlation spectroscopy) This technique was devised by Dadok to allow uniform excitation of a limited region of the spectrum. It involves a rapid linear frequency sweep on the time-scale of T_1 of the region of interest. The key principle is that a linear sweep has a constant power spectrum over the range it sweeps, or is a good approximation to this principle if the sweep is between two discrete frequencies. Time averaging is achieved in the normal manner by repeating the sweep many times. The output of the spin system is the **convolution** of the input excitation and the NMR spectrum. The latter is therefore retrieved from the rapid scan response by cross-correlation. In other words, the **Fourier transform** of the rapid scan response is multiplied by the complex conjugate (see **complex number**) of the Fourier transform of the excitation. Reverse Fourier transformation then yields the NMR spectrum. It should be mentioned that the signal before the last transformation is analogous to the **free induction decay** of pulsed NMR and can itself be multiplied with various weighting functions. The method is less efficient than pulsed excitation, but its inherent advantage is an increase in effective digital resolution and, since irradiation at the frequency of the solvent resonance can be avoided, dynamic range problems can be circumvented.

FURTHER READING

Dadok, J. and Sprecher, R. F. (1974). *J. Magn. Reson.* **13,** 243.

Correlation time In describing **relaxation** processes in NMR, it is necessary to characterize random molecular motions within the sample, since these motions create fluctuating local magnetic fields which are responsible for the relaxtion. A useful function in describing random motion is the correlation time, τ_c. A global definition of τ_c at this point is difficult since it depends upon the type of motion. For example, in the case of random translational motion, τ_c is defined as the mean time between collisions, whereas in the case of reorientational (rotational) motion, it is defined as the average time for the molecule to rotate by one radian. A more tractable definition can be had by noting that if a molecular exists in a given state for τ_c s, such motion is associated with frequency components centred around τ_c^{-1} Hz.

The molecular correlation time (and hence relaxation) depends upon many factors. Clearly molecular size must have a large influence on the magnitude of τ_c; for small molecules of molecular mass <100, $\tau_c \sim 10^{-12}$–10^{-13} s in aqueous solutions of normal viscosity. Larger molecules (molecular weight >500) are characterized by $\tau_c \sim 10^{-10}$ s, whereas macromolecules may possess a τ_c as large as 10^{-8} s. In addition, τ_c is dependent upon the shape of the molecule. A globular protein (molecular weight ~20 000) might well possess a correlation time of ~10^{-8} s in aqueous solution, whereas a small rod-shaped oligosaccharide (molecular weight 2000) may possess a similar correlation time. Actually, in the latter case, since the molecule is asymmetric, it is difficult to define the correlation time—it depends upon whether the motion being characterized is, for example, rotational motion around the long axis, or whether the molecule is tumbling 'end-over-end'. Further difficulties arise when there is intramolecular motion (see **anisotropic motion**). Here, different parts of the molecule will certainly possess different correlation times, leading to anisotropic relaxation. For these reasons, the correlation time is an exceedingly difficult parameter to measure. For spherical molecules in solution, τ_c is well approximated by the **Stokes–Einstein relation**. In other cases, τ_c is perhaps best estimated experimentally. When the overall motion is isotropic, the ratio of the **spin–lattice relaxation** time to the **spin–spin relaxation** time ($T_1 : T_2$) can be useful. Alternatively, T_1 can be measured at two different frequencies, and τ_c

can be calculated from the Solomon–Bloembergen equations (see spin–lattice relaxation, spin–spin relaxation). When the overall motion is not isotropic, it is necessary to fit the experimental data to one of the suitable theories for the calculation of relaxation times in the presence of anisotropic motion.

FURTHER READING

The concept of the correlation time is explained more fully in any good NMR text. See, for example,
Abragam, A. (1961). *Principles of nuclear magnetism.* Clarendon Press, Oxford.

Cosine transform See **Fourier transform**.

COSY See **correlated spectroscopy**.

Coupling See **dipolar coupling**, **spin coupling**, **strong coupling**, **weak coupling**.

CPMG See **Carr–Purcell–Meiboom–Gill sequence**.

Cross-correlation function The cross-correlation function bears a resemblance to convolution. The cross-correlation between two functions $f(t)$ and $h(t)$ is defined by

C64 $$\rho(t) = \int_{-\infty}^{\infty} f^*(\tau)h(t+\tau)\,\mathrm{d}\tau$$

where * represents the complex conjugate (see **complex number**) of f. The cross-correlation function $\rho(t)$ is a measure of the degree of correlation between two functions. Two unrelated functions will have zero cross-correlation for all τ, whereas two functions between which there is a causal connection may have a finite cross-correlation for some or all values of τ. An example of a device which performs cross-correlation is the **phase-sensitive detector**. The output of this device is proportional to the cosine of the phase angle between two input signals. In NMR one of the input signals is known as the reference, and is a sample of the r.f. used to excite the spin system. The other input signal is the response from the spin system. The output is the cross-correlation between the applied r.f. and the response. This simple example is only valid, however, when the input waveform is a simple harmonic function (e.g. pulsed continuous-wave sinusoidal). When the excitation waveform is stochastic, it is necessary to compute the cross-correlation function. This is simplified by the fact that cross-correlation in one Fourier domain (see **Fourier transform**) is complex conjugate multiplication in the co-domain, i.e.

C65 if $\rho = f(t) * h(t)$ where $*$ denotes cross-correlation then

C66 $$\Gamma = F^*(\nu) . H(\nu)$$

and

C67 $$\Gamma \xrightarrow{\text{FT}} \rho$$ where FT denotes Fourier transformation.

FURTHER READING

Shaw, D. (1984). *Fourier transform NMR spectroscopy* (2nd edn). Elsevier, Amsterdam.

Cross-polarization The study of rare spins (such as ^{13}C) in liquids and solids means that these do not experience significant homonuclear couplings. This is of particular value in NMR of solids since the strong homonuclear **dipolar couplings** are absent. This advantage must be compared with significant loss of signal-to-noise ratio. However, the presence of strong dipolar coupling between rare spins and abundant nuclei (e.g. protons) in solids, or the presence of scalar (J) coupling in liquids can be exploited to provide signal enhancement under appropriate conditions. This process is known as polarization transfer, or cross-polarization. In liquids, polarization transfer was originally achieved by experiments such as **INEPT**. For further information of this and similar experiments in liquids, see **polarization transfer**.

The cross-polarization experiment in solids takes place in three stages: (1) The **spin temperature** of the abundant (I) spin reservoir is lowered, (2) the actual polarization transfer step takes place between the I spin and rare (S) spin reservoirs, and (3) the S spins are observed. There are several mechanisms by which step (2) can be achieved, one of the most widely used being spin-lock polarization transfer. The pulse sequence relevant to this approach is shown in Fig. C27. The 90°x pulse applied to

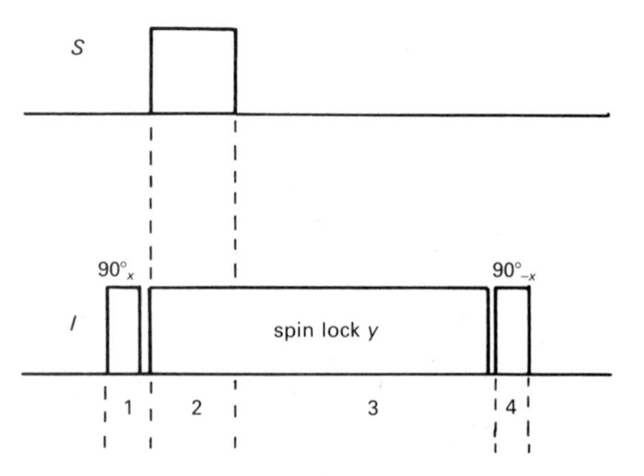

Fig. C27. Pulse sequence for spin-lock polarization transfer. Steps 1, 2, 3, and 4 are described in the text.

the I spin system serves to lower the spin-temperature of these spins. Energy matching of the I and S spins is then generated by the spin-lock fields applied simultaneously to both spin types. It can be shown that the polarization transfer rate is a maximum when the precession frequencies of I and S in their respective rotating frames are equal: $\gamma_I B_{1I} = \gamma_S B_{1S}$. This is known as the **Hartmann–Hahn condition**. The spin-lock field on the S spins is turned off. However, by maintaining the spin lock on the I spins during detection of the S spins, the **free induction decay** will not be influenced by the heteronuclear dipolar coupling. Hence Fourier transformation of the free induction decay will give a dipolar decoupled spectrum of S. At the end of the spin lock period on I, a $90°{-}x$ pulse is applied to flip any remaining coherent I spin magnetization back along the z axis (step 4). The enhancement of the S spin signal is of the order of γ_I/γ_S, i.e. about four for a ^1H–^{13}C experiment. However, a further advantage is that it is possible to accumulate several spectra without waiting for the abundant spins to repolarize. This is known as multiple-contact cross-polarization and is possible because the cross-polarization process does not remove all of the abundant spin magnetization. Since T_1's in the solid state can be extremely long, the saving in time is a considerable advantage, and increases the effective sensitivity of the experiment. A further advantage is that the whole process can be repeated with a time given by $\sim 5T_{1I}$, as opposed to $\sim 5T_{1S}$, and T_1 for protons is smaller than T_1 for ^{13}C. The overall improvement in signal-to-noise-ratio considering all these advantages can be several thousands.

FURTHER READING

A discussion of cross-polarization can be found in any good text in solid state NMR. See for example

Gerstein, B. C. and Dybrowki, C. R. (1985). *Transient techniques in NMR of solids*. Academic Press, London.

Cross-relaxation Cross-relaxation is a mechanism whereby a spin is relaxed by **dipolar coupling** to its neighbour or neighbours.

Consider two spins I and S, which are not scalar (J) coupled (see **spin coupling**). Solomon has derived the following equations for the time decay of the z magnetization, $\langle I_z \rangle$ and $\langle S_z \rangle$, of the two spins coupled by cross-relaxation:

$$\frac{d\langle I_z \rangle}{dt} = -\rho_I(\langle I_z \rangle - I_0) - \sigma_{IS}(\langle S_z \rangle - S_0) \quad \text{C68}$$

$$\frac{d\langle S_z \rangle}{dt} = -\rho_S(\langle S_z \rangle - S_0) - \sigma_{SI}(\langle I_z \rangle - I_0). \quad \text{C69}$$

Here, S_0 and I_0 are the equilibrium values of the magnetization of the respective spins, ρ is the direct relaxation rate of the spin with the lattice, and σ is the cross-relaxation rate. The cross-relaxation terms determine that (C68) and (C69) are a pair of coupled differential equations. The cross-relaxation rate is equal to the difference between the double-quantum and zero-quantum transition probabilities (see **spin–lattice, spin–spin relaxation**) per unit time for the two-spin systems:

$$\sigma = W_2 - W_0. \tag{C70}$$

Since the magnitudes of W_2 and W_0 depend upon the **correlation time**, σ may be either positive or negative in sign. In addition, since σ is responsible for the **nuclear Overhauser effect** (NOE), the same correlation time dependence determines the sign of the NOE. In macromolecules, W_0 becomes much larger than W_2, and cross-relaxation becomes a very efficient process. The magnetization of a given spin then diffuses over a large number of spins, and this is termed **spin diffusion**. This is an unfortunate event for the biological NMR spectroscopist, since the selectivity of the NOE is lost under these circumstances. For a detailed analysis of ρ and σ, see **spin–lattice relaxation**.

FURTHER READING

The classic paper is
Solomon, I. (1955). *Phys. Rev.* **99,** 559.
For a discussion of cross-relaxation in proteins see
Kalk, A. and Berendesen, H. J. C. (1976). *J. Magn. Reson.* **24,** 343.

Cyclically ordered phase sequence (CYCLOPS) In a receiver system equipped with **quadrature detection**, artefacts may be introduced into the spectrum which are generated from non-orthonormal receiver channels, i.e. the phase relationship between signals entering the channels is not 90° and/or the gains of the channels are not equal. The result is an 'image' or 'ghost' which is particularly visible when an intense resonance line is present in the spectrum. The ghost signal is observed at the conjugate frequency to the strong resonance line on the opposite side of the **carrier**. The artefact can be eliminated with the aid of a Cyclically Ordered Phase Sequence (CYCLOPS) applied to the transmitter, with appropriate data routing in the computer. The purpose of the latter is to achieve a rotation of the receiver phase. In practice, CYCLOPS consists of four 90° phase rotations of the transmitter frequency, with similar-rotations for the receiver. Artefacts due to **d.c. offset** are also removed by this procedure. To illustrate the efficacy of CYCLOPS, compare Figs. (C28) and (C29). The spectrum in Fig. C28 is a single scan of a 99% solution of D_2O. The spectrum in Fig. C29 results from four scans using the same sample, thus allowing for full CYCLOPS correction. It is obvious that with CYCLOPS implemented, signal averaging should only

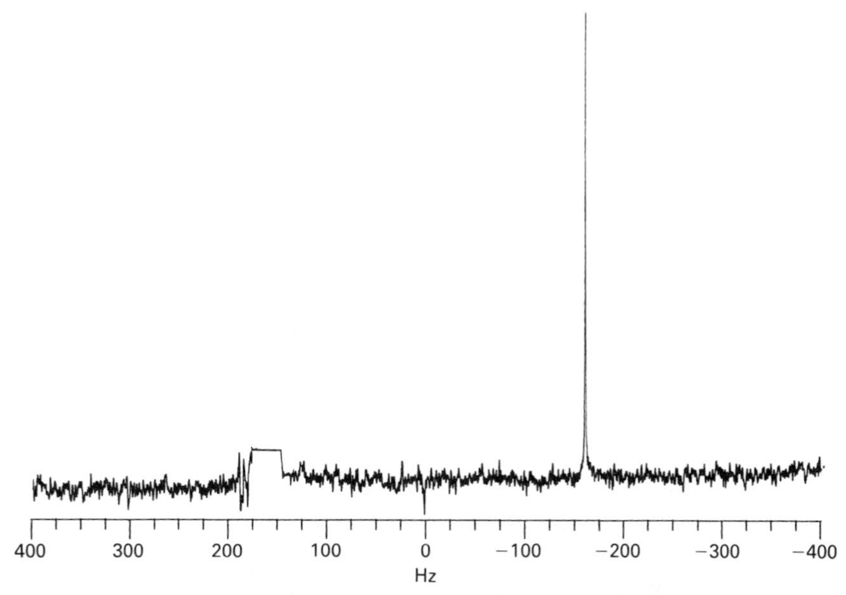

Fig. C28. A single scan of a sample of D_2O. The residual water in the sample gives a strong resonance line (shown truncated) with an artefact on the opposite side of the carrier, due to the imbalance between receiver channels. A zero-frequency artefact is also visible due to the presence of a small d.c. offset.

be terminated at an integral multiple of four scans. When used with multiple pulse experiments with varying phase relationships, any phase cycling required by the experiment should be completed, followed by implementation of CYCLOPS to all pulses and to the receiver. This of course results in a fourfold increase in the number of scans required.

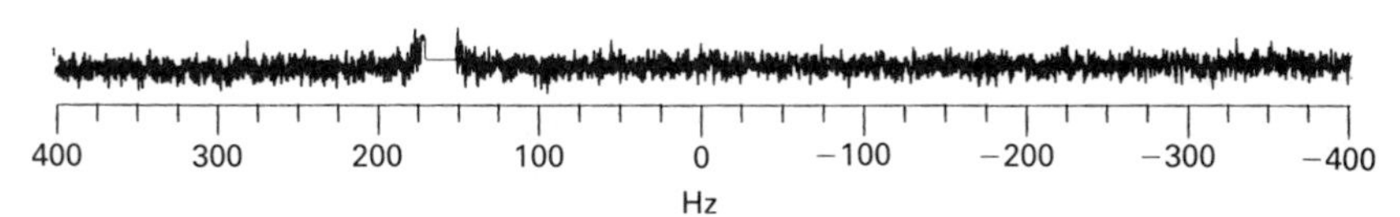

Fig. C29. The same sample with four scans. In this case the CYCLOPS phase cycle has completed, and the artefacts are no longer visible.

FURTHER READING

For a description of CYCLOPS. see
Hoult, D. I. (1978). *Progr. NMR Spectr.* **12,** 41.

CYCLOPS See **cyclically ordered phase sequence**.

D

Damped oscillator The signal induced in the receiver coils of an NMR spectrometer due to the magnetization derived from a group of equivalent spins S can be described by the following equation:

D1 $$M = \cos \omega_S t \,.\, \exp(-t/T_2)$$

where ω_S is the Larmor frequency of the spins, t is the acquisition time, and T_2 is the **spin–spin relaxation** time of the spins. The cosine term describes the oscillatory signal induced in the receiver coils (see Fig. D1a), and the exponential function describes its decay (see Fig. D1b). The product of these functions gives a function known as a damped oscillator (see Fig. D1c). In the case of the NMR experiment, this damped oscillator is known as the free **free induction decay**. In NMR of liquids, **Fourier transformation** of a function such as that shown in Fig. D1c generates a characteristic **lineshape**, known as a Lorentzian line.

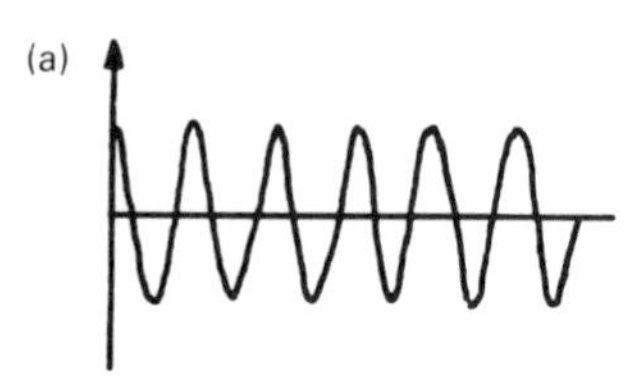

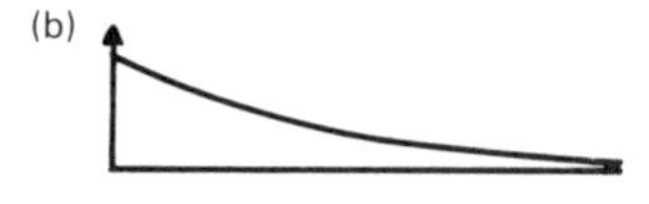

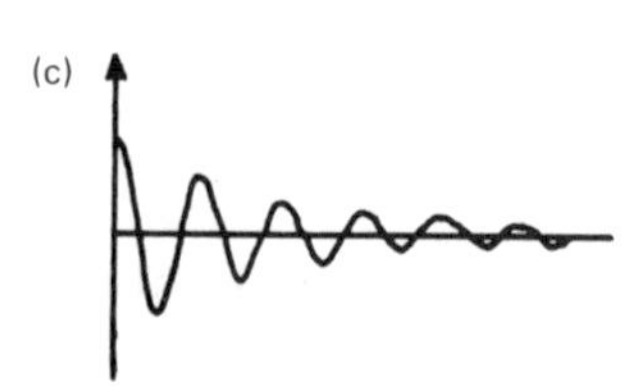

Fig. D1. (a) The function $\cos \omega_s t$ vs. t; (b) The function $\exp(-t/T_2)$ vs. t; (c) The product $\cos \omega_s t \,.\, \exp(-t/T_2)$ vs. t.

DANTE See **delays alternating with nutation for tailored excitation**.

D.c. offset Ideally, the **free induction decay** stored in the memory of the acquisition computer will not contain a direct current (d.c.) component. However, under certain circumstances, e.g. if the **quadrature detection** amplifiers have different d.c. offsets at their output, then correspondingly the free-induction decay will contain a d.c. component. However, this will only arise if an insufficient number of scans is collected such that **CYCLOPS** phase cycling does not complete one cycle. The effect of a d.c. offset upon the free-induction decay is to generate a 'spike' at zero frequency in the NMR spectrum. This arises simply from the fact that the Fourier transform of a continuous d.c. level is a **delta function**. Since acquisition only extends over a finite time, we find that the frequency domain artefact is only an approximation to a delta function. The appearance of such an artefact is shown in Fig. D2.

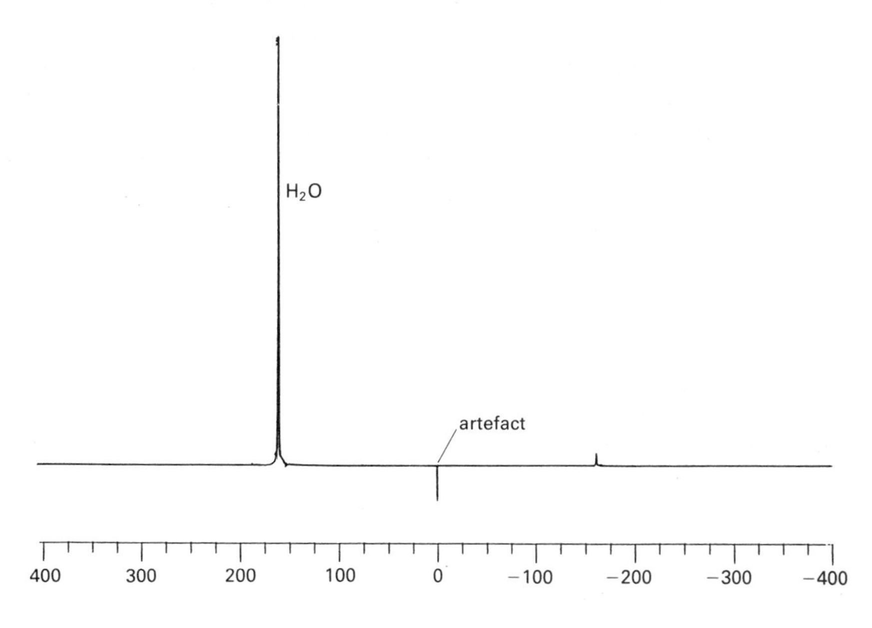

Fig. D2. A zero-frequency artefact in this NMR spectrum of H_2O arises from the presence of a d.c. level in the corresponding free induction decay.

Deconvolution See **convolution**.

Decoupling See **spin decoupling**, **broadband decoupling**, **gated decoupling**, **off-resonance decoupling**.

Delays alternating with nutation for tailored excitation (DANTE) The DANTE sequence is a method for the selective excitation of resonances in the NMR spectrum. It is a regular sequence of short, intense r.f. pulses, which are repeated at a specific rate $\nu = 1/t$. For a series of N such pulses, the pulse width is sufficently small such that each pulse flips the spin magnetization through a very small angle ϕ/N (see **classical formalism**) so that on-resonance the effect is a rotation through ϕ radians. Nuclei which are **offset** by a frequency Δf from resonance experience precession between pulses through an angle $\beta = 2\pi\,\Delta f t$. The following pulse therefore acts upon nuclei with a different precession phase, so that the flip-angle created by each subsequent pulse is not additive. If the offset is large, i.e. $\beta \gg \phi/N$, magnetization vectors describe small cyclic trajectories about the z axis (see **classical formalism**). Little transverse magnetization is thus created at these large offsets. If the number of pulses N is very large, the sequence approximates to a single soft pulse of flip-angle ϕ. However, an important difference between DANTE and a soft pulse is the presence of sidebands at certain discrete offsets due to the condition $\beta = (2\pi n + \beta)$ where n is a small integer. Here, the spin magnetization completes n full revolutions plus β about the z axis, and the cumulative effect of the pulses is again additive. If one of these sidebands is used for the irradiation, then the irradiation frequency can be finely adjusted by varying ν. In addition, the pulsewidth t_{p} and the number of pulses N are also adjustable. The net flip angle at resonance is then given by

$$\phi = \gamma B_1 N t_p.$$

FURTHER READING

Morris, G. A. and Freeman, R. (1978). *J. Magn. Reson.* **29,** 433.

Delta function The delta function, otherwise known as the impulse function, is defined as

$$\delta(t - t_0) = 0, \qquad t \neq t_0, \tag{D2}$$

$$\int_{-\infty}^{\infty} \delta(t - t_0)\,\mathrm{d}t = 1. \tag{D3}$$

That is, the δ function is defined as having undefined magnitude at the time of occurrence and zero elsewhere. The area under the function is unity. This concept is fundamental throughout physics. for example, many will be familiar with the Dirac delta function which is found in quantum mechanics, and is thus found in quantum mechanical descriptions of NMR. A further example of the use of delta functions in NMR is the concept of the impulse response, i.e. the response of the spin system to a delta function (an impulse). Obviously it is difficult to relate an impulse to a physical signal. We can think of it as a pulse waveform of very large magnitude and infinitely small duration such that the area of the pulse is unity.

FURTHER READING

Bracewell, R. M. (1965). *The Fourier transform and its applications.* McGraw-Hill, New York.

Density matrix The use of classical vectors to describe NMR phenomena (see **classical formalism**) is an extremely valuable method with which to 'visualize' certain NMR experiments. However, a large number of NMR experiments, particularly those involving two-dimensional techniques, cannot be described adequately in the classical sense. A variety of alternative quantum mechanical formalisms exist with which to describe these experiments (see e.g. **product operator formalism**, **single-transition operator**, **spherical tensor operator**). Each of these is of particular value in certain circumstances. There is, however, one formalism, the density matrix formalism, which is of universal applicability and from which the above alternatives are derived. Once the energy levels of a system of N spins are fully known (by determining the **eigenvalues** of the **Hamiltonian**), the density matrix provides a complete description of the state of the spin system. Now, just as we are interested in the time evolution of the magnetization vector in the classical formalism, we are interested in the time evolution of the density matrix in the present formalism. Since the density matrix is not a classical device, its time evolution does not correspond with any classical equations. In fact, the time evolution of the density matrix is governed by the **Liouville–von Neumann equation**;

D4 $$\frac{\mathrm{d}\sigma}{\mathrm{d}t} = -\mathrm{i}\hbar^{-1}[\mathcal{H}, \sigma]$$

where $\hbar = h/2\pi$, $[\mathcal{H}, \sigma]$ is the **commutator** of $\mathcal{H}$ and σ, and $\mathcal{H}$ is the Hamiltonian under which the density matrix evolves. The value of $\mathcal{H}$ will vary, depending upon whether an r.f. pulse is applied to the system, or whether a free precession period is involved. In each case a different Hamiltonian can be formulated. If $\mathcal{H}$ does not vary with time, then (D4) can be integrated to give a value for σ at time t, $\sigma(t)$, in terms of its value at $t = 0$, $\sigma(0)$:

D5 $$\sigma(t) = \exp(-\mathrm{i}\mathcal{H}t)\sigma(0)\exp(\mathrm{i}\mathcal{H}t).$$

In other words, if we wanted to find $\sigma(t)$ after the application of an r.f. pulse to $\sigma(0)$, then we would perform the operations shown on the right-hand side of (D5), inserting for $\mathcal{H}$ the Hamiltonian corresponding to the r.f. pulse. In this case the exponential operators in (D5) are

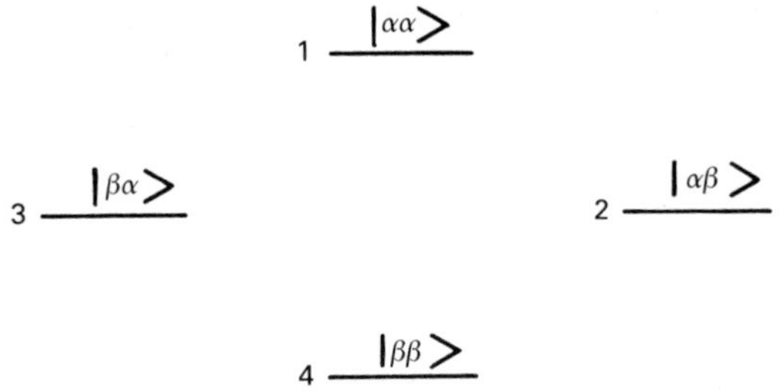

Fig. D3. The basis states of a loosely coupled two-spin system.

sometimes called **rotation operators**. The transformation shown in (D5) consists essentially of the multiplication of three matrices, one corresponding to $\exp(-i\mathcal{H}t)$, another to $\sigma(0)$, and finally one corresponding to $\exp(i\mathcal{H}t)$. The determination of the matrix forms of $\exp(-i\mathcal{H}t)$ and $\exp(i\mathcal{H}t)$ is described under **matrix representation**. In order to illustrate the principles further, let us use the density matrix formalism to examine the effect of a single 90° pulse on a weakly coupled two-spin $\frac{1}{2}$ system *IS* (Fig. D3) which is initially at thermal equilibrium. First, we obviously need to derive a matrix form for $\sigma(0)$. For a system of N spins, σ is an $N \times N$ matrix. It is an Hermitian matrix, i.e. the elements σ_{rc} and σ_{cr} are complex conjugates. The diagonal elements of the matrix are identical to the populations of the states. In contrast, the off-diagonal elements show the occurrence of coherence 'in progress' between two states. Using the **bra-ket notation** for the basis states in Fig. D3, we can assign the population numbers P_1, P_2, P_3, P_4 to each state as shown. Assuming the spin system is at thermal equilibrium, the density matrix $\sigma(0)$ can be represented as follows;

D6
$$\begin{array}{cc} & \begin{array}{cccc} |\alpha\alpha\rangle & |\alpha\beta\rangle & |\beta\alpha\rangle & |\beta\beta\rangle \end{array} \\ \sigma(0) = & \begin{bmatrix} P_1 & 0 & 0 & 0 \\ 0 & P_2 & 0 & 0 \\ 0 & 0 & P_3 & 0 \\ 0 & 0 & 0 & P_4 \end{bmatrix} \begin{array}{l} |\alpha\alpha\rangle \\ |\alpha\beta\rangle \\ |\beta\alpha\rangle \\ |\beta\beta\rangle. \end{array} \end{array}$$

Here, each row and column of $\sigma(0)$ is labelled with the basis states to show how each element of the matrix is related to either coherence (off-diagonal elements, of which there are none at thermal equilibrium) or populations (diagonal elements). This notation will be dropped in the following calculations. The effect of the r.f. pulse is derived by multiplying $\sigma(0)$ by the rotation operators as defined by (D5). At this point it must be emphasized that the right-hand side of (D5) must be evaluated as written, i.e. the matrices must be multiplied in the prescribed order. Assuming that we applied an r.f. pulse of flip angle θ along the x axis of the **rotating frame**, then the corresponding rotation operator for the pulse is given by

D7 $$R_{+x} = \exp\{-iF_x\theta\} = \exp\{-i(I_x + S_x)\theta\}$$

where I_x and S_x are the x component **angular momentum** operators for the two spins. The matrix representation of (D7) is

D8 $$\exp\{-iF_x\theta\} = \begin{bmatrix} c^2 & -isc & -isc & -s^2 \\ -isc & c^2 & -s^2 & -isc \\ -isc & -s^2 & c^2 & -isc \\ -s^2 & -isc & -isc & c^2 \end{bmatrix},$$

where $s = \sin(\theta/2)$ and $c = \cos(\theta/2)$. The matrix of $\exp\{iF_x\theta\}$ (the inverse of $\exp\{-iF_x\theta\}$) is found by changing the signs of the imaginary elements. If, now, we assume $\theta = 90°$, (D8) becomes

D9 $$\exp\{-iF_x\theta\} = \tfrac{1}{2}\begin{bmatrix} 1 & -i & -i & -1 \\ -i & 1 & -1 & -i \\ -i & -1 & 1 & -i \\ -1 & -i & -i & 1 \end{bmatrix}.$$

Therefore, using (D5), $\sigma(t)$ is evaluated as follows:

$$\sigma(t) = \tfrac{1}{2}\begin{bmatrix} 1 & -i & -i & -1 \\ -i & 1 & -1 & -i \\ -i & -1 & 1 & -i \\ -1 & -i & -i & 1 \end{bmatrix} \cdot \begin{bmatrix} P_1 & 0 & 0 & 0 \\ 0 & P_2 & 0 & 0 \\ 0 & 0 & P_3 & 0 \\ 0 & 0 & 0 & P_4 \end{bmatrix} \cdot \tfrac{1}{2}\begin{bmatrix} 1 & +i & +i & -1 \\ +i & 1 & -1 & +i \\ +i & -1 & 1 & +i \\ -1 & +i & +i & 1 \end{bmatrix}$$

D10 $$= \tfrac{1}{4}\begin{bmatrix} P_1 + P_2 & +iP_1 - iP_2 & +iP_1 + iP_2 & -P_1 + P_2 \\ +P_3 + P_4 & +iP_3 - iP_4 & -iP_3 - iP_4 & +P_3 - P_4 \\ -iP_1 + iP_2 & P_1 + P_2 & P_1 - P_2 & +iP_1 + iP_2 \\ -iP_3 + iP_4 & +P_3 + P_4 & -P_3 + P_4 & -iP_3 - iP_4 \\ -iP_1 - iP_2 & P_1 - P_2 & P_1 + P_2 & +iP_1 - iP_2 \\ +iP_3 + iP_4 & -P_3 + P_4 & +P_3 + P_4 & +iP_3 - iP_4 \\ -P_1 + P_2 & -iP_1 - iP_2 & -iP_1 + iP_2 & +P_1 + P_2 \\ +P_3 - P_4 & +iP_3 + iP_4 & -iP_3 + iP_4 & +P_3 + P_4 \end{bmatrix}.$$

Now, if we assume that the spin system was at thermal equilibrium prior to the pulse, P_1, P_2, P_3, and P_4 can be related to the net populations of states using the Boltzmann Law (see **Boltzmann distribution**):

$$P_1 = 1 - \delta, \qquad P_2 = P_3 = 0, \qquad P_4 = 1 + \delta,$$

(D10) thus becomes

D11
$$\sigma(t) = \tfrac{1}{2}\delta \begin{bmatrix} 0 & -\mathrm{i} & -\mathrm{i} & 0 \\ \mathrm{i} & 0 & 0 & -\mathrm{i} \\ \mathrm{i} & 0 & 0 & -\mathrm{i} \\ 0 & \mathrm{i} & \mathrm{i} & 0 \end{bmatrix}.$$

Note here that off-diagonal elements have been generated; these elements, which label transitions between states, tell us that coherence is 'ongoing' between the states which each element labels. If we refer to Fig. D3 and (D6) it is clear that the off-diagonal elements in (D11) connect states such as $|\alpha\alpha\rangle \rightarrow |\alpha\beta\rangle$. A transition between these states is called a single-quantum transition, and each non-zero element in (D11) corresponds with single-quantum coherence. This is the quantum analogue of observable transverse magnetization which would be found after application of a 90° pulse in the **classical formalism**. In order to see how we can obtain an expression for observable magnetization using the density matrix formalism, we must allow $\sigma(t)$ to evolve in time in the absence of the r.f. pulse, i.e. during the acquisition period. If we assume the two-spin system is loosely coupled (see **weak coupling**), then the **Hamiltonian** under which $\sigma(t)$ evolves in the absence of the pulse is composed in the simplest case of two terms, $\mathcal{H}_Z$ and $\mathcal{H}_J$. The Hamiltonian $\mathcal{H}_Z$ is the Zeeman Hamiltonian representing the interaction of the spins in the B_0 field, whereas the spin-coupling Hamiltonian $\mathcal{H}_J$ represents the scalar (J) coupling between the two nuclei. As in the treatment of $\sigma(0)$ evolving under the Hamiltonian corresponding to an r.f. pulse, we treat the evolution of $\sigma(t)$ under $\mathcal{H} = \mathcal{H}_Z + \mathcal{H}_J$ according to (D5):

D12
$$\begin{aligned} \sigma(t') &= \exp\{-\mathrm{i}\mathcal{H}t\}\sigma(t)\exp\{\mathrm{i}\mathcal{H}t\} \\ &= \exp\{-\mathrm{i}(\mathcal{H}_Z + \mathcal{H}_J)t\}\sigma(t)\exp\{\mathrm{i}(\mathcal{H}_Z + \mathcal{H}_J)t\}. \end{aligned}$$

Now, if the basis states we are using are eigenstates of the Hamiltonian (see **eigenfunction**), then the matrix representations of the exponential operators in (D12) are always diagonal. Since the **product basis** we used in formulating our problem (Fig. D3) is indeed the eigenbasis for two weakly coupled spins, then the matrix representation of $\exp\{-\mathrm{i}(\mathcal{H}_Z + \mathcal{H}_J)t\}$ is simply given by

D13
$$\begin{aligned} &\exp\{-\mathrm{i}(\mathcal{H}_Z + \mathcal{H}_J)t\} \\ &= \begin{bmatrix} \exp\{-\mathrm{i}E_1 t\} & 0 & 0 & 0 \\ 0 & \exp\{-\mathrm{i}E_2 t\} & 0 & 0 \\ 0 & 0 & \exp\{-\mathrm{i}E_3 t\} & 0 \\ 0 & 0 & 0 & \exp\{-\mathrm{i}E_4 t\} \end{bmatrix} \end{aligned}$$

where E_1, E_2, E_3, E_4 are the energies of the eigenstates (the eigenvalues of the Hamiltonian) labelled 1, 2, 3, 4 in Fig. D3. Given that the exponential operators in (D12) are diagonal, the operations described in (D12) essentially tell us that we must multiply all elements in the rth row by $\exp\{iE_r t\}$, and all the elements in the cth column by $\exp\{-iE_c t\}$. This requires an element σ_{rc} to acquire an oscillation $\omega_{rc} = (E_r - E_c)$. Thus, $\sigma(t')$ can be immediately written down by performing these multiplications upon each element in $\sigma(t)$:

D14

$$\sigma(t') = \tfrac{1}{2}i\delta \begin{bmatrix} 0 & -\exp\{i\omega_{12}t\} & -\exp\{i\omega_{13}t\} & 0 \\ \exp\{-i\omega_{21}t\} & 0 & 0 & -\exp\{i\omega_{24}t\} \\ \exp\{-i\omega_{31}t\} & 0 & 0 & -\exp\{i\omega_{34}t\} \\ 0 & \exp\{-i\omega_{42}t\} & \exp\{-i\omega_{43}t\} & 0 \end{bmatrix}.$$

The reader may care to derive (D14) explicitly from (D12) using (D13) and its inverse. Incidentally, note that (D14) is indeed Hermetian since σ_{cr} is the complex conjugate (see **complex number**) of σ_{rc}. Note also that elements such as σ_{41} and σ_{23} remain zero. These elements correspond to **double-quantum coherence** and **zero-quantum coherence** respectively (see **multiple-quantum coherence**), neither of which is excited in single pulse experiments in spin $\frac{1}{2}$ nuclei.

The description is almost complete, since $\sigma(t')$ shows the form of the density matrix at the end of the acquisition period. However, one final step is required to extract the observable magnetization: We must form the trace (see Appendix 3) of the product of the operator $F_x = I_x + S_x$ with $\sigma(t')$ if the receiver **phase** is along the axis, or the trace of the product of $F_y = iI_y + iS_y$ with $\sigma(t')$ if the receiver phase is along the y axis. If we arbitrarily choose the former the observable magnetization is formally given by

D15

$$M_x = \mathrm{Tr}\{F_x \,.\, \sigma(t')\}$$

where F_x is in the **matrix representation**

D16

$$F_x = \tfrac{1}{2}\begin{bmatrix} 0 & 1 & 1 & 0 \\ 1 & 0 & 0 & 1 \\ 1 & 0 & 0 & 1 \\ 0 & 1 & 1 & 0 \end{bmatrix}.$$

If (D15) is evaluated explicitly, it will become clear that an equivalent expression can be formulated for M_x:

D17

$$M_{x_{rc}} = 2\,|F_{x_{rc}}|\,.\,\mathrm{Re}\{\sigma_{rc}\}$$

where Re denotes the real part (i.e. excluding terms in i). Using (D17), the observable x magnetization is therefore

D18
$$\begin{aligned} M_x &= M_{x_{12}} + M_{x_{13}} + M_{x_{24}} + M_{x_{34}} \\ &= \text{Re}\,\sigma_{12} + \text{Re}\,\sigma_{13} + \text{Re}\,\sigma_{24} + \text{Re}\,\sigma_{34}. \end{aligned}$$

Note at this point that even if the elements σ_{24} and σ_{23} were non-zero, they would not contribute to observable magnetization, as indeed they should not, as they correspond to **'forbidden' transitions**. In other words (D15) (or D17) is simply a recipe to extract the observable (single-quantum) **magnetization**.

Finally, on evaluating (D18) using (D14) we obtain

D19
$$\begin{aligned} M_x &= -\text{Re}\,\delta\text{i}(\exp\{\text{i}\omega_{12}t\} + \exp\{\text{i}\omega_{13}t\} + \exp\{\text{i}\omega_{24}t\} + \exp\{\text{i}\omega_{34}t\}) \\ &= -\text{Re}\,\delta\text{i}(\cos\omega_{12}t + \text{i}\sin\omega_{12}t + \cos\omega_{13}t + \text{i}\sin\omega_{13}t + \cos\omega_{24}t \\ &\qquad + \text{i}\sin\omega_{24}t + \cos\omega_{34}t + \text{i}\sin\omega_{34}t) \\ &= \delta(\sin\omega_{12}t + \sin\omega_{13}t + \sin\omega_{24}t + \sin\omega_{34}t). \end{aligned}$$

An analogous expression can be derived for M_y:

D20
$$\begin{aligned} M_y &= -\text{i}\,\text{Im}\,\delta\text{i}(\exp\{\text{i}\omega_{12}t\} + \exp\{\text{i}\omega_{13}t\} + \exp\{\text{i}\omega_{24}t\} + \exp\{\text{i}\omega_{34}t\}) \\ &= \delta(\cos\omega_{12}t + \cos\omega_{13}t + \cos\omega_{24}t + \cos\omega_{34}t) \end{aligned}$$

where Im denotes the imaginary part (i.e. terms in i).

The sine terms in (D19) tell us that four dispersion-mode lines will be observed if the receiver is aligned along the x axis. These lines occur at ω_{12}, ω_{13}, ω_{24}, ω_{34} after **Fourier transformation**. Similarly, four absorption–mode lines occur at ω_{12}, ω_{13}, ω_{24}, ω_{24} with the receiver aligned along the y axis (cosine terms). Now, given that $\omega_{12} = E_1 - E_2$, $\omega_{13} = E_1 - E_3$, $\omega_{24} = E_2 - E_4$, $\omega_{34} = E_3 - E_4$, we can determine the resonance frequencies of the four lines from the energies of the four states (the **eigenvalues** of the **Hamiltonian** $\mathcal{H} = \mathcal{H}_Z + \mathcal{H}_J$). These are:

D21
$$\begin{aligned} E_4 &= -\tfrac{1}{2}(\nu_I + \nu_S) + \tfrac{1}{4}J_{IS} \\ E_3 &= -\tfrac{1}{2}(\nu_I - \nu_S) - \tfrac{1}{4}J_{IS} \\ E_2 &= \tfrac{1}{2}(\nu_I - \nu_S) - \tfrac{1}{4}J_{IS} \\ E_1 &= \tfrac{1}{2}(\nu_I + \nu_S) + \tfrac{1}{4}J_{IS}. \end{aligned}$$

Thus,

D22
$$\begin{aligned} \omega_{12} &= \nu_S + \tfrac{1}{2}J_{IS} \\ \omega_{13} &= \nu_I + \tfrac{1}{2}J_{IS} \\ \omega_{24} &= \nu_I - \tfrac{1}{2}J_{IS} \\ \omega_{34} &= \nu_S - \tfrac{1}{2}J_{IS}. \end{aligned}$$

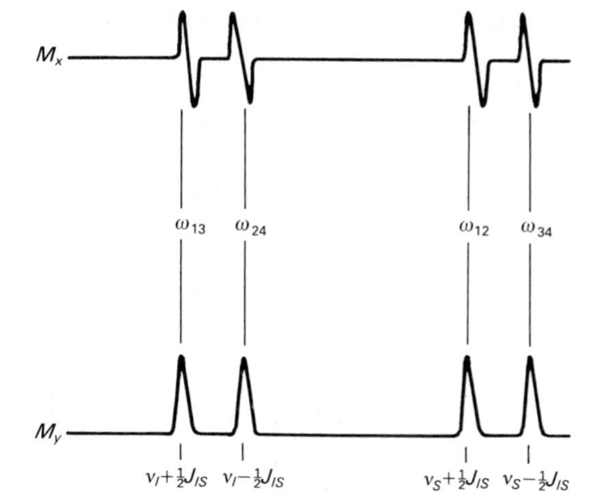

Fig. D4. The x (M_x) and y (M_y) components of the magnetization resulting from the density matrix calculations described above.

We are now in a position to draw the spectra of the two-spin system according to (D19) and (D20) (Fig. D4). All the lines are of the same intensity since the sine and cosine terms in (D19) and (D20) are scaled by the same factor, δ.

Instead of evaluating M_x and M_y from (D14), we could have continued by evolving $\sigma(t')$ under further Hamiltonians by the application of additional pulses and/or delays.

The calculation we have just performed serves to illustrate the application of the density matrix formalism for a one-pulse experiment on a two-spin scalar coupled system. It is hoped that the reader will not recoil from the apparent complexity of this approach. It is tedious, but is nevertheless not difficult to calculate the result for more complex spin systems. In some cases, it is much simpler to employ one of the alternative formalisms (see **product operator formalism**), and certainly for weakly coupled systems the density matrix formalism is more cumbersome. When the weak coupling approximation cannot be assumed, however, the density matrix formalism is invaluable (see **strong coupling**).

FURTHER READING

For a description of density operator techniques, see:

Fano, U. (1957). *Rev. Mod. Phys.* **29,** 74.

See also,

Ernst, R. R., Bodenhausen, G. and Wokaun, A. A. (1987) *Principles of NMR in one and two dimensions,* Chapter 2. Clarendon Press, Oxford.

The concept of the density matrix is particularly well dealt with in

Slichter, C. P. (1978). *Principles of magnetic resonance,* (2nd edn). Springer-Verlag, Berlin.

DEPT See **distortionless enhancement by polarization transfer**.

Detector The Larmor frequencies of nuclei which are of interest to spectroscopists are much too large to allow direct acquisition by computers. This problem is overcome by subtracting from the various frequencies emanating from the preamplifier, (or **intermediate frequency** amplifier, depending upon the spectrometer) the frequency of the transmitter carrier (the reference). This is achieved using a detector. The simplest conceivable detector in NMR is a diode. If the signal from the preamplifier is given by $A \sin \omega_s t$, and the reference by $B \sin \omega_r t$, then the current through the diode is given by

$$I = I_0\left[\exp\left[\frac{ev}{KT}\right] - 1\right] \tag{D23}$$

where K is Boltzmann's constant, T is the absolute temperature, I_0 is a constant, and v is the applied voltage. Expanding the exponent in (D23) gives

$$I = I_0\left[\frac{ev}{KT} + \frac{1}{2!}\frac{(ev)^2}{KT} + \ldots\right] \tag{D24}$$

with $v = A \sin \omega_S t + B \sin \omega_r t$. The contribution to I from the second-order term can be extracted after some trigonometry:

$$v^2 = \frac{A^2 + B^2}{2} - \frac{A^2}{2}\cos 2\omega_s t - \frac{B^2}{2}\cos 2\omega_r t + AB\cos(\omega_s - \omega_r)t - AB\cos(\omega_s + \omega_r)t. \tag{D25}$$

The current through the diode thus contains the desired difference frequency. The other frequencies, being much higher, are easily filtered out. However, a term in $A^2 + B^2$ remains, which is non-linear in both A and B, and so a simple diode introduces distortion. In addition, the output of a diode detector is not sensitive to the **phase** difference between the two input signals, which is unfortunate since many NMR experiments depend upon this requirement. Frequency changing is therefore invariably achieved using **phase-sensitive detectors** rather than diodes.

Diagonal peak See **correlated spectroscopy**.

Difference spectroscopy In biological NMR, difference spectroscopy is often used to simplify the extremely complex spectra which arise from studies of macromolecules. The principle of the technique is the subtraction of a spectrum which is perturbed in some manner by the experimenter from a 'reference' or unperturbed spectrum. Depending upon the precise manner in which the spectrum is perturbed, important information can be obtained about the system under study. Two techniques are of particular value to the biological spectroscopist. The first, **spin-decoupling** difference spectroscopy (SDDS), correlates scalar coupled spins. The resonance derived from the spin of interest is selectively irradiated (see **gated decoupling**) with r.f. energy at its Larmor frequency during the acquisition period. The resonance is thus required to be reasonably well resolved. This spectrum is then subtracted from the reference which is the unperturbed spectrum. In keeping with the theory of spin decoupling, for sufficient r.f. field strength, resonances derived from nuclei scalar coupled to the perturbed nucleus will also be perturbed. These perturbations will be visible even in crowded spectral regions using SDDS.

The second technique which finds frequent use in biological NMR is nuclear Overhauser effect difference spectroscopy (NOEDS). It is related to SDDS in that a chosen resonance is irradiated with a selective r.f. pulse. However, this pulse is applied before acquisition begins. The resulting difference spectrum correlates through-space coupled nuclei. NOEDS, like SDDS, is often of value in assignment. However, the distance dependence of the **nuclear Overhauser effect** can be exploited to define inter-residue through-space connectivities, and is the principal structural tool available to the biological spectroscopist.

Although simple and effective, difference spectroscopy often gives disappointing results due to poor subtraction of 'unperturbed' resonances. This is often due to poor experimental design. A principal cause of subtraction artefacts is the **Bloch–Siegert shift**. This is avoided by ensuring that the decoupler offset is shifted to a region which is clear of resonances in the reference spectrum rather than gating it off. A second cause of poor subtraction is spectrometer frequency instability. Although this should not generally be a problem with most modern spectrometers, it is particularly prevalent when linewidths are small. Obviously, the problem will be least severe if the minimum time elapses between acquisition of the perturbed spectrum and the reference. It is common practice to collect several scans with the decoupler on-resonance (perturbed spectrum), followed by an equivalent number off-resonance (reference), in order to complete one cycle of **CYCLOPS**. Indeed, the difference spectrum is very poor unless this requirement is met. However, an alternative method is to switch CYCLOPS off, and to subtract alternate scans, i.e. one scan on-resonance subtracted from one scan off-resonance. Difference spectra are often markedly improved using this technique, and of course artefacts normally removed by CYCLOPS are equally well eliminated during subtraction of the two spectra.

Digital resolution The digital resolution employed in a given experiment depends simply upon the number of data points which span a given

sweep-width. In one-dimensional NMR, digital resolution primarily affects the spectral resolution for obvious reasons, but in the case of very sharp lines, insufficient digital resolution can distort the intensities also. In **two-dimensional NMR**, digital resolution is of crucial importance in determining crosspeak intensity (see **correlated spectroscopy**). These considerations suggest that the maximum digital resolution available should be used. This is to a large extent true, but the acquisition of (say) 32 k data points with ±500 Hz sweep-width results in an acquisition time of 16 s. This may be prohibitively long, particularly in the case of two-dimensional NMR, and additionally generates a very large dataset. Less than optimal digital resolution is thus often employed in two-dimensional NMR, followed by post-acquisition **zero-filling**. The minimum usable digital resolution is often defined by the experiment. For example, a simple pulse and collect procedure upon a sample with long T_2's requires the acquisition time to be sufficiently long to prevent the **free-induction decay** from being truncated (see **truncation artefacts**). Since the sweep-width is also defined to a certain extent by the sample, the digital resolution is defined by both the sweep-width and by the acquisition time, because all three are obviously inextricably linked by the sampling theorem.

Dipolar coupling The presence of a group of spins around a given spin may result in a number of interactions. One of the more important interactions is that of a spin with the dipolar field produced by other spins. The classical interaction energy E between two magnetic moments μ_1 and μ_2 is

D26 $$E = \frac{\mu_1 \cdot \mu_2}{r^3} - \frac{3(\mu_1 \cdot r)(\mu_2 \cdot r)}{r^5}$$

where r is the vector joining μ_1 to μ_2. A quantum mechanical **Hamiltonian** can be formulated by treating μ_1 and μ_2 as operators:

D27 $$\mu_1 = \gamma_1 \hbar \mathbf{I}_1,$$

D28 $$\mu_2 = \gamma_2 \hbar \mathbf{I}_2.$$

The general dipolar Hamiltonian for N spins then becomes

D29 $$\mathcal{H}_\mathrm{d} = \tfrac{1}{2} \sum_{j=1}^{n} \sum_{k=1}^{n} \left[\frac{\mu_j \cdot \mu_k}{r_{jk}^3} - \frac{3(\mu_j \cdot r_{jk})(\mu_k \cdot r_{jk})}{r_{jk}^5} \right].$$

For the case of two spins, I and S, (D29) can be rewritten as an approximate dipolar Hamiltonian

D30 $$\mathcal{H}_\mathrm{d}^0 = \frac{1}{2} \frac{\gamma_I \gamma_S \hbar^2}{r^3} (1 - 3\cos^2\theta)(3I_z S_z - \mathbf{I} \cdot \mathbf{S})$$

where θ is the angle between the internuclear vector of length r and the applied field. Note that in liquids and gases, all possible values of θ exist due to reorientational motion. The average value of $\cos^2\theta$ is thus $\frac{1}{3}$, and the dipolar coupling averages to zero. However, at any particular time, the dipolar field is not necessarily zero, and thus it can contribute to **relaxation**. In solids, $3\cos^2\theta$ does not average, and very broad lines result from the non-zero dipolar coupling (see **solid state NMR** and **powder spectrum**).

Direct product See Appendix 3.

Dispersion-mode lineshape See **lineshape**.

Distortionless enhancement by polarization transfer (DEPT) The DEPT experiment is an improved version of the **INEPT** experiment. The simplest DEPT sequence is shown in Fig. D5. In contrast to the INEPT experiment, the 90° pulse on the S spins precedes the last pulse of flip-angle β on the I spins. Using the **product operator formalism**, it is convenient to analyse this experiment for a two-spin system IS, where I corresponds for example to protons and S to ^{13}C. Beginning with a system at thermal equilibrium, a 90° pulse on the I spins creates transverse magnetization solely for this nucleus:

D31 $$I_z + S_z \xrightarrow{(\pi/2)I_x} -I_y + S_z.$$

The spin system then evolves under Zeeman terms of the **Hamiltonian** corresponding to spin I (the S-spin terms having no effect on I_y or S_z) and the spin-coupling term

D32 $$-I_y + S_z \xrightarrow{\omega_I I_z + \pi J\tau 2I_zS_z} -I_y \cos\omega_I\tau \cos\pi J_{IS}\tau + 2I_xS_z \cos\omega_I\tau \sin\pi J_{IS}\tau$$
$$+ I_x \sin\omega_I\tau \cos\pi J_{IS}\tau + 2I_yS_z \sin\omega_I\tau \sin\pi J_{IS}\tau.$$

It is usual in experiments such as DEPT and INEPT to choose a value of

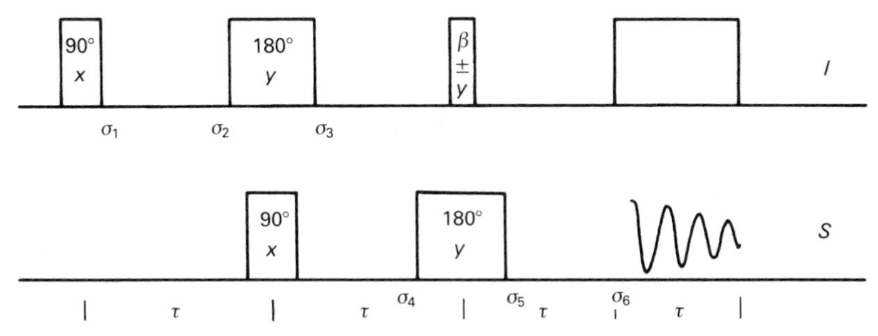

Fig. D5. Pulse sequence for the acquisition of DEPT spectra. See text for details.

τ which maximizes the antiphase component of the magnetization. This value is clearly $\tau = 2J_{CH}^{-1}$, which gives for the density operator just before the second pulse on the I spins:

D33 $$\sigma_2 = 2I_xS_z \cos \omega_I\tau + 2I_yS_z \sin \omega_I\tau.$$

After the second pulse on the I spins (π) and the first pulse on the S spins ($\pi/2$) the density operator thus takes the form

D34 $$2I_xS_z \cos \omega_I\tau + 2I_yS_z \sin \omega_I\tau \xrightarrow{\pi I_y} \xrightarrow{(\pi/2)S_x}$$
$$+ 2I_xS_y \cos \omega_I\tau - 2I_yS_y \sin \omega_I\tau = \sigma_3.$$

The salient aspects of the DEPT experiment centre around the multiple-quantum coherence which has been created by the $\pi/2$ pulse on the S spins. Since this does not evolve under spin couplings during the second τ period, the state of the spin system can be described by

D35 $$\sigma_4 = 2I_xS_y$$

where we have omitted the Zeeman evolution term in τ, to clarify the following expressions. After the final $\pm y$ pulse of flip angle β on the I spins, together with the y pulse (π) on the S spins, the state of the density matrix is given by

D36 $$2I_xS_y \xrightarrow{\pm\beta I_y} \xrightarrow{\pi S_y} 2I_xS_y \cos \beta \mp 2I_zS_y \sin \beta = \sigma_5.$$

The observable term, $2I_zS_y \sin \beta$ now evolves during τ to give in phase magnetization during the detection period, when heteronuclear (I spin) decoupling can be applied. The (π) S_y pulse has no effect on a two-spin system. However, in CH_2 and CH_3 groups, the application of the final two pulses creates a different functional dependence upon the flip-angle β. A similar product operator analysis gives for the state of spin system after the final pulses:

D37
$$\mathrm{CH} \mp 2I_zS_y \sin \beta$$
$$\mathrm{CH_2} \mp 4I_zI'_zS_x \sin \beta \cos \beta$$
$$\mathrm{CH_3} \mp 8I_zI'_zI''_zS_y \sin \beta \cos^2 \beta.$$

From these expressions it is straightforward to design an experiment to separate signals from CH, CH_2, and CH_3 groups by suitable linear combinations of spectra obtained with different values of β. Suitable values might be, for example, $\beta = \pi/4$, $\pi/2$ and $3\pi/4$ in separate experiments.

The editing of CH_n groups has been refined to allow for variations n the magnitude of J_{CH} using experiments such as SEMUT-GL. The merits of the various sequences are described in the original literature.

FURTHER READING

Bendall, M. R. and Pegg, D. T. (1983). *J. Magn. Reson.* **53,** 272.

Doddrell, D. M., Pegg, D. T., and Bendall, M. R. (1982). *J. Magn. Reson.* **48,** 323.

Ernst, R. R., Bodenhausen, G. and Wokaun, A. A. (1987) *Principles of NMR in one and two dimensions,* Chapter 4. Clarendon Press, Oxford, and references therein.

The SEMUT sequences are described in

Bildsøe, H., Dønstrup, S., Jakobsen, H. J., and Sørensen, O. W. (1983). *J. Magn. Reson.* **53,** 154.

Sørensen, O. W., Dønstrup, S., Bildsøe, H. and Jakobsen, H. J. (1983). *J. Magn. Reson.* **55,** 347.

Double-quantum coherence Consider a spin system composed of two scalar coupled spins $\frac{1}{2}$ I and S. We can draw an energy-level diagram with all possible transitions (Fig. D6). Each of the single-quantum transitions gives rise to a resonance line in the NMR spectrum of the two-spin system. However, two further transitions, W_{IS}^0 and W_{IS}^2, which are known as the zero-quantum transition and double-quantum transition respectively, do not induce a signal in the NMR receiver. They are members of a class known as **forbidden transitions**. Since they cannot be directly detected, they are not observed in simple pulse-and-collect experiments. However, under certain circumstances, it is possible to detect indirectly double-quantum coherence using multiple-pulse sequences. This gives rise to the important **two-dimensional NMR** experiments **double-quantum correlated spectroscopy** and **double-quantum filtered correlated spectroscopy**.

Since multiple-quantum effects can only be fully understood quantum mechanically, the **classical formalism** can give no simple physical picture of the above experiments. Formally, double-quantum coherence is associated with particular off-diagonal elements of the **density matrix** of states. For a two-spin system such as that shown in Fig. D6, the density matrix can be illustrated as in Fig. D7. Eight off-diagonal elements correspond

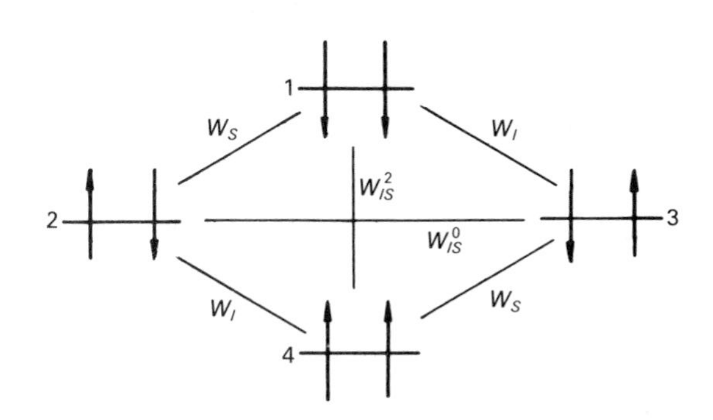

Fig. D6. Energy levels and transitions of a coupled two-spin system *IS*.

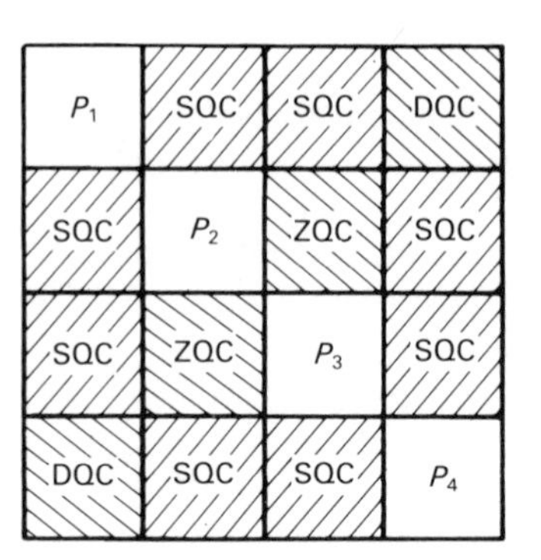

Fig. D7. Elements of the density matrix for a coupled two-spin system. ZQC, SQC, and DQC represent zero-quantum, single-quantum, and double-quantum coherences respectively, and the *P*'s represent the populations of states in Fig. D6.

to allowed single-quantum transitions, two correspond to double-quantum coherence, and two to zero-quantum coherence. Thus, during the course of an experiment, if the elements σ_{41} and σ_{14} are non-zero, this corresponds to an ongoing coherence between states 1 and 4, in other words double-quantum coherence. Equivalently, double-quantum coherence is expressed in the **product operator formalism** by linear combinations of the type $\frac{1}{2}(2I_xS_x - 2I_yS_y)$ and $\frac{1}{2}(2I_xS_y + 2I_yS_x)$. This is demonstrated explicitly for double quantum correlated spectroscopy and double-quantum filtered correlated spectroscopy.

Double-quantum correlated spectroscopy Double-quantum correlated spectroscopy is a technique which allows a two-dimensional representation of the NMR spectrum, in which one axis displays the normal single-quantum transition frequencies, and the orthogonal axis displays the double-quantum transition frequencies. In NMR of liquids, the order-selective detection scheme (see **multiple-quantum coherence**) is generally used to 'selectively' detect double-quantum coherence. This is most easily deomonstrated by explicit calculation. The pulse sequence relevant to this experiment is shown in Fig. D8. For the suppression of undesired coherence, ϕ is cycled through $K\pi/2$ ($K = 0, 1, 2, 3$) (see **phase cycling**) while the signals are alternately added and subtracted. Let us examine the result firstly for $K = 0$, i.e. $\phi = 0$. For a two-spin system *IS*, the density matrix at equilibrium (σ_0) is given in the **product operator formalism** by

D38 $$\sigma_0 = I_z + S_z.$$

The excitation sequence comprised of the two 90° pulses and the 180° pulse can be concisely described in the product operator notation by the following transformations:

$$\xrightarrow{\pi/2(I_x+S_x)} \xrightarrow{\pi J_{IS}2\tau 2I_zS_z} \xrightarrow{\pi/2(I_x+S_x)} \xrightarrow{\phi(I_z+S_z)}$$

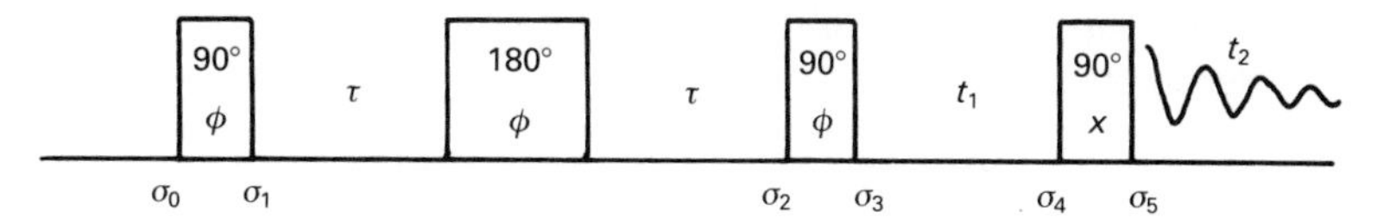

Fig. D8. Pulse sequence for the acquisition of double-quantum correlated spectra.

which simplifies to

D39 $$\xrightarrow{\pi J_{IS} 2\tau 2I_y S_y} \xrightarrow{\phi(I_z+S_z)}$$

where the arrows are the usual shorthand notation for **unitary transformations**. The first transformation in (D39) deals with the two pulses and the evolution period, whereas the second takes care of the phase shifts. The density operator just before the evolution period is thus given by

D40 $$I_z + S_z \xrightarrow{\pi J_{IS} 2\tau 2I_y S_y} \xrightarrow{\phi(I_z+S_z)}$$
$$(I_z + S_z) \cos \pi J_{IS} 2\tau + (2I_x S_y + 2I_y S_x) \sin \pi J_{IS} 2\tau = \sigma_3.$$

The second term on the right-hand side of (D40) represents pure double-quantum coherence. It has been created by the application of the two 90° pulses, the first creating a non-equilibrium density matrix. The 180° pulse causes a refocusing of the chemical shift terms, hence the absence of any $\omega_I I_z + \omega_S S_z$ terms in (D39). In other words, the spin system evolves from σ_1 to σ_3 under an average **Hamiltonian** dominated by $\mathcal{H}_J = \pi J_{IS} 2\tau 2I_z S_z$. As an aside, we can readily show that the term $2I_x S_y + 2I_y S_x$ in (D40) corresponds to double-quantum coherence by expanding it in terms of raising and lowering operators (see **shift operators**):

D41 $$I_x = \tfrac{1}{2}(I^+ + I^-) \qquad S_x = \tfrac{1}{2}(S^+ + S^-)$$
$$I_y = \frac{1}{2\mathrm{i}}(I^+ - I^-) \qquad S_y = \frac{1}{2\mathrm{i}}(S^+ - S^-).$$

By explicit multiplication,

D42 $$2I_x S_y + 2I_y S_x = \frac{1}{2\mathrm{i}}(I^+ S^+ - I^- S^-).$$

At this point we note that the transformation $\xrightarrow{\phi(I_z+S_z)}$ has no effect in (D40) since ϕ is zero. We can now enquire how the terms on the right-hand side of (D40) behave as ϕ is cycled through $\pi/2$, π, and $3\pi/2$ radians. The first term is obviously invariant for any ϕ, since z magnetization is unaffected by a rotation about the z axis. With regard to the second term, we can use the following equation to derive the effect of the phase shift upon the double-quantum term (see **product operator formalism**):

D43 $$(\mathrm{PQT})_x \xrightarrow{\phi I_z} (\mathrm{PQT})_x \cos p\phi + (\mathrm{PQT})_y \sin p\phi$$

In other words, a p-quantum coherence experiences a phase shift p-fold greater than that applied. Thus, if $\phi = \pi/2$, then double-quantum coherence is shifted in phase by π radians. The double-quantum term in (D40) will therefore be invariant for $K = 0$ and 2 ($\phi = 0$ and π) and will change sign for $K = 1$ and 3 ($\phi = \pi/2$ and $3\pi/2$). This explains why the data will eventually be alternately added and subtracted with alternate values of K; the double-quantum term in (D40) adds with each K, whereas the first term subtracts. Actually there is a simple physical interpretation of the p-fold sensitivity to phase shifts of p-quantum coherence. Such coherences are associated with transition frequencies which are approximately p-fold greater than 'observable' single-quantum transition frequencies. It is easy to visualize the fact that a phase shift ϕ at frequency f becomes a $p\phi$ phase shift at frequency pf (see **phase**).

Having created a spin system in a non-equilibrium state described by a density matrix containing pure double-quantum coherence, the latter is now allowed to evolve during t_1 as it must if we are eventually to observe the double-quantum frequencies in ω_1. Double-quantum coherence in an isolated two-spin system is actually insensitive to the scalar coupling between the nuclei, but precesses under the influence of the sum of the chemical shifts according to the following equation (see **product operator formalism**):

D44 $$\begin{aligned}(\mathrm{DQC})_x \xrightarrow{(\omega_I I_z + \omega_S S_z)t_1} &(\mathrm{DQC})_x \cos(\omega_I + \omega_S)t_1 \\ &+ (\mathrm{DQC})_y \sin(\omega_I + \omega_S)t_1.\end{aligned}$$

Applying this equation to σ_3,

D45 $$\begin{aligned}&(2I_xS_y + 2I_yS_x)\sin \pi J_{IS}2\tau \xrightarrow{(\omega_I I_z + \omega_S S_z)t_1} \\ &\quad[(2I_xS_y + 2I_yS_x)\cos(\omega_I + \omega_S)t_1 \\ &\qquad - (2I_xS_x - 2I_yS_y)\sin(\omega_I + \omega_S)t_1]\sin \pi J_{IS}2\tau = \sigma_4\end{aligned}$$

where it will be remembered that the term on the left-hand side of (D45) is the only surviving term from σ_3 after the application of the phase cycle. Note that none of the terms contained in σ_4 (right-hand side of D45) can give rise to observable magnetization. In common with all multiple-quantum experiments, we must apply a further pulse in order to convert the terms in σ_4 into **observable** magnetization. This is known as the mixing pulse. After a $\pi/2$ mixing pulse, assumed to be along the x axis, we obtain σ_5;

$$[(2I_xS_y + 2I_yS_x)\cos(\omega_I + \omega_S)t_1 - (2I_xS_x - 2I_yS_y)\sin(\omega_I + \omega_S)t_1]\sin \pi J_{IS}2\tau \xrightarrow{\pi/2(I_x+S_x)} (2I_xS_z + 2I_zS_x)\cos(\omega_I + \omega_S)t_1 \sin \pi J_{IS}2\tau = \sigma_5 \quad \text{D46}$$

where only the cosine modulated term is converted into observable magnetization, or rather, evolves into observable magnetization during t_2:

$$\begin{aligned}(2I_xS_z + 2I_zS_x)\cos(\omega_I + \omega_S)t_1 \sin \pi J_{IS}2\tau &\xrightarrow{\pi J_{IS}t_2 2I_zS_z} \xrightarrow{(\omega_I I_z + \omega_S S_z)t_2} \\ &+ I_y \cos(\omega_I + \omega_S)t_1 \sin \pi J_{IS}2\tau \sin \pi J_{IS}t_2 \cos \omega_I t_2 \\ &- I_x \cos(\omega_I + \omega_S)t_1 \sin \pi J_{IS}2\tau \sin \pi J_{IS}t_2 \sin \omega_I t_2 \\ &+ S_y \cos(\omega_I + \omega_S)t_1 \sin \pi J_{IS}2\tau \sin \pi J_{IS}t_2 \cos \omega_S t_2 \\ &- S_x \cos(\omega_I + \omega_S)t_1 \sin \pi J_{IS}2\tau \sin \pi J_{IS}t_2 \sin \omega_S t_2\end{aligned} \quad \text{D47}$$

where only observable terms are retained on the right-hand side of (D47). If the receiver phase is along the $+x$ axis, (actually it will be cycled along x axis to alternately add and subtract data), only the terms in I_x and S_x need be considered. After some trigonometry, we obtain for the observable magnetization

$$\begin{aligned}\langle M_x \rangle = &-I_x \cos(\omega_I + \omega_S)t_1 \,.\, \tfrac{1}{2}[\cos(\omega_I t_2 - \pi J_{IS}t_2) \\ &-\cos(\omega_I t_2 + \pi J_{IS}t_2)] \sin \pi J_{IS}2\tau \\ &-S_x \cos(\omega_I + \omega_S)t_1 \,.\, \tfrac{1}{2}[\cos(\omega_S t_2 - \pi J_{IS}t_2) \\ &-\cos(\omega_S t_2 + \pi J_{IS}t_2)] \sin \pi J_{IS}2\tau.\end{aligned} \quad \text{D48}$$

After two-dimensional Fourier transformation, we obtain the spectrum for the two-spin system shown in Fig. D9. A pair of crosspeaks is obtained with an intensity proportional to $\sin \pi J_{IS}2\tau$. These peaks are in antiphase absorption with a splitting J_{IS} in ω_2, and as singlets at $(\omega_I + \omega_S)$ in ω_1. Since there is amplitude modulation during t_1 $(\cos(\omega_I + \omega_S)t_1)$ the presentation shown in (D9) is that which would be obtained by employing a real cosine transform (see **Fourier transform**) with respect to t_1, and only signals at $+\omega_1$ are shown. However, signals are in fact found at $\pm\omega_1$, which are the **coherence transfer echo** and **antiecho** components respectively. This may be understood in terms of the identity $\cos \theta = \frac{1}{2}(e^{i\theta} + e^{-i\theta})$. With a mixing pulse $= \pi/2$ radians, these components are of equal intensity. However, for a mixing pulse with flip-angle $\neq 90°$, these components have different intensities. To see how this arises it is necessary to refer to the state of the density operator before the mixing pulse. The relevant equation is (D45). If we apply a $\pi/2$ mixing pulse, we

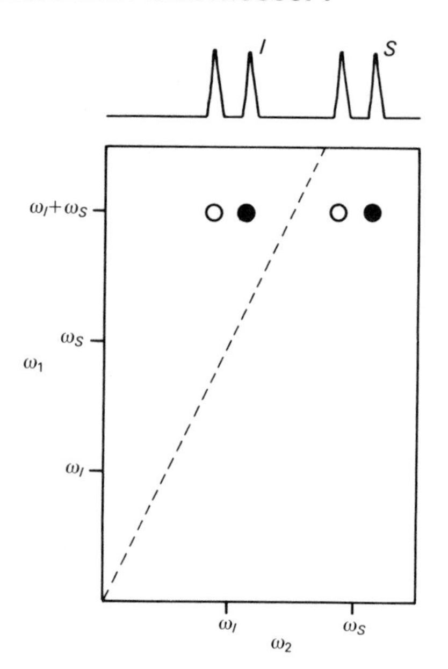

Fig. D9. Theoretical double-quantum spectrum of a coupled two-spin system *IS*. Open and filled circles represent positive and negative intensities.

have already seen that the cosine component on the right-hand side of (D45) gives rise to (D46). With a mixing pulse $\neq\pi/2$, we find that the sine component on the right-hand side of (D45) is also partially converted into observable magnetization. This imparts a partial **phase modulation** during t_1, resulting in unequal intensities for the coherence transfer echo and antiecho components. We can see this explicitly if we re-evaluate (D46) from (D45), setting the mixing pulse to an arbitrary flip-angle β:

$$\begin{aligned}
&[(2I_xS_y + 2I_yS_x)\cos(\omega_I+\omega_S)t_1 - (2I_xS_x \\
&\quad -2I_yS_y)\sin(\omega_I+\omega_S)t_1]\sin\pi J_{IS}2\tau \\
&\xrightarrow{\beta(I_x+S_x)} (2I_xS_y\cos\beta + 2I_xS_z\sin\beta + 2I_yS_x\cos\beta \\
&\quad +2I_zS_x\sin\beta)\cos(\omega_I+\omega_S)t_1\sin\pi J_{IS}2\tau \\
&\quad -(2I_xS_x - 2[(I_y\cos\beta + I_z\sin\beta)(S_y\cos\beta \\
&\quad +S_z\sin\beta)])\sin(\omega_I+\omega_S)t_1\sin\pi J_{IS}2\tau.
\end{aligned} \tag{D49}$$

After evolution during t_2, the observable terms in I_x and S_x are

$$\begin{aligned}
\langle M_x\rangle = &-I_x\sin\pi J_{IS}t_2\sin\beta\cos(\omega_I+\omega_S)t_1\sin\pi J_{IS}2\tau\sin\omega_It_2 \\
&- S_x\sin\pi J_{IS}t_2\sin\beta\cos(\omega_I+\omega_S)t_1\sin\pi J_{IS}2\tau\sin\omega_St_2 \\
&- I_x\sin\pi J_{IS}t_2\cos\beta\sin\beta\sin(\omega_I+\omega_S)t_1\sin\pi J_{IS}2\tau\cos\omega_It_2 \\
&- S_x\sin\pi J_{IS}t_2\cos\beta\sin\beta\sin(\omega_I+\omega_S)t_1\sin\pi J_{IS}2\tau\cos\omega_St_2.
\end{aligned} \tag{D50}$$

We now find two terms in both I_x and S_x, one containing the t_1 dependence $\cos(\omega_I + \omega_S)t_1 \sin\beta$ and the other $\sin(\omega_I + \omega_S)t_1 \cos\beta \sin\beta$. For appropriate β, therefore, we obtain a linear combination of sine and cosine terms which will generate phase modulation with consequent echo or antiecho selection. We note immediately that the ideal linear combination requires $\sin\beta = \cos\beta \sin\beta$, and so we cannot obtain complete selection. In practice, we find that for $\beta = 135°$, $\sin\beta \approx 0.7$, and $\cos\beta \sin\beta \approx -0.5$, which gives good selectivity for the echo component. Remembering that $\cos\theta = \frac{1}{2}(e^{i\theta} + e^{-i\theta})$ and $\sin\theta = \frac{1}{2}i(e^{i\theta} - e^{-i\theta})$, we can insert the numerical values for $\sin\beta$ and $\sin\beta \cos\beta$, giving

$$\cos(\omega_I + \omega_S)t_1 \sin\beta \rightarrow (0.7/2)(\exp\{i(\omega_I + \omega_S)t_1\} + \exp\{-i(\omega_I + \omega_S)t_1\}) \quad \text{D51}$$

$$\sin(\omega_I + \omega_S)t_1 \sin\beta \cos\beta \rightarrow (-0.5/2i)(\exp\{i(\omega_I + \omega_S)t_1\} - \exp\{-i(\omega_I + \omega_S)t_1\}). \quad \text{D52}$$

Addition of these components (for they are both components of $\langle M_x \rangle$) gives a numerical selection of the echo component by a factor of 6, together with an increase in crosspeak intensity of 1.2. It is therefore possible to place the transmitter offset in the middle of the spectrum, since the signs of the precession frequencies in ω_1 are reasonably well discriminated. At this point some may be wondering why it is necessary to take such a circuitous route to achieve echo selection in this experiment, when a simple phase shift is required in experiments such as ^1H–^1H **correlated spectroscopy** (see **phase modulation**). Apart from the small increase in sensitivity, the simple answer is that we would require 45° phase shifts in the present experiment to achieve the same result. Although this is entirely feasible, the above is a simple and reasonable effective alternative. However, if use is to be made of phase-sensitive data processing (see **phase-sensitive experiments**), a 45° phase shift must of course be generated.

Before leaving the theoretical details, we should mention that in extended coupling networks, the double absorption lineshape as calculated above and illustrated in Fig. D9 is distorted by additional dispersion-mode contributions—true absorption-mode lineshapes are only produced when total spin coherence is considered for the system of interest. However, this added complication does not place undue restrictions upon the technique in complicated spin systems. To complete the analysis we provide a phase cycling procedure for double-quantum correlated spectroscopy, assuming phase-sensitive manipulation of the data:

P1	P2	P3	P4	Rx	
X	X	X	X	+	location 1
Y	Y	Y	X	−	
$-X$	$-X$	$-X$	X	+	
$-Y$	$-Y$	$-Y$	X	−	
$X+\psi$	$X+\psi$	$X+\psi$	X	+	location 2
$Y+\psi$	$Y+\psi$	$Y+\psi$	X	−	
$-X+\psi$	$-X+\psi$	$-X+\psi$	X	+	
$-Y+\psi$	$-Y+\psi$	$-Y+\psi$	X	−	

where $\psi = 45°$. This sequence is repeated four times, incrementing **CYCLOPS phase cycling** at each eighth transient giving a minimum of $32n$ scans per t_1 increment.

The rather tedious theoretical analysis described above serves to illustrate the basic principles of double-quantum correlated spectroscopy. We can now describe some useful applications. The original application of the technique is the determination of connectivities in the carbon skeleton of organic molecules, the so-called **INADEQUATE** experiment. This application depends simply upon the technique as we have described it above. When the number of coupled spins in the system of interest is greater than two, more information is available. This is most often the case in biological NMR, where we are interested in compounds such as amino acid residues, sugars, lipids, and nucleic acid bases. All of these may have very complicated coupling networks. The applications of double-quantum correlated spectroscopy to extended networks fall nicely into three groups; the detection of direct scalar connectivities, remote connectivities, and magnetic equivalence. We can illustrate each of these applications with the simple **spin systems** A–M–X (where $J_{AX} = 0$) and A_2X, and their 'simulated' double-quantum spectra. Consider firstly the phase-sensitive double-quantum correlated spectrum of the A–M–X system (Fig. D10). If we define $J_{AM} \neq 0$ and $J_{MX} \neq 0$ then, in analogy to the two-spin IS system discussed above, we should find resonances at $\omega_1 = \omega_M + \omega_X$ and $\omega_1 = \omega_A + \omega_M$. This is indeed the case. Note that each pair of crosspeaks is 'bisected' by the skew diagonal $\omega_1 = 2\omega_2$. This characteristic pattern shows that A–M and M–X are directly scalar connected. In contrast, we find a single crosspeak at $\omega_1 = \omega_A + \omega_X$. Since we have defined $J_{AX} = 0$, this crosspeak obviously does not show that A and X are directly scalar coupled. If, however, we extrapolate the ω_1 coordinate of the crosspeak onto the skew diagonal, the ω_2 coordinate at this point is at the midpoint of ω_A and ω_X. This type of pattern shows that A and X are remotely scalar connected via a common coupling partner, in this case M.

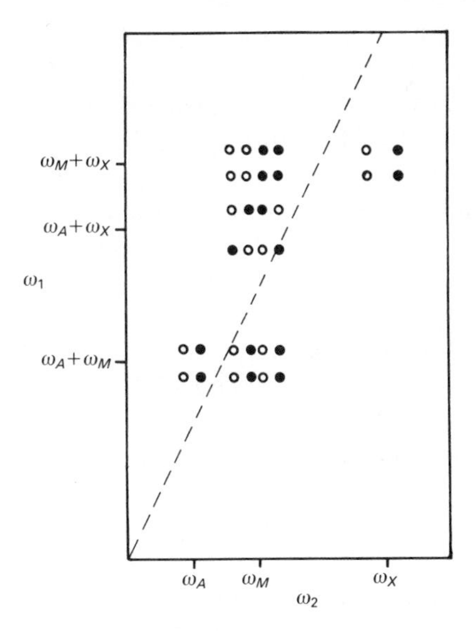

Fig. D10. Theoretical double-quantum spectrum of an *AMX* system with $J_{AM} \neq 0$, $J_{MX} \neq 0$, $J_{AX} = 0$. Lineshapes are mixed phase.

In order to see how double-quantum spectroscopy can give information regarding magnetic equivalence it is necessary to consider spin systems such as A_2X, whose double-quantum spectrum is shown in Fig. D11. As in Fig. D10, direct connectivity between A and X is demonstrated by the pair of crosspeaks at ω_A and ω_X symmetrically disposed about the skew diagonal. In addition, we find a single crosspeak at $\omega_1 = 2\omega_A$. When

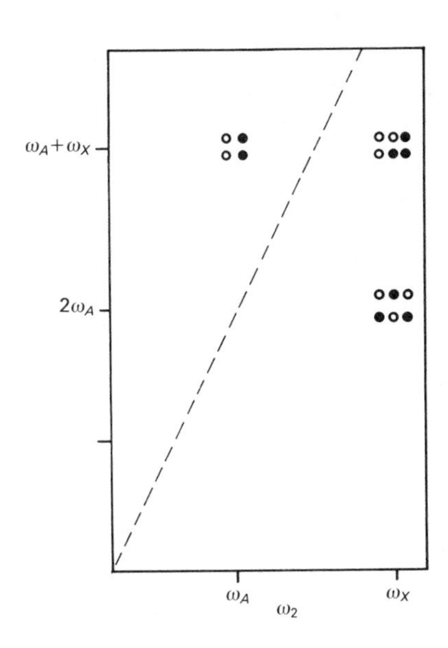

Fig. D11. Theoretical double-quantum spectrum of an A_2X system. Lineshapes are of composite phase.

extrapolated to the skew diagonal as before, the corresponding ω_2 frequency corresponds to that of ω_A. This pattern demonstrates that there are at least two equivalent nuclei with Larmor frequency ω_A. We would need to filter through a higher coherence order in order to determine whether two or three equivalent nuclei were present.

It should be clear that the characteristic crosspeak patterns described above are very useful in the assignment of residues in macromolecules, and double-quantum spectroscopy is of particular value in protein NMR. By analysis of remote connectivities, it can be established whether amide and β-protons belong to the same spin system or not. In addition, the degeneracy of β-proton chemical shifts can be demonstrated, and it is possible to distinguish glycine amide protons from all others. None of this information is in general available from **correlated spectroscopy**.

FURTHER READING

For a detailed analysis of multiple quantum experiments see

Braunschweiler, L., Bodenhausen, G., and Ernst, R. R. (1983). *Mol. Phys.* **48,** 535.

See also

Ernst, R. R., Bodenhausen, G., and Wokaun, A. A. (1987) *Principles of NMR in one and two dimensions,* Chapter 8. Clarendon Press, Oxford, and references therein.

Double-quantum filtered correlated spectroscopy (DQFCOSY) This experiment is related to **double-quantum correlated spectroscopy**. The two-dimensional spectrum is similar in appearance to that obtained in **correlated spectroscopy** (COSY), although the spectrum is simpler since the spin system is first filtered through double-quantum coherence. In many ways this experiment has advantages over conventional COSY, which is perhaps best illustrated by theoretical analysis of a simple example, a weakly coupled spin $\frac{1}{2}$ system IS. The pulse sequence relevant to this experiment is shown in Fig. D12. The phase ϕ is cycled through $K\pi/2$ radians ($K = 0, 1, 2, 3$) in a manner exactly analogous to that used

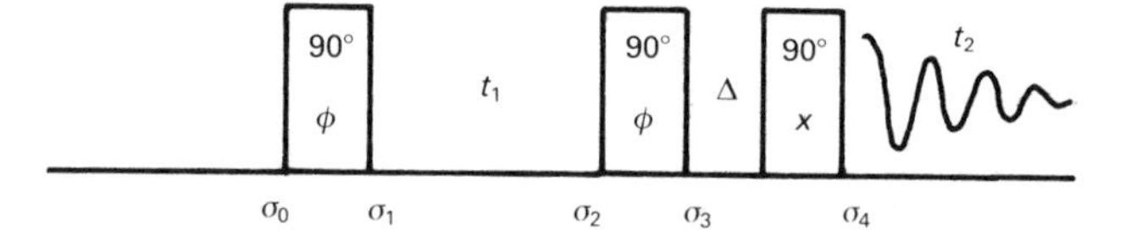

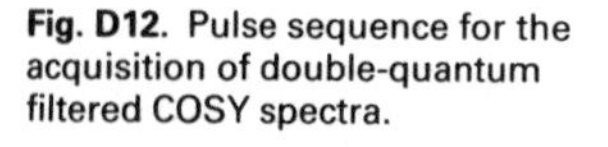

Fig. D12. Pulse sequence for the acquisition of double-quantum filtered COSY spectra.

in double-quantum correlated spectroscopy. The purpose of this cycling is to achieve order-selective detection of **double-quantum coherence** between the second and third r.f. pulses. If we begin the analysis with $\phi = 0$, the state of the spin system after the second pulse is defined by σ_3, in the **product operator formalism**:

$$\begin{aligned}\sigma_3 = &[-I_z \cos \omega_I t_1 + I_x \sin \omega_I t_1 - S_z \cos \omega_S t_1 + S_x \sin \omega_S t_1] \cos \pi J_{IS} t_1 \\ &- [2I_x S_y \cos \omega_I t_1 + 2I_y S_x \cos \omega_S t_1 + 2I_z S_y \sin \omega_S t_1 \\ &+ [2I_y S_z \sin \omega_S t_1] \sin \pi J_{IS} t_1.\end{aligned} \tag{D53}$$

This expression is analogous to that derived in the analysis of **correlated spectroscopy**. In common with the rules laid out under the product operator formalism, it is permissible to expand the two-spin coherence terms into their zero-quantum and double-quantum coherence components:

$$\begin{aligned}\sigma_3 = &[-I_z \cos \omega_I t_1 + I_x \sin \omega_I t_1 - S_z \cos \omega_S t_1 + S_x \sin \omega_S t_1] \cos \pi J_{IS} t_1 \\ &+ \{\tfrac{1}{2}[(2I_x S_y + 2I_y S_x) - (2I_y S_x - 2I_x S_y)] \cos \omega_I t_1 \\ &+ \tfrac{1}{2}[(2I_x S_y + 2I_y S_x) + (2I_y S_x - 2I_x S_y)] \cos \omega_S t_1 \\ &+ 2I_z S_y \sin \omega_I t_1 + 2I_y S_z \sin \omega_S t_1\} \sin \pi J_{IS} t_1.\end{aligned} \tag{D54}$$

During the phase cycle, all terms except those corresponding to double-quantum coherence cancel, in analogy with double-quantum correlated spectroscopy:

$$\sigma_3 = \{\tfrac{1}{2}(2I_x S_y + 2I_y S_x) \cos \omega_I t_1 + \tfrac{1}{2}(2I_x S_y + 2I_y S_x) \cos \omega_S t_1\} \sin \pi J_{IS} t_1. \tag{D55}$$

Unlike double-quantum correlated spectroscopy, double-quantum coherence is not allowed to evolve, but is immediately reconverted to observable single-quantum magnetization by the third (mixing) pulse. The delay Δ allows for a clean shift in r.f. **phase** when ϕ does not equal zero, i.e. when the transmitter phase is not along the $+x$ axis. Assuming a mixing pulse of phase $+x$, we obtain for the density operator after the third pulse

$$\begin{aligned}\sigma_4 = &\{\tfrac{1}{2}(2I_x S_z + 2I_z S_x) \cos \omega_I t_1 \\ &+ \tfrac{1}{2}(2I_x S_z + 2I_z S_x) \cos \omega_S t_1\} \sin \pi J_{IS} t_1.\end{aligned} \tag{D56}$$

Each term in σ_4 now evolves during t_2 to generate observable magnetization:

$$\{\tfrac{1}{2}(2I_xS_z + 2I_zS_x)\cos\omega_I t_1 + \tfrac{1}{2}(2I_xS_z + 2I_zS_x)\cos\omega_S t_1\}\sin\pi J_{IS}t_1$$

$$\xrightarrow{\pi J_{IS}t_2 2I_zS_z}\xrightarrow{(\omega_I I_z + \omega_S S_z)t_2}$$

$$\begin{aligned}
&+\tfrac{1}{2}I_y \sin\pi J_{IS}t_2 \cos\omega_I t_1 \sin\pi J_{IS}t_1 \cos\omega_I t_2\\
&-\tfrac{1}{2}I_x \sin\pi J_{IS}t_2 \cos\omega_I t_1 \sin\pi J_{IS}t_1 \sin\omega_I t_2\\
&+\tfrac{1}{2}S_y \sin\pi J_{IS}t_2 \cos\omega_I t_1 \sin\pi J_{IS}t_1 \cos\omega_S t_2\\
&-\tfrac{1}{2}S_x \sin\pi J_{IS}t_2 \cos\omega_I t_1 \sin\pi J_{IS}t_1 \sin\omega_S t_2\\
&+\tfrac{1}{2}I_y \sin\pi J_{IS}t_2 \cos\omega_S t_1 \sin\pi J_{IS}t_1 \cos\omega_I t_2\\
&-\tfrac{1}{2}I_x \sin\pi J_{IS}t_2 \cos\omega_S t_1 \sin\pi J_{IS}t_1 \sin\omega_I t_2\\
&+\tfrac{1}{2}S_y \sin\pi J_{IS}t_2 \cos\omega_S t_1 \sin\pi J_{IS}t_1 \cos\omega_S t_2\\
&-\tfrac{1}{2}S_x \sin\pi J_{IS}t_2 \cos\omega_S t_1 \sin\pi J_{IS}t_1 \sin\omega_S t_2.
\end{aligned} \quad \text{D57}$$

If the receiver phase is along the $+x$ axis, after some trigonometry we find for the observable magnetization:

$$\begin{aligned}
\langle M_x\rangle = &-\tfrac{1}{2}I_x[\tfrac{1}{2}\sin(\pi J_{IS}t_1 + \omega_I t_1) - \tfrac{1}{2}\sin(\omega_I t_1 - \pi J_{IS}t_1)]\\
&\quad[\tfrac{1}{2}\cos(\omega_I t_2 - \pi J_{IS}t_2) - \tfrac{1}{2}\cos(\omega_I t_2 + \pi J_{IS}t_2)]\\
&-\tfrac{1}{2}S_x[\tfrac{1}{2}\sin(\pi J_{IS}t_1 + \omega_I t_1) - \tfrac{1}{2}\sin(\omega_I t_1 - \pi J_{IS}t_1)]\\
&\quad[\tfrac{1}{2}\cos(\omega_S t_2 - \pi J_{IS}t_2) - \tfrac{1}{2}\cos(\omega_S t_2 + \pi J_{IS}t_2)]\\
&-\tfrac{1}{2}I_x[\tfrac{1}{2}\sin(\pi J_{IS}t_1 + \omega_S t_1) - \tfrac{1}{2}\sin(\omega_I t_1 - \pi J_{IS}t_1)]\\
&\quad[\tfrac{1}{2}\cos(\omega_I t_2 - \pi J_{IS}t_2) - \tfrac{1}{2}\cos(\pi J_{IS}t_2 + \omega_I t_2)]\\
&-\tfrac{1}{2}S_x[\tfrac{1}{2}\sin(\omega_S t_1 + \pi J_{IS}t_1) - \tfrac{1}{2}\sin(\omega_S t_1 - \pi J_{IS}t_1)]\\
&\quad[\tfrac{1}{2}\cos(\omega_S t_2 - \pi J_{IS}t_2) - \tfrac{1}{2}\cos(\omega_S t_2 + \pi J_{IS}t_2)].
\end{aligned} \quad \text{D58}$$

After two-dimensional **Fourier transformation**, the 'phase-sensitive' spectrum will appear as in Fig. D13. Here all resonances are presumed to be of the absorption mode. This is actually not the case according to (D58), where we have sinusoidal components with respect to t_1. However, a 90° linear **phase correction** will restore the absorption mode in this dimension, which is the preferred presentation. Alternatively, we could have chosen observable terms in I_y by setting the receiver phase along the y axis. Figure D13 is notable for its resemblance to the COSY spectrum of an IS spin system. Note, however, that the diagonal peaks, like the crosspeaks, are in antiphase absorption. By comparison, the diagonal peaks in conventional COSY are in phase dispersion (see **lineshape**), which is an undesirable lineshape, giving poor resolution due to long dispersion tails. The present experiment thus provides a useful gain in resolution, which is particularly advantageous when searching for crosspeaks close to the diagonal. A further advantage of the antiphase

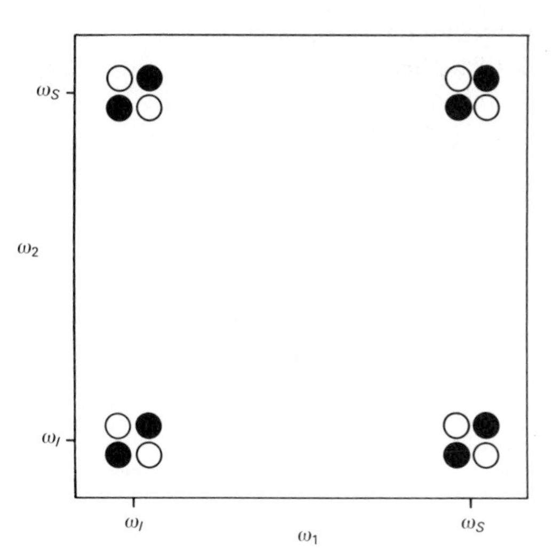

Fig. D13. Theoretical phase-sensitive double-quantum filtered COSY spectrum of a coupled two-spin system *IS*. Open and filled circles represent positive and negative intensities.

nature of the diagonal peaks is that for a given digital resolution, any cancellation of intensity which might occur in the crosspeaks (see **correlated spectroscopy**) is reflected in the diagonal peaks, and thus the latter are not the dominant signals in terms of intensity. Finally, it is obvious that singlets (e.g. solvent resonances) cannot generate double-quantum coherence (they are uncoupled), and hence cannot pass the double-quantum filter. To a large extent, therefore, solvent signals are eliminated from the spectrum. In practice, instrument instabilities prevent complete attenuation of these signals. The advantages described above are offset by a decrease in overall sensitivity of the experiment. Equation (D58) shows that all resonances appear with half the intensity found in conventional COSY experiments. This disadvantage must be compared against the advantages when determining an overall strategy for a given sample. To complete our analysis, we give the phase cycling procedure for double-quantum filtered COSY, assuming phase-sensitive analysis of the data:

P1	P2	P3	R_x	
X	X	X	+	memory location 1
Y	Y	X	−	
$-X$	$-X$	X	+	
$-Y$	$-Y$	X	−	
Y	X	X	+	memory location 2
$-X$	Y	X	−	
$-Y$	$-X$	X	+	
X	$-Y$	X	−	

This procedure is repeated four times while simultaneously incrementing **CYCLOPS phase cycling** at each eighth transient, giving a minimum of 32n scans per t_1 increment.

Since DQFCOSY does not achieve significant spin-filtering, its main application is as a companion to the conventional COSY experiment. However, we should note that for spin systems of biological interest, the lineshapes in double-quantum filtered COSY will be more complex than those calculated for a two-spin system due to additional coupling pathways. Thus, although crosspeaks will always be in antiphase absorption, diagonal peaks will inherit some dispersive character. This is analogous to the lineshape distortions found in **double-quantum correlated spectroscopy**. However, in practice these dispersive contributions are not severe, and DQFCOSY gives a very worthwhile improvement in resolution over the basic COSY experiment.

FURTHER READING

For an early application of double-quantum filtered COSY see:

Piantini, U., Sorensen, O. W., and Ernst, R. R. (1982). *J. Am. Chem. Soc.* **104,** 6800.

A practical application of double-quantum filtered COSY applied to proteins is

Rance M., Sorensen, O. W., Bodenhausen, G., Wagner, G., Ernst, R. R., and Wuthrich, K. (1983). *Biochem. Biophys. Res. Comm.* **117,** 479.

DOUBTFUL The term DOUBTFUL is an acronym for *DOUBL*e quantum *T*ransitions for *F*inding *U*nresolved *L*ines. It is an ingenious method for the selective detection of magnetically isolated two-spin systems in the presence of spectral overlap. The key principle in this experiment is the behaviour of double-quantum coherence between the two spins during evolution under their spin coupling. The pulse sequence is identical to that used for **double-quantum correlated spectroscopy** and **INADEQUATE** (Fig. D14).

Double-quantum coherence is created between the two spins by the 90°–180°–90° pulse sandwich. During the t_1 period, this coherence is modulated by the algebraic sum of the chemical shift terms, but is not affected by the coupling between the two nuclei since they are actively involved in the transition. Now if the carrier is positioned midway between the resonances of the two spins, the algebraic sum of their

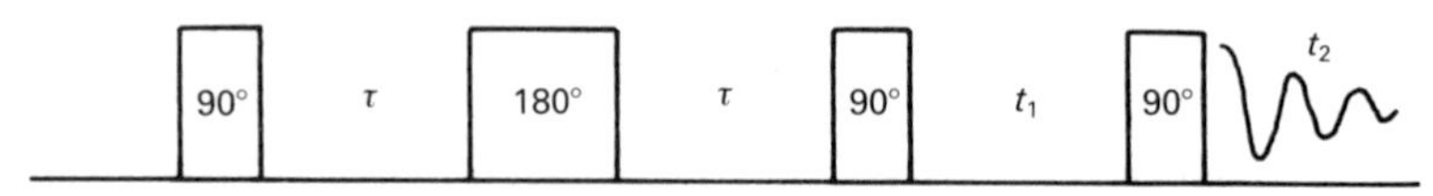

Fig. D14. Pulse sequence for the acquisition of spectra filtered using DOUBTFUL.

chemical shifts will be zero, and the intensity of neither resonance will be modulated during t_1. In contrast, the resonance intensities of other resonances in the spectrum will undergo complex sinusoidal and/or cosinusoidal oscillations due to both non-zero sums of the chemical shifts, together with modulation under spin-coupling terms for systems containing more than two coupled spins. If, therefore, a series of experiments is co-added for various t_1 values (rather than stored in separate locations as is normal in two-dimensional NMR), the average intensities of all resonances except the desired two-spin system will tend to zero. For best results, the t_1 values and their increments must be chosen carefully. The disadvantage of this approach towards multiple-quantum filtration (see **multiple-quantum filter**) lies in the fact that the two-spin systems must be magnetically isolated to avoid evolution during t_1 under spin coupling to a 'passive' spin, i.e. a spin which is not actively involved in the transition.

FURTHER READING

DOUBTFUL was first described by

Hore, P. J., Zuiderweg, E., Nicolay, K., Dijkstra, K., and Kaptein, R. (1982). *J. Am. Chem. Soc.* **104,** 4286.

DQFCOSY See **double-quantum filtered correlated spectroscopy**.

Dyson expression The time development of a quantum mechanical spin system under the Hamiltonian

D59 $$\mathcal{H} = \mathcal{H}_1 + \mathcal{H}_2 + \mathcal{H}_3 + \ldots + \mathcal{H}_n$$

is given by the solution of the **Liouville–von Neumann equation**

D60 $$\dot{\sigma} = -\mathrm{i}\hbar^{-1}[(\mathcal{H}_1 + \mathcal{H}_2 + \mathcal{H}_3 + \ldots + \mathcal{H}_n), \sigma]$$

where $\mathcal{H}_n > \mathcal{H}_{n+1}$.

The solution of (D60) is simple only if the $\mathcal{H}$'s commute (see **commutator**) and are time independent. In the cases that they are not, we can employ **average Hamiltonian theory** to simplify the calculation. In this, the goal is to express a complex time dependent Hamiltonian in the form of a single, manageable exponential. We achieve this by transforming to an interaction representation

$$\alpha(t) = U_1(t)\tilde{\sigma}(t)U_1^{-1}(t)$$

where $U_1(t)$ can be defined by the Dyson expression

D61 $$U_1(t) = T\exp\left[-\mathrm{i}\int_0^t \mathcal{H}_1(t')\,\mathrm{d}t'\right].$$

T is the Dyson time ordering operator. It takes any product of time-dependent operators and places them in order of decreasing time from left to right. This allows us to make the expansion

D62

$$U_1(t) = T\Big[1 - \mathrm{i}\int_0^t \mathrm{d}\tau\,\mathcal{H}(\tau) - (\mathrm{i}^2/2!)\int_0^t \mathrm{d}\tau\int_0^t \mathrm{d}e\,\mathcal{H}(\tau)\mathcal{H}(e) - (\mathrm{i}^3/3!)\int_0^t \mathrm{d}\tau\int_0^t \mathrm{d}e\int_0^t \mathrm{d}\phi\,\mathcal{H}(\tau)\mathcal{H}(e)\mathcal{H}(\phi) + \ldots\Big].$$

Thus the Dyson expression gives a means of determining the time evolution operator at any time t. As an alternative the Magnus expansion could be applied (see **average Hamiltonian theory**).

FURTHER READING

Gerstein, B. C. and Dybowski, C. R. (1985). *Transient techniques in NMR of solids*. Academic Press, London.

Dyson time ordering operator See **Dyson expression**.

E

Eigenbasis When we perform quantum mechanical calculations upon spin systems in order to predict the results of NMR experiments, it is necessary to begin with a basis set (see **basis state**) with which to describe the spin system of interest. We can then extract the necessary information by solving the **Liouville–von Neumann equation** using the appropriate **Hamiltonian** operator. In this manner, it is possible to follow the time evolution of the **density matrix** under the various Hamiltonians operative in our chosen experiment. The complexity of this calculation depends upon our choice of wavefunctions for the basis set. For example, in the case of a scalar coupled two-spin $\frac{1}{2}$ system (IS), the basis set might be composed of the four product functions $|\alpha\alpha\rangle$, $|\alpha\beta\rangle$, $|\beta\alpha\rangle$, and $|\beta\beta\rangle$ (see **basis state**). If the two spins are loosely coupled, i.e. the scalar coupling constant (J) is very much less than the frequency of separation of the resonances, then this set of product functions is the best choice for the basis set. To see why this is so we must consider the Hamiltonian under which the spin system will evolve. This Hamiltonian will be composed of the usual Zeeman and scalar coupling terms:

E1 $$\mathcal{H} = \mathcal{H}_Z + \mathcal{H}_J = \omega_I I_z + \omega_S S_z + J_{IS} I_z S_z.$$

If we now form the **matrix representation** of $\mathcal{H}$, using the product functions described above, we obtain

E2 $$\mathcal{H} = \begin{bmatrix} \frac{1}{2}(\omega_I + \omega_S) + \frac{1}{4}J_{IS} & 0 & 0 & 0 \\ 0 & \frac{1}{2}(\omega_I - \omega_S) - \frac{1}{4}J_{IS} & 0 & 0 \\ 0 & 0 & \frac{1}{2}(\omega_S - \omega_I) - \frac{1}{4}J_{IS} & 0 \\ 0 & 0 & 0 & -\frac{1}{2}(\omega_S + \omega_I) + \frac{1}{4}J_{IS} \end{bmatrix}$$

Since the product functions are **eigenfunctions** of the **Hamiltonian**, the matrix representation of $\mathcal{H}$ is diagonal. The importance of this is that the corresponding **exponential operator** of $\mathscr{H}$ is also diagonal:

$$\exp\{-\mathrm{i}\mathscr{H}t\} = \begin{bmatrix} \exp\{-\mathrm{i}\mathscr{H}_{11}t\} & 0 & 0 & 0 \\ 0 & \exp\{-\mathrm{i}\mathscr{H}_{22}t\} & 0 & 0 \\ 0 & 0 & \exp\{-\mathrm{i}\mathscr{H}_{33}t\} & 0 \\ 0 & 0 & 0 & \exp\{-\mathrm{i}\mathscr{H}_{44}t\} \end{bmatrix} \tag{E3}$$

and this simplifies calculations involving $\exp\{-\mathrm{i}\mathscr{H}t\}$ (see **density matrix**). In this example, the product functions $|\alpha\alpha\rangle$, $|\alpha\beta\rangle$, $|\beta\alpha\rangle$, $|\beta\beta\rangle$, being eigenfunctions of the Hamiltonian, are known as the eigenbasis.

In the case where the spins *IS* are strongly coupled, $\mathscr{H}$ becomes more complex, and it is necessary to find alternative functions to form the eigenbasis (see **strong coupling**).

Eigenfunction If we consider a single spin $\frac{1}{2}$ in a magnetic field, it can have one of two possible orientations (Fig. E1). To each orientation we can assign a wavefunction or **basis state**. If we now consider the results of the application of the angular momentum operators (see **angular momentum**) upon these states, we obtain the well-known relations

$$\begin{aligned} I_x|\alpha\rangle &= \tfrac{1}{2}|\beta\rangle, & I_y|\alpha\rangle &= \tfrac{1}{2}\mathrm{i}|\beta\rangle, & I_z|\alpha\rangle &= \tfrac{1}{2}|\alpha\rangle \\ I_x|\beta\rangle &= \tfrac{1}{2}|\alpha\rangle, & I_y|\beta\rangle &= -\tfrac{1}{2}\mathrm{i}|\alpha\rangle, & I_z|\beta\rangle &= -\tfrac{1}{2}|\beta\rangle. \end{aligned} \tag{E4}$$

Of these equations, those in I_z are of particular relevance. Mathematically, these can be said to be interpretable as **eigenvalue** equations. That is, the result of operating upon a given function by I_z generates a number (the eigenvalue) and leaves the original function unchanged. Under these conditions, the function in question is called the **eigenfunction**, and the corresponding state is called the eigenstate. More specifically, $|\alpha\rangle$ and $|\beta\rangle$ are eigenfunctions of I_z, and their corresponding eigenvalues are $+\frac{1}{2}$ and $-\frac{1}{2}$ respectively.

A more complex example illustrates that the above result still holds.

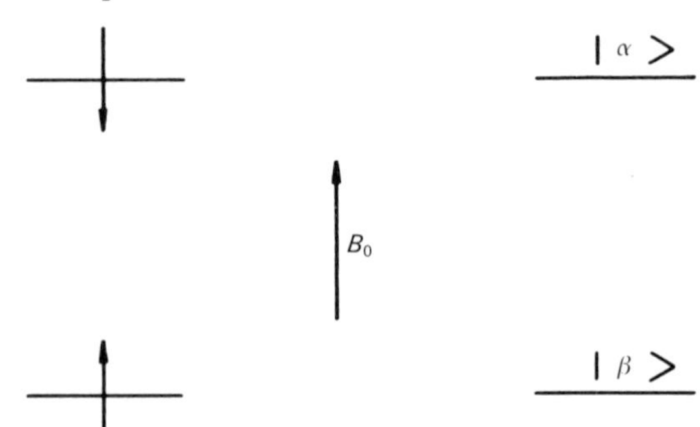

Fig. E1. A single spin $\frac{1}{2}$ can have two orientations in a magnetic field. We can ascribe a wavefunction to each orientation as shown.

For example, consider the **Hamiltonian** for a weakly coupled two-spin $\frac{1}{2}$ system *IS* in a magnetic field,

E5 $$\mathscr{H} = \omega_I I_z + \omega_S S_z + J_{IS} I_z S_z .$$

From the above it should be obvious that the simple product functions $|\alpha\alpha\rangle$, $|\alpha\beta\rangle$, $|\beta\alpha\rangle$, and $|\beta\beta\rangle$, for the two-spin system must be eigenfunctions of $\mathscr{H}$, and their corresponding eigenvalues are easily extracted:

E6 $$\begin{aligned} \mathscr{H}\,|\alpha\alpha\rangle &= \tfrac{1}{2}(\omega_I + \omega_S) + \tfrac{1}{4}J_{IS}\,|\alpha\alpha\rangle, \\ \mathscr{H}\,|\alpha\beta\rangle &= \tfrac{1}{2}(\omega_I - \omega_S) - \tfrac{1}{4}J_{IS}\,|\alpha\beta\rangle, \\ \mathscr{H}\,|\beta\alpha\rangle &= \tfrac{1}{2}(\omega_S - \omega_I) - \tfrac{1}{4}J_{IS}\,|\beta\alpha\rangle, \\ \mathscr{H}\,|\beta\beta\rangle &= -\tfrac{1}{2}(\omega_I + \omega_S) + \tfrac{1}{4}J_{IS}\,|\beta\beta\rangle. \end{aligned}$$

However, for the full isotropic Hamiltonian, which we must use when we encounter strongly coupled systems (see **strong coupling**), the product functions are not eigenfunctions of $\mathscr{H}$.

Eigenstate See **eigenfunction**.

Eigenvalue In NMR, the eigenvalues of a given set of **eigenfunctions** are of particular importance, since they are the energies of the states to which each eigenfunction corresponds. In the simple case of a loosely coupled two-spin $\frac{1}{2}$ system *IS*, the eigenvalues are easily extracted for each state (see **eigenfunction**). This is because the product functions are eigenfunctions of the **Hamiltonian**, and the **matrix representation** of the latter is diagonal, with its eigenvalues comprising the diagonal elements. More generally, the eigenvalues of a given Hamiltonian cannot be derived as easily, since the simple product functions will not be eigenfunctions of the Hamiltonian. The key principle in this case is to diagonalize the matrix representation of the Hamiltonian, when the eigenvalues will again comprise the diagonal elements. This in turn requires that we find new basis functions which are eigenfunctions of the Hamiltonian. This can be achieved by using the **variational method**. Equivalently, the eigenvalues can be found by transforming the Hamiltonian from the product-base into the eigenbase (see **eigenbasis**):

E7 $$\mathscr{H}_{\text{eigenbase}} = U\mathscr{H}_{\text{product base}}U^{-1}$$

where U is a matrix which transforms the product base into the eigenbase. An example of this procedure is described under **strong coupling**.

Emission line NMR, in common with most forms of spectroscopy, is detected by the absorption of energy from an applied perturbation. From this definition arises the term absorption line. In NMR such a line arises from the absorption of energy by spins in the low spin state, resulting in their transition to the high spin state. However, in certain non-equilibrium NMR experiments, a net excess of spins exists in the high spin state (a situation characterized by negative **spin temperature**). As the spin-state populations return to their equilibrium values, energy is emitted resulting in so-called emission lines in the NMR spectrum. The characteristic property of these is their negative intensity. They can in fact be very intense in experiments involving **chemically induced dynamic nuclear polarization**. They are also very common in many two-dimensional NMR experiments, such as **correlated spectroscopy**. In these experiments no net **coherence transfer** is obtained, and the familiar antiphase (see **phase**) nature of crosspeaks is due to absorption (positive) and emission (negative) lines: energy is absorbed across one transition and is re-emitted across another.

Ensemble average In NMR, the observed signals originate from the whole ensemble of a large number of spins, which leads to 'classical' behaviour. Under these circumstances we can in principle write an equation for the **expectation value** for the operator A corresponding to an observable (see **bra-ket notation**);

E8 $$\langle A\rangle = \langle \psi | A | \psi \rangle.$$

If each spin in the ensemble is prepared in an identical state $|\psi\rangle$, then (E8) is a correct expression for $\langle A\rangle$. In general, however, $|\psi\rangle$ is different between spins in the ensemble, and we must introduce the concept of an ensemble average. The wavefunction $|\psi\rangle$ of an isolated spin can be expanded in terms of the **orthonormal** eigenfunctions $|n\rangle$;

E9 $$|\psi\rangle = \sum_{n} |n\rangle \langle n | \psi_n\rangle$$

where $|n\rangle\langle n|$ is a coefficient. If (E9) is now substituted into (E8), we obtain

E10 $$\langle A\rangle = \sum_{nn'} \langle \psi_n | n\rangle \langle n | A | n'\rangle \langle n' | \psi_{n'}\rangle.$$

If we now replace $|\psi\rangle$ by its ensemble average over all spins, rearrangement of (E10) gives

E11 $$\overline{\langle A\rangle} = \sum_{nn'} \langle n | A | n'\rangle \langle n' \overline{| \psi_{n'}\rangle \langle \psi_n |} n\rangle.$$

We see that the ensemble averaging is restricted to the **density matrix** $\overline{|\psi_{n'}\rangle\langle\psi_n|}$. The density matrix thus provides us with a means by which the statistical-mechanical nature of the spin system can be dealt with, and from which the values of ensemble **observables** can be extracted easily. Throughout this text, the density matrix is given the symbol σ, and so (E11) becomes

E12 $$\overline{\langle A \rangle} = \sum_{nn'} \langle n | A | n' \rangle \langle n' | \sigma | n \rangle = \mathrm{Tr}(A\sigma)$$

where Tr denotes the trace of the matrix (see Appendix 3). Equation (E12) gives us an expression for the **expectation value** of the operator A.

Evolution In all Fourier transform NMR experiments, whether a simple pulse-and-collect sequence or a complex two-dimensional experiment, data are collected in the time domain. At the very least, therefore, we are interested in the time evolution of the spin system during the acquisition period, since this will govern the appearance of the NMR spectrum after **Fourier transformation**. More generally, we are interested in the time evolution of the spin system during other times in more complex experiments. Quantum mechanically, the behaviour of the spin system during a given time period depends upon the corresponding **Hamiltonian** which is operative during this period. We can then follow the time evolution of the **density matrix** of spin states under this Hamiltonian, from which the state of the spin system as a whole can be computed. The time evolution of the density matrix is governed by the **Liouville–von-Neumann equation**, which, for a time-independent Hamiltonian (i.e. the effect of the Hamiltonian is constant throughout the time interval of interest) can be integrated to give a value for the density matrix ($\sigma(0)$) at time $t(\sigma(t))$:

E13 $$\sigma(t) = \exp\{-\mathrm{i}\mathcal{H}t\}\sigma(0)\exp\{\mathrm{i}\mathcal{H}t\}$$

where $\mathcal{H}$ is the Hamiltonian operative during the time interval $0 \rightarrow t$. The **exponential operators** in (E13) plot the time evolution of $\sigma(0)$, and are sometimes called **propagators**. These can be obtained in their **matrix representation**, allowing (E13) to be solved explicitly to derive a matrix for $\sigma(t)$, from which the **observable** magnetization (should we wish to detect the magnetization at this point) can be extracted.

Exchange See **chemical exchange**.

Exchange spectroscopy (two-dimensional exchange spectroscopy) The fundamental principles and the experimental strategy of exchange spectroscopy are formally identical to those described under **nuclear Overhauser effect spectroscopy** (NOESY). The relevant pulse sequence is shown in Fig. E2. In the case of symmetrical two-site chemical exchange between two species A and B of equal concentration, we can

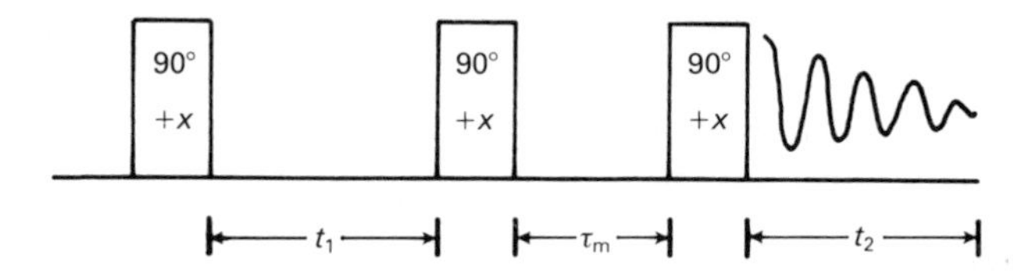

Fig. E2. Pulse sequence for two-dimensional exchange spectroscopy. See text for details.

define an exchange rate $k = k_{ab} = k_{ba}$. Assuming equal **spin–lattice relaxation** rates $R_{A1} = R_{B1} = R_1$, and equal transverse relaxation $T_{A2} = T_{B2} = T_2$, the transverse components in t_1 are described in the limit of slow exchange by

E14 $$M_A(t_1) = M_{A0} \exp(i\omega_A t_1 - t_1/T_2),$$

E15 $$M_B(t_1) = M_{B0} \exp(i\omega_B t_1 - t_1/T_2).$$

A second pulse with the same phase as the first creates longitudinal magnetization at $\tau_m = 0$:

E16 $$M_{zA} = -M_{A0} \cos \omega_A t_1 \exp(-t_1/T_2),$$

E17 $$M_{zB} = -M_{B0} \cos \omega_B t_1 \exp(-t_1/T_2).$$

Any remaining transverse components are destroyed by phase cycling or homospoil procedures (see **nuclear Overhauser effect spectroscopy**).

The z components in (E16) and (E17) migrate from one site to another due to chemical exchange during the mixing period τ_m, while the magnetization is attenuated due to spin–lattice relaxation during this same period. The magnetization at the end of the mixing period is therefore given by

E18 $$M'_{zA} = M_{zA}\,\tfrac{1}{2}[1 + \exp(-2k\tau_m)] \exp(-\tau_m/T_1) + M_{zB}\,\tfrac{1}{2}[1 - \exp(-2k\tau_m)] \exp(-\tau_m/T_1),$$

E19 $$M'_{zB} = M_{zA}\,\tfrac{1}{2}[1 - \exp(-2k\tau_m)] \exp(-\tau_m/T_1) + M_{zB}\,\tfrac{1}{2}[1 + \exp(-2k\tau_m)] \exp(-\tau_m/T_1).$$

The final pulse converts these components into observable magnetization. In analogy to the NOESY experiment, crosspeaks in the two-dimensional spectrum correlate resonances corresponding to chemically exchanging species. The amplitudes of diagonal and crosspeaks depend upon the equilibrium magnetization M_{A0} and M_{B0} and upon the mixing coefficients, which can be extracted from the following equations:

E20 $$a_{AA} = a_{BB} = \tfrac{1}{2}[1 + \exp(-2k\tau_m)] \exp(-\tau_m/T_1),$$
$$a_{AB} = a_{BA} = \tfrac{1}{2}[1 - \exp(-2k\tau_m)] \exp(-\tau_m/T_1).$$

The exchange rate in the present case can be determined in the initial rate approximation from the ratio of the peak intensities:

E22
$$a_{AA}/a_{AB} = [1 + \exp(-2k\tau_{\mathrm{m}})]/[1 - \exp(-2k\tau_{\mathrm{m}})] \simeq [1 - k\tau_{\mathrm{m}}]/k\tau_{\mathrm{m}}.$$

The expressions described here can be generalized to N-site exchange, but their complexity entails numerical solution such as that shown for three spins under **nuclear Overhauser effect spectroscopy**.

FURTHER READING

For detailed theoretical descriptions of exchange spectroscopy, see

Macura, S. and Ernst, R. R. (1980). *Mol. Phys.* **41,** 95.
Ernst, R. R., Bodenhausen, G., and Wokaun, A. A. (1987). *Principles of NMR in one and two dimensions.* Chapter 9 and references therein. Clarendon Press, Oxford.

Expectation value In the microscopic world of quantum mechanics, the result of an observation may not correspond with the expected 'classical' behaviour. Consider a single spin $\frac{1}{2}$. If we could measure either the x or y component of its **magnetization**, we would get one of two results, $+\frac{1}{2}\hbar$ or $-\frac{1}{2}\hbar$. If we repeated the measurement, the result would not always be the same. We rationalize this by noting that the possible results of an observation are the **eigenvalues** of the **observable** operator. If now, we took an average over a very large number of measurements, then we would obtain the 'classical' result. Hence an NMR sample containing a multitude of spins behaves 'classically'. We introduce the term 'expectation value' to represent this average over many measurements. The expectation values of any operator A corresponding to an observable can be calculated from the wavefunction for the system as follows:

E22
$$\langle A \rangle = \int \psi^* A \psi \, \mathrm{d}\tau$$

where * represents the complex conjugate (see **complex number**), and the integral extends over all space. In the compact **bra-ket notation** of Dirac, (E22) may be rewritten as

E23
$$\langle A \rangle = \langle \psi | A | \psi \rangle.$$

In general, NMR spectroscopists do not compute expectation values according to (E23). This is because we represent the state of the spin system using the **density matrix** (σ), which is a means by which we can specify the state of the spin system as a whole without explicit reference to the state of the individual spins. We can then define an ensemble expectation value for any operator A corresponding to an observable:

E24
$$\langle A \rangle = \mathrm{Tr}(A\sigma),$$

where Tr denotes trace (see Appendix 3). Thus, if we wanted to know the x component of the spin magnetization at time t, (E24) would become

E25 $$\langle F_x \rangle = M_x = \mathrm{Tr}(F_x \sigma(t)).$$

See also **ensemble average**.

Exponential operator The exponential function of a variable can be expanded into the well-known series

E26 $$e^x = 1 + x + (x^2/2!) + (x^3/3!) + \ldots.$$

In NMR, we often define a similar function, where x is an operator F,

E27 $$e^F = 1 + F + (F^2/2!) + (F^3/3!)\ldots.$$

The exponential operator in (E27) is of central importance in NMR theory. For example, consider the integrated **Liouville–von Neumann** equation for the evolution of the **density matrix** under a time-independent **Hamiltonian**;

E28 $$\sigma_{(t)} = \exp\{-\mathrm{i}\mathcal{H}t\}\sigma_{(0)}\exp\{\mathrm{i}\mathcal{H}t\}.$$

Here, we find two exponential operators on the right-hand side of (E28). The form of this operator depends upon the Hamiltonian under which the density matrix has evolved. If for example, we had applied an r.f. pulse of flip-angle α to a spin along the x axis of the **rotating frame**, then the exponential operators would take the form $\exp\{-\mathrm{i}I_x\alpha\}$ and $\exp\{\mathrm{i}I_x\alpha\}$ where I_x is an **angular momentum** operator. In order to gain a deeper understanding of these functions it is convenient to examine them in their expanded form. Using (E27) we can write

E29 $$\exp\{\mathrm{i}I_x\alpha\} = 1 + \mathrm{i}I_x\alpha + \frac{(\mathrm{i}I_x\alpha)^2}{2!} + \frac{(\mathrm{i}I_x\alpha)^3}{3!} + \frac{(\mathrm{i}I_x\alpha)^4}{4!} + \ldots$$

E30 $$= 1 + \mathrm{i}I_x\alpha - \frac{I_x^2\alpha^2}{2!} - \frac{\mathrm{i}I_x^3\alpha^3}{3!} + \frac{I_x^4\alpha^4}{4!} + \ldots.$$

Using the rules defined in Appendix 1, (E30) can be rewritten as

E31 $$\exp\{\mathrm{i}I_x\alpha\} = \mathbf{1}\left(1 - \frac{\alpha^2}{4.2!} + \frac{\alpha^4}{16.4!} - \frac{\alpha^6}{64.6!}\ldots\right) + 2\mathrm{i}I_x\left(\alpha - \frac{\alpha^3}{8.3!} + \frac{\alpha^5}{32.5!}\ldots\right)$$

where $\mathbf{1}$ is the **identity operator**. The first term on the right-hand side of (E31) can be related to a Taylor series for cosine, and the second term to a Taylor series for sine. Therefore we can write

E32 $$\exp\{\mathrm{i}I_x\alpha\} = \cos(\alpha/2)\mathbf{1} + 2\mathrm{i}\sin(\alpha/2)I_x.$$

This equation allows us to generate the **matrix representation** of

$\exp\{iI_x\alpha\}$. Furthermore, for this simple case, we gain physical insight into its properties: consider the result of I_x (see **angular momentum**) when it operates upon either the $|\alpha\rangle$ or $|\beta\rangle$ state of the spin (see **basis state**):

E33
$$\left.\begin{aligned} I_x\,|\alpha\rangle &= \tfrac{1}{2}\,|\beta\rangle \\ I_x\,|\beta\rangle &= \tfrac{1}{2}\,|\alpha\rangle. \end{aligned}\right\}$$

From (E33) it should be clear that the exponential operator in (E32) expresses a 'probability' $\cos(\alpha/2)$ that the state of the spin will remain unchanged, and a probability $\sin(\alpha/2)$ that the spin will 'flip'. It is not easy to form a mental picture such as this for exponential operators corresponding to Hamiltonians with more terms. However, since expansions such as (E32) are a prerequisite to obtaining the matrix representations of all exponential operators, it is instructive to show how equations like (E32) are constructed for more complex operators. If, instead of a one-spin system, we had applied a non-selective pulse to a system of two non-identical spins $\frac{1}{2}$ I and S, the exponential operator would take the form $\exp\{i(I_x + S_x)\alpha\}$ (which is usually written as $\exp\{iF_x\alpha\}$). At this stage we come to a delicate point. Although exponential operators behave in general as exponential functions (compare e.g. E26 and E27), problems can arise if the exponent contains non-commuting (see **commutator**) operators. For example, although $\exp\{A + B\} = e^A e^B$ if A and B are simple functions, $\exp\{A + B\} \neq e^A e^B$ if A and B are non-commuting operators. If we consider carefully the two-spin exponential operator above, we note that I_x and S_x do commute, since they each operate on different spins. It is therefore permissible to write

E34
$$\exp\{i(I_x + S_x)\alpha\} = \exp\{iI_x\alpha\}\,.\,\exp\{iS_x\alpha\}.$$

Using (E32), (E34) can obviously be written as

E35
$$\begin{aligned} \exp\{i(I_x + S_x)\alpha\} &= (\cos(\alpha/2)\mathbf{1}_I + 2i\sin(\alpha/2)I_x) \\ &\quad (\cos(\alpha/2)\mathbf{1}_S + 2i\sin(\alpha/2)S_x) \\ &= \cos^2(\alpha/2)\mathbf{1}_I\mathbf{1}_S - 4\sin^2(\alpha/2)I_xS_x + 2i\sin(\alpha/2) \\ &\quad \cos(\alpha/2)\mathbf{1}_IS_x + 2i\sin(\alpha/2)\cos(\alpha/2)\mathbf{1}_SI_x. \end{aligned}$$

Again this is the starting point for the generation of $\exp\{i(I_x + S_x)\alpha\}$ into its matrix representation. Equations such as (E35) can be formulated for any number of spins as long as the operators in the exponent commute. A common example of an exponent containing non-commuting operators is the exponential operator corresponding to free precession of two scalar coupled spins $\frac{1}{2}$ I and S under a Hamiltonian consisting of Zeeman and full scalar coupling terms, $\mathcal{H}_{IS} = \mathcal{H}_Z + \mathcal{H}_J = \omega_I I_z + \omega_S S_z + 2\pi J\mathbf{I}_I\mathbf{I}_S$. The scalar coupling term $2\pi J\mathbf{I}_I\,.\,\mathbf{I}_S = 2\pi J(I_xS_x + I_yS_y + I_zS_z)$ contains non-commuting operators and hence we cannot use an equation such as (E34) to simplify the expansion of the exponential operator $\exp[i(\omega_I I_z + \omega_S S_z + 2\pi J\mathbf{I}_I \cdot \mathbf{I}_S)t]$. However, if the two spins are weakly coupled, the truncated Hamiltonian becomes $\mathscr{H}_{IS} = \omega_I I_z + \omega_S S_z + 2\pi J I_z S_z$ (see **weak coupling**). Now all terms commute, and it would be a straightforward task to expand $\exp[i(\omega_I I_z + \omega_S S_z + 2\pi J I_z S_z)t]$. In fact it is not necessary to calculate this expansion explicitly; provided the basis functions (see **basis state**) are **eigenfunctions** of the Hamiltonian $\mathscr{H}_{IS}$, then the matrix representation of $\exp\{i\mathscr{H}_{IS}t\}$ will always be diagonal. Evaluation of equations such as (E28) containing $\mathscr{H}_{IS}$ is then straightforward (see **density matrix**). For this reason, when calculating expressions for strongly coupled systems (when $\mathscr{H}_{IS}$ is not truncated, see **strong coupling**), it is normal practice to work in the **eigenbasis** of the strongly coupled system to simplify the task of obtaining a matrix representation for $\exp\{i\mathscr{H}_{IS}t\}$.

Exponential weighting See **apodization**.

Extreme narrowing Random reorientational and translational motions in liquids are responsible in part for the 'high-resolution' capability of NMR in this phase (see **averaging**). However, the rates of such motion can have an important influence upon the spectrum. In general, we find that rapid motion gives rise to narrower lines. In liquids, this is primarily due to the dependence of **relaxation** upon the rate of motion characterized by the **correlation time** τ_c. Since linewidth in the liquid state is given by

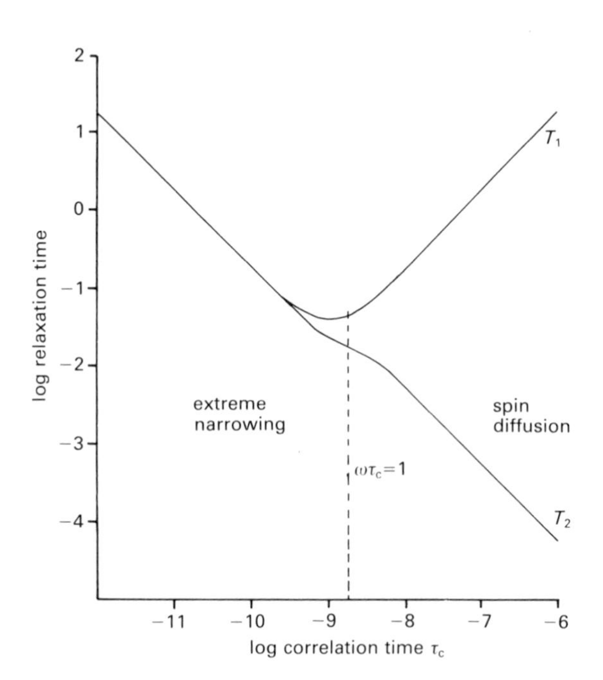

Fig. E3. Plots of T_1 and T_2 vs. correlation time τ_c at 200 MHz.

$1/(\pi T_2^*)$ (see **relaxation**), it follows that the motional dependence of T_2 is transferred to the linewidth. If we plot the magnitude of both T_1 and T_2 vs. correlation time for a given Larmor frequency ω, assuming dipole–dipole relaxation, we obtain curves such as those shown in Fig. E3. We find that T_1 passes through a minimum at $\omega\tau_c \approx 1$. **Spin–lattice relaxation** is most efficient at this point. It is possible to define two distinct limits in Fig. E3. First, it is noted that in the region $\omega\tau_c \ll 1$, $T_1 = T_2$. This is known as the extreme narrowing limit. Conversely, when $\omega\tau_c \gg 1$, we speak of the **spin–diffusion** limit. Virtually all macromolecules of interest in biological NMR have motions in the spin-diffusion limit, whereas small molecules (molecular weight <500) are characterized by motions in the extreme narrowing limit. A detailed analysis of the motional dependence of T_1 and T_2 upon molecular motion can be found under the heading **relaxation**. However, at this point it is instructive to consider qualitatively the important aspects of extreme narrowing. Both relaxation parameters are described by spectral density functions which describe the frequency components of the motion. The spin–lattice relaxation rate is determined by the functions $J(\omega)$ and $J(2\omega)$, whereas the **spin–spin relaxation** rate is characterized by an additional term $J(0)$:

$$\begin{aligned}(1/T_1) &= J(\omega) + J(2\omega)\\ (1/T_2) &= J(0) + J(\omega) + J(2\omega).\end{aligned} \qquad \text{E36}$$

The arguments 0, ω, and 2ω describe spectral densities at zero frequency, at ω, and at 2ω respectively. Intuitively, we might expect that for fast motions, $J(0)$ will not be large, and this is indeed the case. The magnitude of T_2 then approaches T_1. In addition, since $\omega\tau_c \ll 1$ by definition for fast motions, the spectral density functions are proportional to the correlation time, and hence T_1 and T_2 decrease linearly with τ_c. The extreme narrowing limit has important implications regarding the magnitude of the **nuclear Overhauser effect**.

F

Fast exchange See **chemical exchange**.

Field gradients The imposition of magnetic or r.f. field gradients, linear or otherwise, can be of great value to the experimenter. For example, the generation of a linear magnetic field gradient is the basis of NMR **imaging**. With regard to high-resolution NMR, field gradients can be most useful in the selection of **coherence transfer pathways**. This depends upon the characteristic **phase** properties of the desired coherence (see **phase coherence**) and the generation of echoes (see **coherence transfer echo**, **spin echo**, **rotary echo**) in inhomogeneous magnetic or r.f. fields. A simple example is the selective detection of **zero-quantum coherence** using a homospoil pulse. A further example is the deliberate imposition of a strong magnetic field gradient in order to separate the **coherence transfer echo** and **antiecho** in **two-dimensional NMR** without the use of phase cycling procedures. This procedure can be extended to allow the selective detection of certain orders of **multiple-quantum coherence**. In this case, the method relies upon the fact that formation of a P-order multiple-quantum echo (or, equivalently, the destruction of coherence) occurs P times faster than a single-quantum echo. Actually, selection of coherence order can also be achieved by exploiting the effects of r.f. field inhomogeneity by using inhomogeneous **z-pulses**. This has the considerable advantage that no special hardware is required to generate the field gradients. As an example, we can analyse an experiment which uses inhomogeneous z-pulses to select double-quantum coherence (Fig. F1). This is a simple sequence for the creation of even orders of multiple-quantum coherence by the first three pulses followed by immediate reconversion into single-quantum coherence (observable magnetization) by the last pulse. A common method to achieve selection of **double-quantum coherence** is to phase cycle (see **phase cycling**) the first three pulses, and to alternate the phase of the receiver by 0 and 180°. If instead we apply an inhomogeneous z-pulse just before the last pulse for n seconds, various orders of multiple-quantum coherence will in effect defocus at a rate dependent upon the coherence order; a P-order coherence will defocus P times faster than single-quantum coherence. After reconversion to single-quantum coherence by the last pulse, the z-pulse is again applied for pn seconds. Thus, if we wished to detect

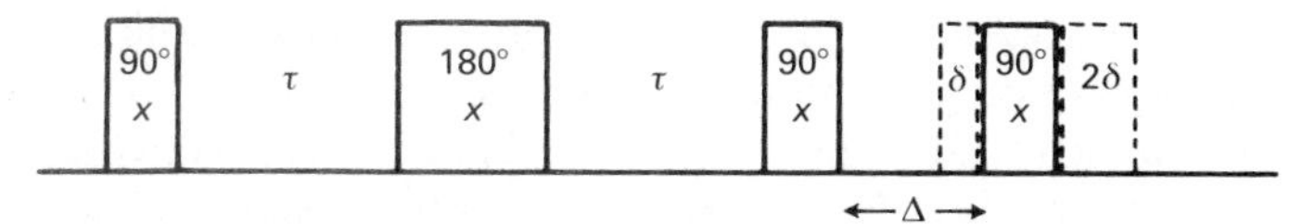

Fig. F1. Pulse sequence for the acquisition of NMR spectra filtered through double-quantum coherence using inhomogeneous *Z* pulses (illustrated by broken lines).

selectively magnetization derived from double-quantum coherence, the second *z*-pulse must be $2n$ seconds long. In that time, double-quantum coherence which defocused during the first *z*-pulse will exactly refocus as single quantum coherence at the end of the second *z*-pulse. This response is a combined rotary echo and coherence transfer echo. Importantly, for a sufficient inhomogeneous r.f. field, all other coherence orders are not refocused during the second *z*-pulse, and order selection is attained. The obvious advantage of the *z*-pulse method over phase cycling is that order selection could be achieved in a single scan. In addition, *z*-pulses achieve true order selection, whereas phase cycling to select *p*-quantum coherence is often also transparent to certain higher orders. However, the latter constraint is generally not problematic in biological NMR, and the lower sensitivity of the *z*-pulse method in comparison with phase cycling detracts slightly from its application to biological systems.

FURTHER READING

For a description of inhomogeneous r.f. fields applied to the selection of coherence transfer pathways, see

Counsell C. J. R., Levitt, M. H., and Ernst, R. R. (1985). *J. Magn. Reson.* **64,** 470.

Filter See **multiple-quantum filter**, **Z-filter**.

Flip-angle effects Flip-angle effects are intensity perturbations of multiplets in one- or two-dimensional NMR spectra which are dependent upon the flip-angle of the r.f. pulse or pulses. They can occur in any spin system which is not in an equilibrium state. In one-dimensional NMR flip-angle effects are often a nuisance, since they can complicate the interpretation of **nuclear Overhauser effect** experiments. In two-dimensional NMR studies, they can often be used to advantage. A good example is the discrimination of the **coherence transfer echo** and **antiecho** in **double-quantum correlated spectroscopy**. However, one of the original applications of the flip-angle effect was in the simplification of ^{1}H–^{1}H **correlated spectroscopy** (COSY) spectra. If the flip-angle of the mixing pulse in a COSY experiment is not 90°, then interesting effects occur with respect to the intensities of resonance lines in a given multiplet in both diagonal peaks and crosspeaks. A brief theoretical discourse will help to illustrate this. Consider a COSY experiment on a loosely coupled spin system *IS*. It is necessary only to analyse the resonance intensities of a given multiplet to illustrate the effect. Choosing arbitrarily the diagonal peak arising from spin *I*, a **product operator formalism** analysis of COSY for an *IS* spin system gives the following terms for I_y (see **correlated spectroscopy** (COSY):

$$I_{\mathrm{DIA}} = \tfrac{1}{2} I_y[\sin(\omega_I + \pi J_{IS})t_1 + \sin(\omega_I - \pi J_{IS})t_1] \times \tfrac{1}{2}[\sin(\omega_I + \pi J_{IS})t_2 + \sin(\omega_I - \pi J_{IS})t_2] \quad \text{F1}$$

where both pulses are 90°. All resonances in this diagonal peak have the same intensity. This can be proven by expanding the sinusoidal oscillations in (F1) into their coherence transfer echo and antiecho components in t_1, using the identity $\sin\theta = \frac{1}{2\mathrm{i}}(\exp\{\mathrm{i}\theta\} - \exp\{-\mathrm{i}\theta\})$:

$$\begin{aligned} I_{DIA} = I_y \frac{1}{4\mathrm{i}} &[\exp\{\mathrm{i}(\omega + J)t_1\} - \exp\{-\mathrm{i}(\omega + J)t_1\} \\ &+ \exp\{\mathrm{i}(\omega - J)t_1\} - \exp\{-\mathrm{i}(\omega - J)t_1\}] \\ &\times \frac{1}{4\mathrm{i}}[\exp\{\mathrm{i}(\omega + J)t_2\} - \exp\{-\mathrm{i}(\omega + J)t_2\} \\ &+ \exp\{\mathrm{i}(\omega - J)t_2\} - \exp\{-\mathrm{i}(\omega - J)t_2\} \end{aligned} \quad \text{F2}$$

where $\omega = \omega_I$ and $J = \pi J_{IS}$. If we now assume **quadrature detection** ('frequency discrimination') in t_2, and selective detection of the coherence transfer echo (see **phase modulation**) during t_1, it is sufficient to consider the following terms:

$$\begin{aligned} I_{DIA} = -I_y \tfrac{1}{16}[&-\exp\{-\mathrm{i}(\omega + J)t_1\}\exp\{\mathrm{i}(\omega + J)t_2\} \\ &-\exp\{-\mathrm{i}(\omega + J)t_1\}\exp\{\mathrm{i}(\omega - J)t_2\} \\ &-\exp\{-\mathrm{i}(\omega - J)t_1\}\exp\{\mathrm{i}(\omega + J)t_2\} \\ &-\exp\{-\mathrm{i}(\omega - J)t_1\}\exp\{\mathrm{i}(\omega - J)t_2\}]. \end{aligned} \quad \text{F3}$$

Each of the four exponential products in (F3) gives rise to a single component of the diagonal multiplet of spin *I*. They all have the same intensity. This is consistent with the theoretical plot calculated under **correlated spectroscopy** (COSY). Now let us consider what happens when the flip-angle of the mixing pulse is not 90° but β°. A simple product operator analysis shows that (F3) still holds in this case, but there are three additional contributions to the diagonal peak intensity.

The complete formula is thus as follows:

F4

$$
\begin{aligned}
I_{\mathrm{DIA}}(\beta^\circ) = {} & \tfrac{1}{2}I_y[\sin(\omega_I + \pi J_{IS})t_1 + \sin(\omega_I - \pi J_{IS})t_1] \\
& \times\tfrac{1}{2}[\sin(\omega_I + \pi J_{IS})t_2 + \sin(\omega_I - \pi J_{IS})t_2] \\
& +\cos\beta\tfrac{1}{2}I_y[\sin(\omega_I + \pi J_{IS})t_1 - \sin(\omega_I - \pi J_{IS})t_1] \\
& \times\tfrac{1}{2}[\sin(\omega_I + \pi J_{IS})t_2 - \sin(\omega_I - \pi J_{IS})t_2] \\
& -\cos^2\beta\tfrac{1}{2}I_y[\cos(\omega_I - \pi J_{IS})t_1 - \cos(\omega_I + \pi J_{IS})t_1] \\
& \times\tfrac{1}{2}[\cos(\omega_I - \pi J_{IS})t_2 - \cos(\omega_I + \pi J_{IS})t_2] \\
& -\cos\beta\tfrac{1}{2}I_y[\cos(\omega_I + \pi J_{IS})t_1 + \cos(\omega_I - \pi J_{IS})t_1] \\
& \times\tfrac{1}{2}[\cos(\omega_I + \pi J_{IS})t_2 + \cos(\omega_I - \pi J_{IS})t_2].
\end{aligned}
$$

We can now proceed as in the derivation of (F3) using the additional identity $\cos\theta = \frac{1}{2}(\exp\{\mathrm{i}\theta\} + \exp\{-\mathrm{i}\theta\})$;

F5

$$
\begin{aligned}
I_{\mathrm{DIA}}(\beta^\circ) = {} & -\cos\beta\tfrac{1}{16}\,I_y[-\exp\{-i(\omega + J)t_1\} \\
& \exp\{\mathrm{i}(\omega + J)t_2\} + \exp\{-\mathrm{i}(\omega + J)t_1\} \\
& \exp\{\mathrm{i}(\omega - J)t_2\} + \exp\{-\mathrm{i}(\omega - J)t_1\}\exp\{\mathrm{i}(\omega + J)t_2\} \\
& -\exp\{-\mathrm{i}(\omega - J)t_1\}\exp\{\mathrm{i}(\omega - J)t_2\}] \\
& -\cos^2\beta\tfrac{1}{16}I_y[\exp\{-\mathrm{i}(\omega - J)t_1\}\exp\{\mathrm{i}(\omega - J)t_2\} \\
& -\exp\{-\mathrm{i}(\omega - J)t_1\} \\
& \exp\{\mathrm{i}(\omega + J)t_2\} - \exp\{-\mathrm{i}(\omega + J)t_1\}\exp\{\mathrm{i}(\omega - J)t_2\} \\
& +\exp\{-\mathrm{i}(\omega + J)t_1\}\exp\{\mathrm{i}(\omega + J)t_2\}] \\
& -\cos\beta\tfrac{1}{16}I_y[\exp\{-\mathrm{i}(\omega + J)t_1\}\exp\{\mathrm{i}(\omega + J)t_2\} \\
& +\exp\{-\mathrm{i}(\omega + J)t_1\} \\
& \exp\{\mathrm{i}(\omega - J)t_2\} + \exp\{-\mathrm{i}(\omega - J)t_1\}\exp\{\mathrm{i}(\omega + J)t_2\} \\
& +\exp\{-\mathrm{i}(\omega - J)t_1\}\exp\{\mathrm{i}(\omega - J)t_2\}] \\
& -\tfrac{1}{16}I_y[-\exp\{-\mathrm{i}(\omega - J)t_1\}\exp\{\mathrm{i}(\omega + J)t_2\} \\
& -\exp\{-\mathrm{i}(\omega + J)t_1\}\exp\{\mathrm{i}(\omega - J)t_2\} \\
& -\exp\{-\mathrm{i}(\omega - J)t_1\}\exp\{\mathrm{i}(\omega + J)t_2\} \\
& -\exp\{-\mathrm{i}(\omega - J)t_1\}\exp\{\mathrm{i}(\omega - J)t_2\}].
\end{aligned}
$$

Collecting terms, we now find the following intensities for each component of the multiplet of spin I:

F6

$$
\begin{aligned}
& \exp\{-\mathrm{i}(\omega + J)t_1\}\exp\{\mathrm{i}(\omega + J)t_2\} \rightarrow 1 - \cos^2\beta \\
& \exp\{-\mathrm{i}(\omega + J)t_1\}\exp\{\mathrm{i}(\omega - J)t_2\} \rightarrow 1 + \cos^2\beta - 2\cos\beta \\
& \exp\{-\mathrm{i}(\omega - J)t_1\}\exp\{\mathrm{i}(\omega + J)t_2\} \rightarrow 1 + \cos^2\beta - 2\cos\beta \\
& \exp\{-\mathrm{i}(\omega - J)t_1\}\exp\{\mathrm{i}(\omega - J)t_2\} \rightarrow 1 - \cos^2\beta.
\end{aligned}
$$

The first and fourth terms in (F6) will be on the diagonal after **two-dimensional Fourier transformation**, whreas the second and third will be 'off-diagonal' (at a distance ~J Hz). The intensities of these two types of signal will now be different. For $\beta = 45°$, 60°, and 180° the ratio between the two types as calculated from (F6) is as follows:

$$\beta = 45°, \qquad I_{\mathrm{DIA}}/I_{\mathrm{OFF}} = 5.7,$$

$$\beta = 60°, \qquad I_{\mathrm{DIA}}/I_{\mathrm{OFF}} = 3,$$

$$\beta = 180°, \qquad I_{\mathrm{DIA}} = 0.$$

A contour plot of the diagonal peak derived from spin I might therefore look like Fig. F2. Of particular relevance is the response for $\beta = 45°$. This causes an effective increase in resolution along the diagonal since the off-diagonal contributions are reduced by approximately sixfold. These responses derive from so called parallel transitions, i.e. those not connected by a common energy level (see **connectivity networks**). A similar effect arises in crosspeak multiplets, and Bax and Freeman have shown that this can be used to derive the relative signs of coupling constants depending upon how the crosspeaks are skewed. However, these advantages must be offset against an overall loss in sensitivity for small flip-angles.

An important aspect of flip-angle effects is that while these are most useful in experiments using echo selection, in general they cannot be employed in phase-sensitive experiments. This is because the **coherence transfer echo** and **antiecho** components of the detected magnetization are not equal, as they must be in order for phase-sensitive data processing to function correctly (see **phase-sensitive experiments**). The reader may care to prove for himself that the antiecho contribution, which can be derived from (F2), is not equal to that from the coherence transfer echo as described by (F6). For further examples of flip-angle effects, see **zero-quantum coherence** and **z-filters**.

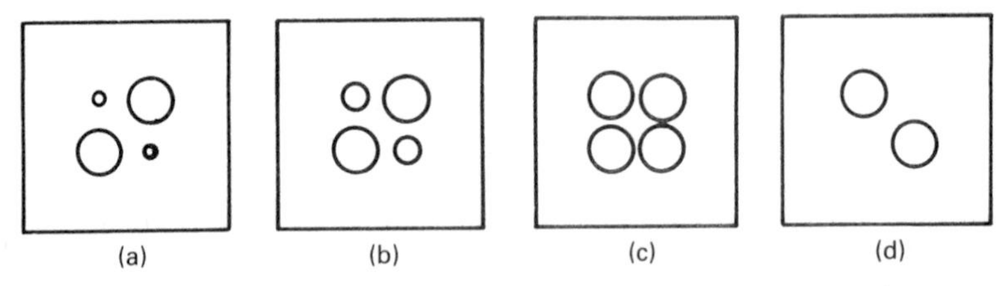

Fig. F2. Diagrammatic representation of a diagonal peak corresponding to a doublet in a COSY spectrum with the flip-angle of the mixing pulse equal to (a) 45°, (b) 60°, (c) 90°, and (d) 180°.

FURTHER READING

For a detailed analysis of flip-angle effects in COSY spectra, see

Bax, A. and Freeman, R. (1981), *J. Magn. Reson.* **44,** 542.

Folding-over The time-domain response of a spin system to an r.f. perturbation is characterized by an interferogram of cosinusoidal or sinusoidal damped oscillations, each derived from an ensemble of equivalent spins. In the **classical formalism** for the description of pulse NMR, each oscillation corresponds to a vector precessing in the rotating frame of coordinates. This precessing **magnetization** induces an e.m.f. in a pair of receiver coils aligned perpendicular to the x axis. However, the induced e.m.f. is not sensitive to the sense of the precession, as shown in Fig. F3. Thus, if the transmitter **carrier** is placed in the centre of the spectral window, the signs of the NMR frequencies will be undetermined, resulting in folding-over. Theoretically, this is described by an amplitude modulation of the induced e.m.f.:

F7 $$S(t) = \cos \omega t = (1/2)(\exp\{\mathrm{i}\omega t\} + \exp\{-\mathrm{i}\omega t\}).$$

The terms $\exp\{\mathrm{i}\omega t\}$ and $\exp\{-\mathrm{i}\omega t\}$ represent the counter-rotating components of the magnetization. This problem can clearly be alleviated if the signs of the NMR frequencies can be determined. This can be achieved by employing **quadrature detection**. Also see **aliasing**.

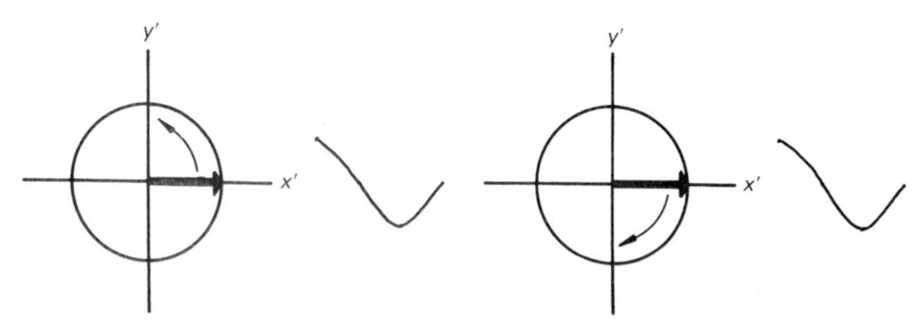

Fig. F3. The signal detected by a single NMR detector oriented along the x' axis of the rotating frame is insensitive to the direction of precession.

Forbidden transitions 'Forbidden' transitions, those for which $\Delta m \neq 1$, are unfortunately so named, since they are only forbidden in the sense that they may not be directly detected. For example, multiple-quantum spectroscopy is an important aspect of modern two-dimensional NMR and multiple-quantum transitions are often described as forbidden. If multiple quantum transitions were truly forbidden, then such experiments would not be possible. In fact the only transitions which can create an observable signal are single-quantum transitions. The corresponding single-quantum coherence (also loosely referred to as **magnetization**) can generate an e.m.f. in the receiver coils of the spectrometer. Conversely, **multiple-quantum coherence**, although present during the detection period of many two-dimensional experiments, does not generate an observable signal. For this reason multiple-quantum experiments require

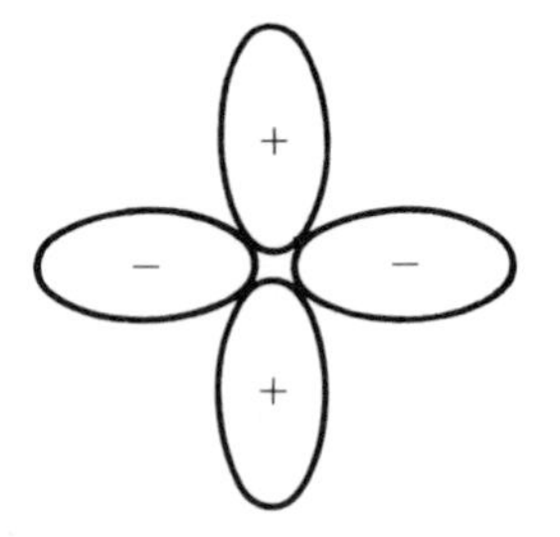

Fig. F4. Representation of double-quantum coherence as a d orbital. The net magnetization induced by this classical object is zero.

as a final step the application of a mixing pulse to create single-quantum coherence. It is difficult to present a classical picture as to why multiple-quantum coherence cannot lead to observable magnetization, since it is very much a quantum mechanical property. One way of visualizing this is to define a class of transverse magnetization with special properties. For example, in the case of double-quantum coherence, this can be described in terms of a 'd-orbital' (Fig. F4). At the quantum mechanical level, we obviously need to include in any formalism a means by which multiple-quantum coherence does not contribute to observable magnetization. In the **density matrix** formalism, this is achieved by calculating the trace of the given observable operator and the density matrix at time t:

$$M_x = \mathrm{Tr}\{F_x \sigma_{(t)}\},$$
$$M_y = \mathrm{Tr}\{F_y \sigma_{(t)}\}. \quad \text{F8}$$

Since the only non-zero elements of F_x and F_y correspond to single-quantum coherence, (F8) extracts those components of the density matrix which correspond with observable magnetization. Correspondingly, in the **product operator formalism**, we make a mental note that only terms in I_x and I_y, for example, can lead to observable magnetization.

Four-dimensional NMR Many of the assignment ambiguities in two-dimensional NMR spectra can be resolved by extension to a third frequency dimension (see **three-dimensional NMR**). Despite the enormous increase in resolution afforded by three-dimensional NMR, assignment ambiguities still exist in heteronuclear three-dimensional NMR spectra of large proteins. It is therefore desirable to increase the dimensionality still further, i.e. to four-dimensional NMR. A four-dimensional NMR experiment is readily conceived by combining three two-dimensional NMR experiments, leaving out the detection period of the first, the preparation and detection periods of the second, and the preparation period of the third. A particularly useful four-dimensional experiment for proteins labelled with ^{13}C and ^{15}N is ^{13}C–^{15}N-edited NOESY (Fig. F5). With this technique, NOEs between NH protons and aliphatic protons are spread out by the chemical shifts of directly-bonded

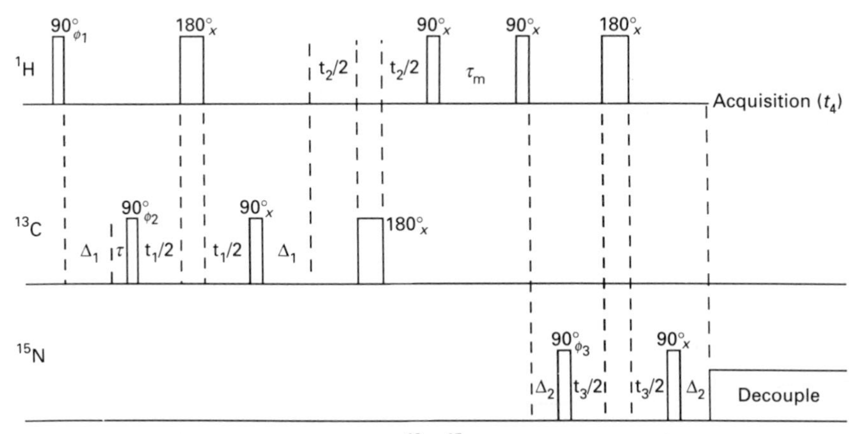

Fig. F5. Pulse sequence for four-dimensional ^{13}C–^{15}N-edited NOESY. The delays Δ_1 and Δ_2 allow for the efficient creation of multiple quantum coherence, and are set to slightly less than $1/(2J_{CH})$ and $1/(2J_{NH})$ respectively in order to minimize relaxation losses. The delay τ is included to compensate for the ^{13}C 180° pulse so that no first order phase correction is required in F_2. The phase cycling used is $\varphi 1 = 4(x)$, $\varphi 2 = 2(x, -x)$, $\varphi 3 = 2(x), 2(-x)$, and receiver $= x, -x, -x, x$. Quadrature detetdion in the t_1, t_2, and t_3 dimensions is achieved by shifting the phases $\varphi 1$, $\varphi 2$, and $\varphi 3$ by 90° in the appropriate manner (see **phase-sensitive experiments**).

^{15}N and ^{13}C atoms, respectively. This experiment resolves extensive ambiguities which may still be present in a three-dimensional ^{15}N edited NOESY experiment (see **three-dimensional NOESY-HMQC**), in which NOEs between NH protons and aliphatic protons are spread into the third dimension by the chemical shift of the directly-bonded ^{15}N atoms. Although this three-dimensional experiment is effective in removal of chemical shift degeneracy of NH protons, severe overlap of aliphatic resonances remains. The relationship between two-dimensional NOESY, three-dimensional NOESY-HMQC, and four-dimensional ^{13}C–^{15}N-edited NOESY is shown in Fig. F6. It is seen that a four-dimensional NMR experiment can be thought of as a series of three-dimensional experiments, where the variable in the fourth dimension is held constant for each. This is entirely analogous to the manner in which a three-dimensional NMR experiment can be visualized in terms of a series of two-dimensional 'slices', and a four-dimensional experiment can indeed also be analysed as a series of slices, each at a particular ^{13}C and ^{15}N chemical shift. Each slice at a particular ^{15}N frequency in the three-dimensional NMR spectrum constitutes a cube within the four-dimensional spectrum in which each cube is subdivided into a further series of slices based on the ^{13}C chemical shift of the ^{13}C atoms directly bonded to the aliphatic protons, which results in greater effective resolution of the latter.

FURTHER READING

Kay, L. E., Clore, G. M., Bax, A., and Gronenborn, A. M. (1990). *Science* **249,** 411.

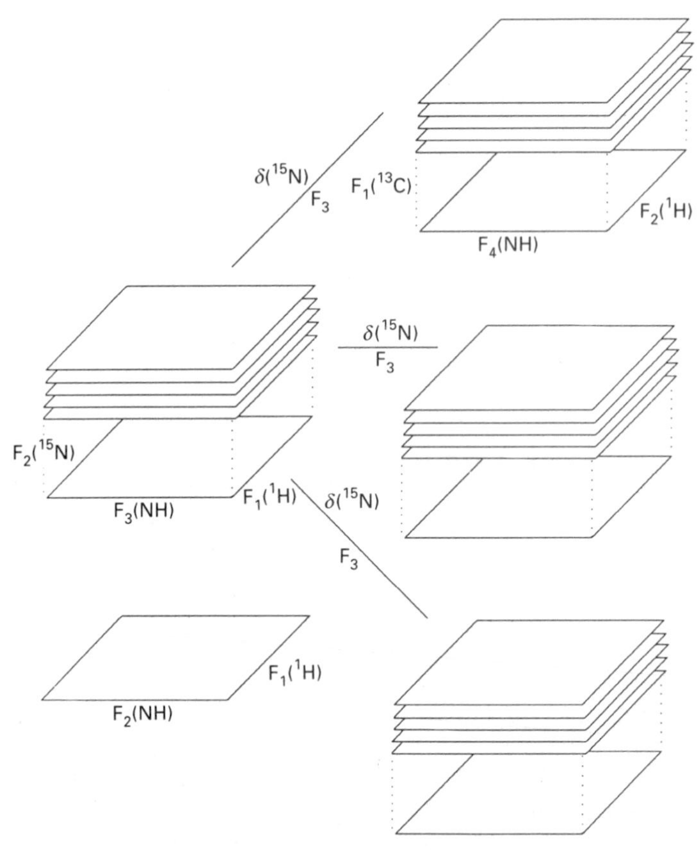

Fig. F6. Schematic illustration of the relationship between two-, three-, and four-dimensional NMR spectra. The comparisons illustrated are between two-dimensional NOESY, three-dimensional NOESY-HMQC, and four-dimensional $^{13}C-^{15}N$-edited NOESY experiments.

Fourier transform In modern-day NMR spectrometers, data are invariably collected in the time domain; i.e., they are stored in the computer memory as a function of time. However, spectroscopists are interested in the frequency-domain response of a spin system since the energy differences between spin states possess chracteristic resonance lines at specific frequencies. In fact the time domain and the frequency domain are inextricably linked, and we can convert between the two using a procedure known as Fourier transformation. The Fourier transform relates the time-domain data $f(t)$ with the frequency-domain data $f(\omega)$ by the following equation:

$$f(\omega) = \int_{-\infty}^{+\infty} f(t) \exp\{i\omega t\} \, dt. \qquad \text{F9}$$

The Fourier transform as written in (F9) is known as the continuous transform, since the limits of integration extend between $-\infty$ and $+\infty$. In practice, Fourier transformation is achieved in NMR by digital computers using the Cooley–Tukey algorithm. Under these circumstances we define the discrete Fourier transform:

$$f(\omega) = \sum_{-t}^{+t} f(t) \exp\{i\omega t\} \, dt \tag{F10}$$

where the integral extends over a finite time. For practical purposes, the result of (F10) can be considered identical to (F9).

The existence of two related domains allows us to define 'Fourier pairs'. Several of these are of particular importance in NMR. For example, the Fourier transform of a time-domain decaying exponential is a Lorentzian line (see **lineshape**) at zero frequency (Fig. F7). This is identical to the well-known relationship between the **free induction decay** and the NMR spectrum. If, instead, the time-domain signal is a decaying sinusoidal or cosinusoidal oscillation (see **damped oscillator**), then again the frequency-domain signal is a Lorentzian line, but offset from zero frequency by an amount equal to the frequency of oscillation of the sinusoidal or cosinusoidal waveform (Fig. F8). A third and equally important example of a Fourier pair is the Fourier transform of an r.f. pulse (Fig. F9). We find that the r.f. pulse is represented by a 'spread' of

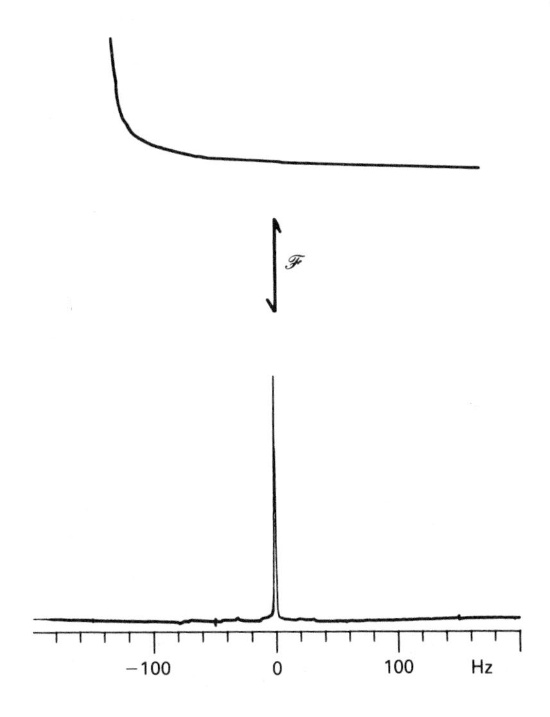

Fig. F7. A decaying exponential gives a Lorentzian line at zero frequency after Fourier transformation.

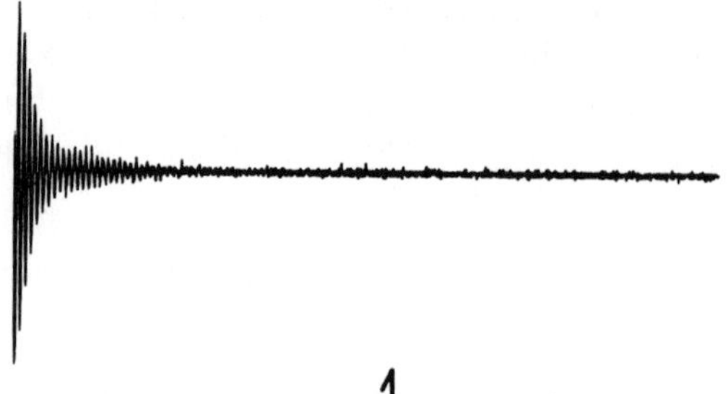

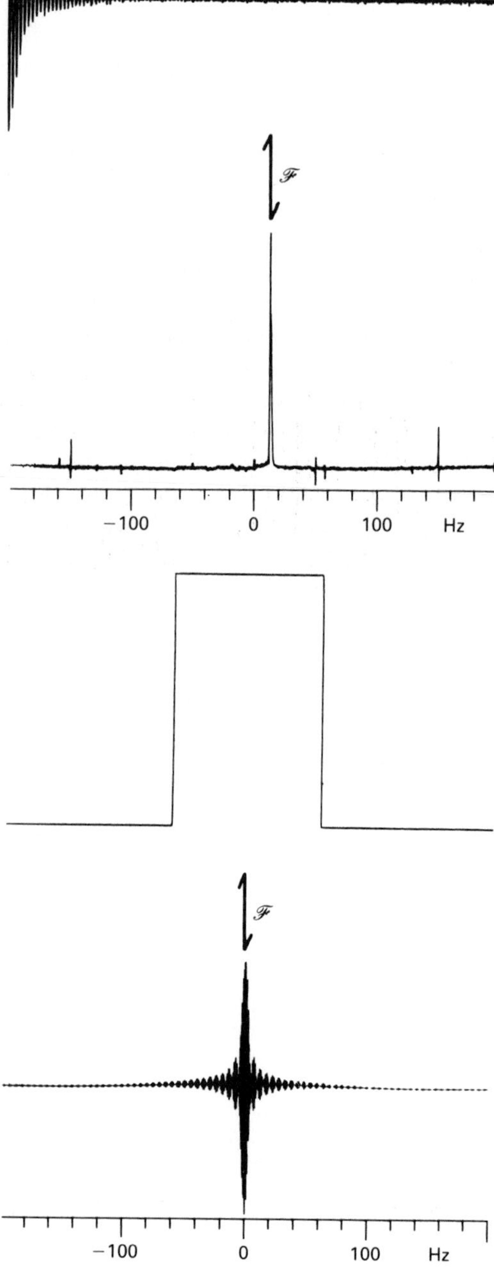

Fig. F8. An exponentially decaying cosinusoid gives a Lorentzian line offset from zero frequency by an amount equal to the frequency of oscillation of the cosinusoid.

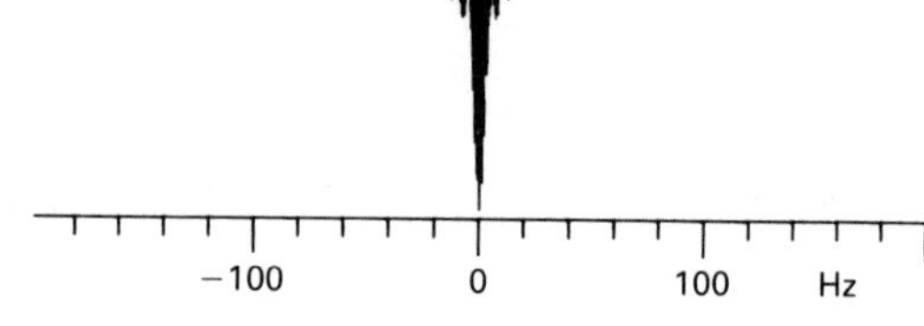

Fig. F9. A long pulse has Fourier components over a relatively narrow frequency range.

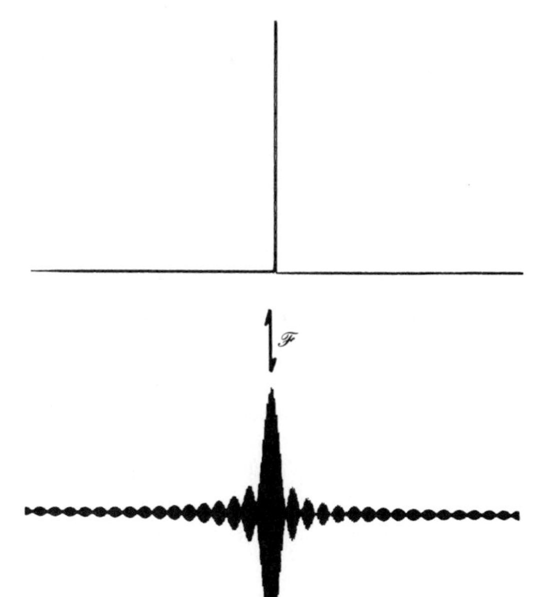

Fig. F10. A narrow pulse has Fourier components over a relatively wide frequency range.

frequencies centred about the r.f. **carrier** frequency. If we reduce the pulse length we find the spread of frequencies is greater (Fig. F10). We could continue until the pulse width was infinitely small (i.e. an impulse or **delta function**) in which case the Fourier transform would be a d.c. level (Fig. F11). Practically, the Fourier pair shown in Fig. F10 is of importance in NMR, since the frequency-domain signal corresponding to

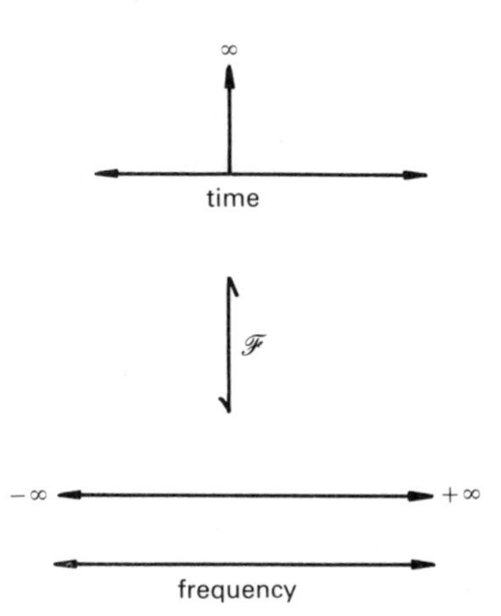

Fig. F11. A delta function has a Fourier partner which is a d.c. level.

a time-domain r.f. pulse tells us the spectral width (see **sweep-width**) over which a given r.f. pulse extends. Obviously a frequency-domain signal such as that shown in Fig. F11 would be ideal, since then uniform excitation over an arbitrary spectral width would be possible. This would however, require infinite power, so we must be satisfied with frequency-domain responses of the form shown in Fig. F10, which algebraically correspond to a function of the form $(\sin x)/x$.

Some may find difficulty with the notion that a time-domain signal has a corresponding frequency-domain partner. However, all of us have experienced this at one time or another. There are many instances in everyday life where pulsed waveforms are created due to the switching of an electric current. An example is the generation of a spark in automobile ignition systems. This very brief d.c. pulse generates frequency components over a very wide spectral width, which can be demonstrated readily with a domestic radio receiver.

In NMR, the Fourier transform of a particular function is important. It is the decaying exponential function

F11 $$f(t) = \exp\{i\omega t\} \exp\{-t/T_2\}.$$

If it is assumed that for $t < 0$, $f(t) = 0$, then the Fourier transform of this function can be expressed simply by

F12 $$\mathrm{FT}\,\{\exp(i\omega t)\exp(-t/T_2)\} = [\mathrm{Abs}\,(\omega^+) + i\,\mathrm{Dis}\,(\omega^+)],$$

where $\mathrm{Abs}\,(\omega^+)$ is the real part or Absorption lineshape and $i\,\mathrm{Dis}\,(\omega^+)$ is the imaginary or dispersion lineshape (see *lineshape*). The Fourier transform of the related function

F13 $$\mathrm{FT}\{\exp(-i\omega t)\exp(-t/T_2)\} = [\mathrm{Abs}(\omega^-) + i\,\mathrm{Dis}(\omega^-)]$$

gives similar lineshapes at negative frequencies. The function $\exp\{i\omega t\}$ can be thought of as a complex analytic signal (in this case **free-induction decay**) of the function $\cos \omega t$ whose quadrature function is $-\sin \omega t$ (see **Hilbert transform**). Equations (F12) and (F13) are thus representative of the Fourier transforms of signals detected in quadrature (see **quadrature detection**). A second function which is important in two-dimensional NMR (or a one-dimensional experiment employing single-phase detection) is the following representing a decaying **amplitude modulation**:

F14 $$f(t) = \cos \omega t \exp(-t/T_2) = \tfrac{1}{2}(\exp(i\omega t) + \exp(-i\omega t))\exp(-t/T_2).$$

Using (F12) and (F13), the Fourier transform of this component is seen to be

F15 $$\mathrm{FT}\{\cos \omega t\} = (\mathrm{Abs}(\omega^+) + i\,\mathrm{Dis}(\omega^+) + \mathrm{Abs}(\omega^-) + i\,\mathrm{Dis}(\omega^-)]$$

giving signals at $\pm\omega$. The signs of the frequencies are thus not discriminated, in contrast to the previous result.

There are two other transforms which are related to the Fourier transform; The cosine transform of a function $f(t)$ is

F16 $$F_{\cos}(s) = 2\int_0^{\infty} f(t) \cos \omega t \, dt$$

which is the same as the Fourier transform if $f(t)$ is an even function (i.e. a function symmetrical about $t = 0$). The sine transform of $f(t)$ is defined by

F17 $$F_{\sin}(s) = 2\int_0^{\infty} f(t) \sin \omega t \, dt.$$

If $f(t)$ is zero to the left of the origin (as found for example in a free induction decay, $f(t) = 0$ for $t < 0$) then

F18 $$F(s) = \tfrac{1}{2}F_{\cos}(s) - \tfrac{1}{2}F_{\sin}(s)$$

and zeroing the imaginary part of a complex free induction decay before Fourier transformation will result in a real cosine transform. Finally, we should mention that in any practical NMR experiment the signal will be digitized so the time-domain signals are series rather than continuous functions. However, for our purposes the detected signals can be considered as continuous functions, and they are treated as such in all discussions of Fourier and related transforms throughout this work.

See also **two-dimensional Fourier transform**.

FURTHER READING

Bracewell, R. M. (1965). *The Fourier transform and its applications*. McGraw-Hill, New York.

Free induction decay In all **Fourier transform** NMR experiments, the response of the spin system to a given perturbation is measured by the induction of an e.m.f. in the receiver coils of the spectrometer by precessing transverse magnetization. This might be a simple sinusoidal or cosinusoidal response from a group of equivalent spins, or a complex interferogram of oscillations with various frequencies derived from a complex spin system. In any case the response of the spin system is 'plotted' as a function of time in the computer memory. Such a response is called the free induction decay. The (frequency-domain) NMR spectrum is obtained from this time-domain free induction decay by Fourier transformation. There is no generalized equation to describe the free induction decay since it depends upon the spin system under investigation. However, the form of the free induction decay is obtained directly from a **density matrix** calculation or its variants by calculation of the **expectation value** of the relevant observable operator:

$$M_x = \langle F_x \rangle = \mathrm{Tr}\{\sigma F_x\},$$
$$M_y = \langle F_y \rangle = \mathrm{Tr}\{\sigma F_y\}. \quad \text{F19}$$

It is common practice to ignore relaxation in such calculations. However, it is always understood that the transverse magnetization decays with a time constant T_2^* (see **spin–spin relaxation** T_2), and the free induction decay thus inherits the same decay constant.

Since the free induction decay represents the time-domain response of the spin system, it is convenient to employ certain weighting functions to it before Fourier transformation, in order to improve either the resolution or the signal-to-noise ratio of the resulting spectrum. The precise weighting function employed depends upon the circumstances, see e.g. **convolution**.

Frequency domain See **Fourier transform**.

Frequency modulation In this method of modulation, the frequency of the **carrier** is varied in sympathy with the input signal which is to be transmitted. If f_{max} is the maximum frequency deviation corresponding to the maximum modulating frequency f_m, we can define a parameter called the modulation index $\beta = f_{max}/f_m$. The equation for the frequency modulated carrier wave is

$$i = I\cos(\omega_c t + \beta \sin \omega_m t) \quad \text{F20}$$

where i is the instantaneous carrier current, ω_c is the carrier frequency, and ω_m is the modulating frequency. This equation can be expanded as an infinite series and becomes

$$\begin{aligned} i = {} & IJ_0\beta \cos \omega_c t - IJ_1\beta[\cos(\omega_c - \omega_m)t - \cos(\omega_c + \omega_m)t] \\ & + IJ_2\beta[\cos(\omega_c - 2\omega_m)t - \cos(\omega_c + 2\omega_m)t)] \\ & - IJ_3\beta[\cos(\omega_c - 3\omega_m)t - \cos(\omega_c + 3\omega_m)t] + \ldots \end{aligned} \quad \text{F21}$$

where J_0, J_1, J_2, J_3 are known as Bessel functions. Equation (F21) shows that we will in theory find an infinite number of sidebands on either side of the carrier. However, the number of significant sidebands depends upon β. Unlike **amplitude modulation** and **phase modulation**, frequency modulation is not an inherent characteristic of NMR experiments. However, special forms of r.f. excitation depend upon the properties of frequency modulation for their function.

G

Gated decoupling (time-shared decoupling) The strong r.f. fields which are necessary for decoupling in homonuclear NMR experiments can present severe leakage problems between transmitter and receiver. To prevent this, it is possible to utilize a technique known as gated decoupling. In this method, the decoupler field is applied in the form of short pulses τ_p during the dwell time between sampling points (Fig. G1). The application of pulsed excitation of course generates modulation sidebands. With small flip-angles of the decoupling field and high repetition rates, it is possible to consider the frequency-domain spectrum of the pulse sequence. The amplitudes a_n of the modulation sidebands at frequencies $\omega_n = \omega_D + 2\pi n/\tau$ for $n = 0, \pm1, \pm2, \ldots$ are given by

G1 $$a_n = B_p \frac{\sin(\pi n \tau_p/\tau)}{\pi n}$$

where B_p is the peak value of the r.f. field, and τ is the interpulse spacing. For a sufficiently high sampling rate $1/\tau$, only one of the pulse modulation sidebands (that at the centre frequency) lies within the spectrum, and all other sidebands may effectively be neglected.

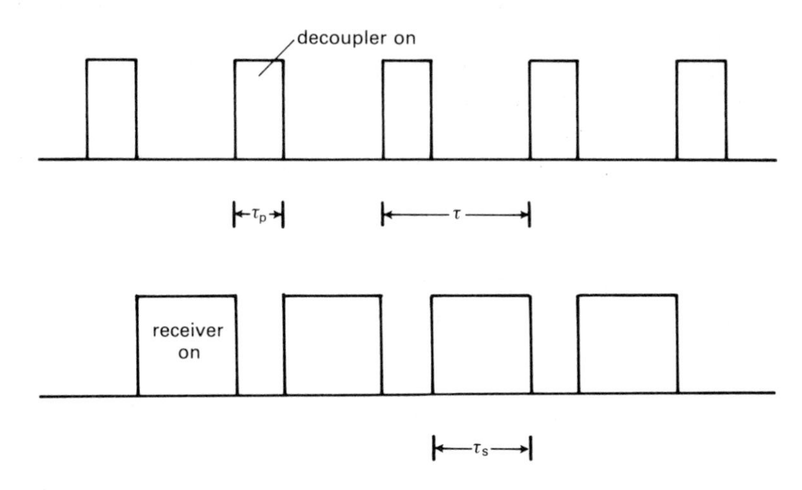

Fig. G1. Illustration of gated decoupling as a series of short pulses applied during the dwell time of the receiver.

Gaussian lineshape See **lineshape**.

Gaussian pulse The excitation spectrum resulting from a rectangular pulse (see **hard pulse**) of amplitude B_1, of **pulse width** t_p and flip-angle $\alpha_0 = \gamma B_1 t_p = \pi/2$ radians, is given in the linear approximation by a sinc function:

$$M_y = M_0 \alpha_0 \operatorname{sinc}\{\alpha_0/\pi \sin\theta\} \tag{G2}$$

where $\tan\theta = B_1/\Delta B$.

In practice, this results in a broad excitation spectrum provided the pulse width is small. However, experiments involving selective excitation require a narrow excitation spectrum. While this can be achieved by lengthening the pulse, this procedure is not ideal. An alternative is to employ an r.f. pulse shaped with a Gaussian envelope (see **lineshape**). In the linear response region, a Gaussian pulse envelope in the time domain gives an excitation function in the frequency domain which is also Gaussian. A Gaussian lineshape has a very desirable property with regard to selective excitation, since the amplitude tails off quite rapidly with respect to frequency.

FURTHER READING

For a discussion of Gaussian pulses, see

Bauer, C., Freeman, R., Frenkiel, T., Keeler, J. and Shaka, A. J. (1984). *J. Magn. Reson.* **58,** 442.

Green function When studying a system in its linear approximation (see **linearity**), it is convenient to define a function with which to describe it. One means by which this can be achieved is to apply a function to the input of the system and to measure the output. The behaviour of any linear system can in fact be characterized in the time domain by the impulse response, or Green function. In other words, if we apply an impulse (see **delta function**) to the system, it will become 'spread out' or convoluted (see **convolution**) by the characteristics of the system. We can describe the response $r(t)$ of the system to a delta function at its input by

$$r(t) = h(t) * \delta(t). \tag{G3}$$

If we **Fourier transform** this equation the corresponding frequency-domain response is given by

$$R(\nu) = h(\nu) \,.\, \delta(\nu). \tag{G4}$$

However, since the transform of $\delta(t)$ is unity then (G4) reduces to

$$R(\nu) = h(\nu) \tag{G5}$$

$h(\nu)$ is called the transfer function of the system, which imparts changes in amplitude and phase at the output with respect to the input. Thus, if we apply a delta function to a system of nuclear spins, the response of the system is the transfer function, which in this particular example is obviously the NMR spectrum. As long as the system is linear, the impulse response provides complete information to calculate the spectrum.

H

Hahn spin echo See **spin echo**.

Hamiltonian A central postulate of quantum mechanics is that any **observable** has a corresponding **operator**. In spectroscopy we are particularly concerned with the 'energy-operator' since this gives us the resonance frequencies and intensities of the resonance lines of spectral lines when it is inserted into the relevant equation. We refer to this 'energy-operator' as a Hamiltonian operator or simply Hamiltonian. The Hamiltonian contains terms which account for all internal and external interactions of the spin system under investigation. An example of an internal interaction is the scalar coupling between spins in solution, to which a scalar coupling Hamiltonian $\mathcal{H}_J$ is assigned. An example of an external interaction is the perturbation of the spin system by r.f. energy, which is represented by another Hamiltonian, $\mathcal{H}_{\text{r.f.}}$. In general, several different external Hamiltonians may operate during the course of an experiment. The state of the spin system as represented by, for example, the **density matrix**, can be calculated from the solution of the **Liouville–von Neumann** equation using the relevant Hamiltonian:

H1 $$\dot{\sigma} = -\mathrm{i}\hbar^{-1}[\mathcal{H}, \sigma].$$

When the Hamiltonian is time-independent over the period $t = 0$ to $t = t$, the solution of (H1) is straightforward:

H2 $$\sigma(t) = \exp\{-\mathrm{i}\mathcal{H}t\}\sigma(0)\exp\{\mathrm{i}\mathcal{H}t\}.$$

An example of the use of (H2) is described under density matrix. When summed, the various terms of the Hamiltonian at a given instant in time are collectively known as the nuclear spin Hamiltonian. It may be composed of some or all of the following:

H3 $$\mathcal{H} = \mathcal{H}_{\text{Z}} + \mathcal{H}_{\text{r.f.}} + \mathcal{H}_{\text{CS}} + \mathcal{H}_{\text{Q}} + \mathcal{H}_{\text{SR}} + \mathcal{H}_D + \mathcal{H}_J$$

where

$\mathcal{H}_{\text{Z}}$ represents external static magnetic fields (Zeeman term)
$\mathcal{H}_{\text{r.f.}}$ represents external r.f. magnetic fields
$\mathcal{H}_{\text{CS}}$ represents induced magnetic fields due to orbital electronic motions (chemical shift)

$\mathcal{H}_Q$ represents electric field gradients (quadrupolar coupling)
$\mathcal{H}_{SR}$ represents moment associated with molecular angular momentum (spin rotation)
$\mathcal{H}_D$ represents magnetic dipolar coupling
$\mathcal{H}_J$ represents indirect coupling through electron spins (scalar, J coupling)

In NMR of liquids, we are primarily concerned with $\mathcal{H}_Z$, $\mathcal{H}_{r.f.}$ and $\mathcal{H}_J$ in practical calculations (see e.g. **density matrix, product operator formalism**). However, we briefly comment upon each term.

1. ZEEMAN HAMILTONIAN, $\mathcal{H}_Z$

The static magnetic field is usually chosen to lie along the positive z axis. This leads to

$$\mathcal{H}_Z = \sum_i \omega_i I_{zi} \tag{H4}$$

where ω_i is the Larmor frequency of spin i, I_{zi} is the z component angular momentum operator for spin i, and the sum runs over all spins.

2. RADIOFREQUENCY HAMILTONIAN, $\mathcal{H}_{r.f.}$

The r.f. field is usually applied perpendicular to the static field. If, for example, the phase of the r.f. is parallel to the x axis then;

$$\mathcal{H}_{r.f.} = B_1(t)\cos(\omega t + \phi(t)) \sum_i \gamma_i I_{xi} \tag{H5}$$

where I_{xi} is the x component angular momentum operator of spin i, and the sum runs over all homonuclear spins. The term $B_1(t)\cos(\omega t + \phi(t))$ implies that the r.f. irradiation can be modulated in both amplitude and phase, but has a constant **carrier** frequency ω. In the simplifying case of an r.f. pulse of constant amplitude and phase along the $+x$ axis, ignoring off-resonance effects we can redefine $\mathcal{H}_{r.f.}$ as

$$\mathcal{H}_{r.f.} = \beta/t \sum_i I_{xi} \tag{H6}$$

where the flip-angle, $\beta = \gamma_i B_1 t$, where t is the length of time for which B_1 is applied. For the great majority of calculations in the present work, $\mathcal{H}_{r.f.}$ is taken according to (H6).

3. CHEMICAL SHIFT HAMILTONIAN, $\mathcal{H}_{CS}$

This can be written in the form

$$\mathcal{H}_{CS} = \hbar \sum_i \gamma^i \mathbf{I}_i \,.\, \sigma_i \,.\, \mathbf{B} \tag{H7}$$

where σ_i is the chemical shielding **tensor**, $\mathbf{I}_i$ is the angular momentum operator for spin i (I_{xi}, I_{yi}, I_{zi}) and **B** is the static magnetic field; $-\sigma_i \cdot \mathbf{B}$ is the magnetic field induced by the electrons at the site of nucleus i.

4. QUADRUPOLAR HAMILTONIAN, $\mathcal{H}_Q$

This Hamiltonian can be written

H8
$$\mathcal{H}_Q = \sum_i \frac{eQi}{6I_i(2I_i - 1)} \sum_{\alpha,\beta} V^i_{\alpha\beta}[\tfrac{3}{2}(I_{\alpha i}I_{\beta i} + I_{\beta i}I_{\alpha i}) - \delta_{\alpha\beta}(\mathbf{I}_i)^2]$$

H9
$$= \sum_i \frac{eQi}{6I_i(2I_i - 1)} \mathbf{I}_i \cdot \mathbf{V}_i \cdot \mathbf{I}_i$$

where eQi and I_i are the nuclear quadrupole moment and the nuclear spin quantum number of the ith nucleus; $V^i_{\alpha\beta}$ is the second (α, β) derivative of the electric potential at the ith nucleus, and $\mathbf{I}_i$ is the angular momentum operator of spin i, (I_{xi}, I_{yi}, I_{zi}).

5. SPIN–ROTATION INTERACTION HAMILTONIAN, $\mathcal{H}_{SR}$

This is given by

H10
$$\mathcal{H}_{SR} = \sum_m \sum_i \mathbf{I}_i \cdot \mathbf{C}_{i,m} \cdot \mathbf{J}_m$$

where $\mathbf{I}_i = (I_{xi}, I_{yi}, I_{zi})$, $\mathbf{C}_i$ is the spin–rotation interaction tensor and $\mathbf{J}_m$ is the molecular angular momentum. This Hamiltonian describes the coupling of nuclear spins i of a molecular m with the magnetic moment associated with the molecular angular momentum. The sum over i runs over all nuclei in the molecule, and the sum over m runs over all molecules of the sample.

6. DIPOLAR HAMILTONIAN, $\mathcal{H}_D$

The dipolar Hamiltonian is given by

H11
$$\mathcal{H}_D = \frac{1}{2} \sum_{j=1}^{N} \sum_{k=1}^{N} \left[\frac{\mu_j \cdot \mu_k}{\mathbf{r}_{jk}^3} - \frac{3(\mu_j \cdot \mathbf{r}_{jk})(\mu_k \cdot \mathbf{r}_{jk})}{\mathbf{r}_{jk}^5} \right]$$

where $\mu_i = \gamma_i \hbar \mathbf{I}_i$ and $\mathbf{r}_{jk} = |r_j - r_k|$. Equation (H11) is sometimes written in tensor notation:

H12
$$H_D = \mathbf{I}_j \cdot \mathbf{D} \cdot \mathbf{I}_k,$$

where $\mathbf{I}_j = (I_{xj}, I_{yj}, I_{zj})$ and **D** is the dipolar coupling tensor. If I_{xj} and I_{yj} are expressed in terms of raising and lowering opeators (see **shift operators**) I_j^+, and I_j^- respectively, and the x, y, z coordinates are expressed in terms of spherical coordinates r, θ, ϕ, $\mathcal{H}_D$ can be rewritten in a form convenient for computing matrix elements (see **matrix**

representation):

$$\mathcal{H}_D = \frac{\gamma_j \gamma_k \hbar^2}{r^3}[A + B + C + D + E + F],$$

where

H13
$$\begin{aligned}
A &= I_{zj} I_{zk}(1 - 3\cos^2\theta), \\
B &= -\tfrac{1}{4}[I_j^+ I_k^- + I_j^- I_k^+](1 - 3\cos^2\theta) \\
C &= -\tfrac{3}{2}[I_j^+ I_{zk} + I_{zj} I_k^+]\sin\theta\cos\theta\exp\{-\mathrm{i}\phi\} \\
D &= -\tfrac{3}{2}[I_j^- I_{zk} + I_{zj} I_k^-]\sin\theta\cos\theta\exp\{\mathrm{i}\phi\} \\
E &= -\tfrac{3}{4} I_j^+ I_k^+ \sin^2\theta\exp\{-2\mathrm{i}\phi\} \\
F &= -\tfrac{3}{4} I_j^- I_k^- \sin^2\theta\exp\{2\mathrm{i}\phi\}.
\end{aligned}$$

7. SPIN COUPLING HAMILTONIAN, $\mathcal{H}_J$

This term may be written

H14
$$\mathcal{H}_J = \gamma^2\hbar^2 \sum_{i<k} \mathbf{I}_i \,.\, \mathbf{J}_{ik} \,.\, \mathbf{I}_k$$

where $\mathbf{I}_i = (I_{xi}, I_{yi}, I_{zi})$ and $\mathbf{J}_{ik}$ is the scalar coupling tensor. $\mathcal{H}_J$ as shown in (H14) is sometimes known as the isotropic spin coupling Hamiltonian. We can expand this Hamiltonian to a form more familiar to the pages of this work:

H15
$$\mathcal{H}_J = \sum_{i<k} J_{ik}(I_{xi} I_{xk} + I_{yi} I_{yk} + I_{zi} I_{zk})$$

where J_{ik} is the spin coupling constant (in Hz or $2\pi J_{ik}$ radians/s) and I_{xi}, I_{yi}, I_{zi} are the x, y and z component **angular momentum** operators respectively for spin i. We also define a **weak coupling** Hamiltonian,

H16
$$\mathcal{H}_j = \sum_{i<k} J_{ik} I_{zi} I_{zk}.$$

In principle, both the dipolar and spin coupling Hamiltonians couple every spin of the sample with all others. For this reason they are sometimes called many-spin Hamiltonians, in contrast to the other five which are sums of single-spin Hamiltonians. See also **average Hamiltonian theory**.

Hard pulse The term 'hard pulse' is often used to describe an r.f. pulse which excites the spin system non-selectively over a given bandwidth. Usually, it is a simple rectangular pulse of short duration t_p. As a first approximation, it will excite the spin system over a bandwidth given by t_p^{-1} Hz. Thus an efficient hard pulse will be of very short duration. The flip-angle (β) of the pulse will however depend upon the strength of the r.f. field β_1 (and thus upon the transmitter power) and upon the magnetogyric ratio (γ) of the nucleus in question:

H17 $$\beta = \gamma \beta_1 t_p$$

In order to generate an efficient 90° hard pulse, therefore, a reasonably large transmitter power (~10 W) is required for protons.

Hartmann–Hahn condition A Fourier transform experiment on a solid polymer has a serious limitation. In the case of ^{13}C NMR, T_1's for solids are of the order of tens of seconds (see **relaxation**). The technique of signal averaging thus becomes very slow. One method by which this can be avoided is to generate the ^{13}C polarization at the expense of protons, which recover more rapidly. This technique is called **cross-polarization** (CP).

Actually, the transfer of polarization from protons to carbons with an applied B_0 is slow, since the frequency (and thus energy) mismatch of the Larmor frequencies is large ($\gamma_H \simeq 4\gamma_C$).

Hartmann and Hahn discovered that CP became much more efficient when the Larmor frequencies were matched by performing a spin-lock experiment (see **spin-locking**) in the doubly rotating frame. This is achieved experimentally by using two r.f. fields, one at the Larmor frequency of the protons and one at the Larmor frequency of carbons. The amplitudes of these fields H_{1H} and H_{1C} respectively, can be separately adjusted to satisfy the Hartmann–Hahn condition:

H18 $$\gamma_H H_{1H} = \gamma_C H_{1C}$$

This allows exactly matched mutual spin flips (flip-flop processes) between carbons and protons. Most importantly the transfer can be repeated after allowing proton repolarization. The length of the spin-lock period is often referred to as the contact time.

The Hartmann–Hahn condition can also be exploited to effect coherence transfer in NMR of liquids. See **homonuclear Hartmann–Hahn spectroscopy**.

FURTHER READING

See the original work of
Hartmann, S. R. and Hahn, E. L. (1962) *Phys. Rev.* **128,** 2042.

More recent work includes
Bertrand, R. D., Moniz, W. B., Garroway, A. N., and Chingas, G. C. (1978). *J. Am. Chem. Soc.* **100,** 5227.

Chingas, G. C., Garroway, A. N., Bertrand, R. D. and Moniz, W. B. (1981). *J. Chem. Phys.* **74,** 127.

Hartmann–Hahn spectroscopy See **homonuclear Hartmann–Hahn spectroscopy**.

Hausdorff formula In any given NMR experiment, the spin system generally evolves during a time period t under a defined **Hamiltonian** ($\mathcal{H}$) which is either intrinsic to the spin system or is 'tailored' by the experimenter by the application of a specific pulse sequence. In any case the state of the spin system as represented by the density operator $\sigma(t)$ at time t can be calculated from the solution of the **Liouville–von Neumann** equation:

H19 $$\sigma(t) = \exp\{-\mathrm{i}\mathcal{H}t\}\sigma(0)\exp\{\mathrm{i}\mathcal{H}t\}$$

if the Hamiltonian is time independent in the period $t = 0$ to $t = t$. If the Hamiltonian contains several terms, it is possible to expand the **exponential operators** in (H19) into a product of exponents:

H20 $$\exp\{-\mathrm{i}(\mathcal{H}_A + \mathcal{H}_B)t\} = \exp\{-\mathrm{i}\mathcal{H}_A t\}\exp\{-\mathrm{i}\mathcal{H}_B t\}.$$

Explicit evaluation of (H19) is then achieved simply by calculating the **matrix representations** of the exponential operators (and their inverses) in (H20). However, it is very important to realize that (H20) is only valid if $\mathcal{H}_A$ and $\mathcal{H}_B$ commute. In the case that they do not, we are left with the problem of calculating the matrix representation of the term on the left-hand side of (H20). One way to overcome this difficulty is to work in the eigenbase of the relevant Hamiltonian (see e.g. **strong coupling**) where matrix representation is always diagonal. An alternative in some cases is to employ the Hausdorff formula. Equation (H19) can then be expanded thus:

H21 $$\begin{aligned}\sigma(t) &= \exp\{-\mathrm{i}\mathcal{H}t\}\sigma(0)\exp\{\mathrm{i}\mathcal{H}t\}\\ &= \sigma(0) - \mathrm{i}t[\mathcal{H}, \sigma(0)] + \frac{(it)^2}{2!}[\mathcal{H}, [\mathcal{H}, \sigma(0)]]\\ &\quad - \frac{(\mathrm{i}t)^3}{3!}[\mathcal{H}, [\mathcal{H}, [\mathcal{H}, \sigma(0)]]] + \ldots.\end{aligned}$$

The successive **commutators** in (H21) appear formidable, but in practice $\sigma(0)$ is often represented by an expansion in terms of product operators, in which case the commutators in (H21) correspond with the well-known commutation relations of **angular momentum** operators. In using (H21) it must be remembered that the solution is valid only if the series converges. Often it is found that the Taylor series for sine and cosine can be extracted, leading to a concise solution for $\sigma(t)$.

Heisenberg representation See **Schrodinger and Heisenberg representation**.

Hermitian matrix See **density matrix**.

Heteronuclear correlation spectroscopy The principles of heteronuclear correlation spectroscopy are precisely analogous to homonuclear correlation spectroscopy (COSY). However, a different experimental regime is required since two nuclear types with different Larmor frequencies are involved. The simplest pulse sequence for heteronuclear correlation spectroscopy is that shown in Fig. H1. It differs from homonuclear COSY only in that the second pulse is applied simultaneously to both nuclei (Fig. H1). We can analyse the pulse sequence in Fig. H1 using the **product operator formalism**. For simplicity a two-spin system *IS* can be examined. It is assumed that spins *I* are the abundant spins and *S* are the rare spins. The *S* spins will eventually be detected. We will show later that the experiment can be performed with detection of abundant spins, giving a large improvement in sensitivity.

The application of a $\pi/2$ pulse upon the *I* spins generates transverse magnetization:

H22 $$I_z + S_z \xrightarrow{(\pi/2)I_x} -I_y + S_z.$$

The density matrix, described in terms of the operators $-I_y$ and S_z, then evolves under the Zeeman and spin coupling terms of the **Hamiltonian**.

H23 $$\begin{aligned} -I_y + S_z \xrightarrow{\omega_I I_z t_1 + \omega_S S_z t_1 \; 2\pi J t_1 2I_z s_z} & -I_y \cos \omega_I t_1 \cos \pi J_{IS} t_1 \\ & + 2I_x S_z \cos \omega_I t_1 \sin \pi J_{IS} t_1 + I_x \sin \omega_I t_1 \cos \pi J_{IS} t_1 \\ & + 2I_y S_z \sin \omega_I t_1 \sin \pi J_{IS} t_1, \end{aligned}$$

where the S_z term is dropped for convenience.

The $(\pi/2)I_x$ and $(\pi/2)S_x$ pulses then effect coherence transfer between

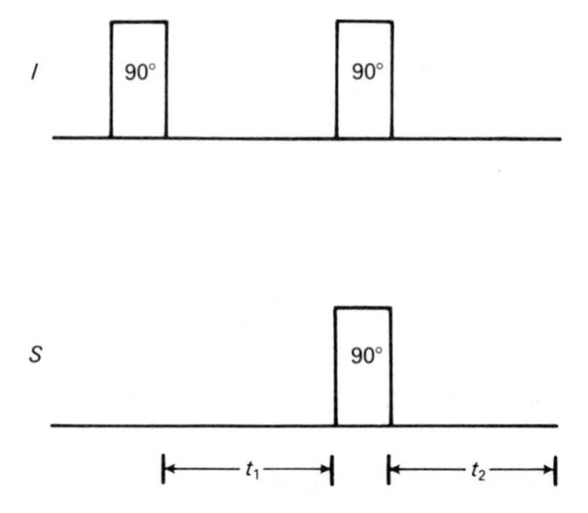

Fig. H1. Simplest pulse sequence for the acquisition of heteronuclear correlated spectra.

spins:

$$-I_y \cos \omega_I t_1 \cos \pi J_{IS} t_1 + 2I_x S_z \cos \omega_I t_1 \sin \pi J_{IS} t_1 + I_x \sin \omega_I t_1 \cos \pi J_{IS} t_1$$

$$+2I_y S_z \sin \omega_I t_1 \sin \pi J_{IS} t_1 \xrightarrow{\pi/2(I_x+S_x)} -I_z \cos \omega_I t_1 \cos \pi J_{IS} t_1$$

$$-2I_x S_y \cos \omega_I t_1 \sin \pi J_{IS} t_1 + I_x \sin \omega_I t_1 \cos J_{IS} t_1 - 2I_z S_y \sin \omega_I t_1 \sin \pi J_{IS} t_1. \quad \text{H24}$$

The term $-2I_zS_y$ represents antiphase magnetization which precesses at the Larmor frequency of spin I (abundant) during t_1, and precesses at the Larmor frequency of spin S (rare) during t_2. It will evolve during t_2 to give observable magnetization. It is thus analogous to a crosspeak in homonuclear COSY experiments, and demonstrates that the correlated nuclei are scalar coupled. However, since a $\pi/2$ pulse is not applied to the S spins before the t_1 period, there are no diagonal peaks in heteronuclear correlation spectroscopy. This is confirmed by the absence of any additional observable S spin terms in (H24). The I_x term is an '**observable**', but will not be detected in this particular experiment since it is outside the receiver bandwidth, which is centred on the S spins. Unfortunately, this simple regime does not allow for broadband I spin decoupling during t_2. Since the observable S magnetization is in antiphase with respect to J_{IS}, the spin multiplets would cancel. It is therefore necessary to modify the pulse sequence in order to effect the highly desirable I spin decoupling. The necessary modification is quite straightforward—one simply allows the antiphase magnetization to refocus before detection. In practice, it is found that delay periods before and after the mixing pulse are beneficial (Fig. H2). The delays allow the coherence to dephase before and to rephase after coherence transfer. If the intervals are chosen as $\tau = \tau' = (2J_{IS})^{-1}$, then the effects of the delays

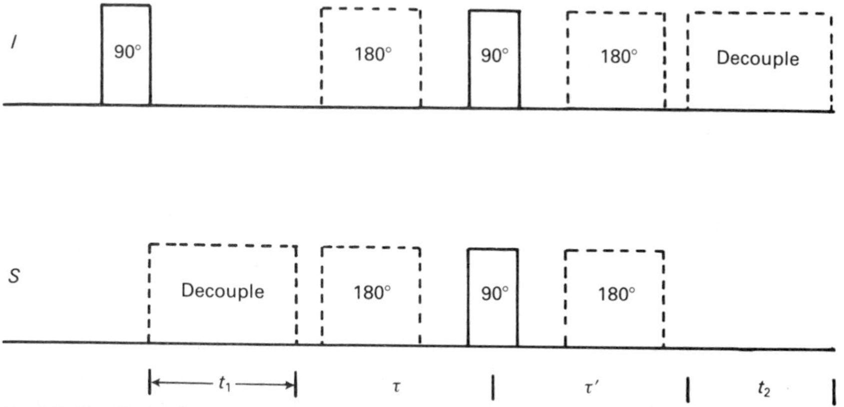

Fig. H2. Modified pulse sequence which allows for heteronuclear decoupling in the evolution and detection periods. The optional π pulses remove offset-dependent phase errors.

are equivalent to $\pi/2$ rotations about the z axis (see **product operator formalism**). In this case the I_x term on the right-hand side of (H24) is relevant, and it is transformed by the $\tau - (\pi/2)(I_x + S_x) - \tau'$ sequence as follows:

H25 $$I_x \xrightarrow{(\pi/2)2I_zS_z} 2I_yS_z \xrightarrow{\pi/2(I_x+S_x)} -2I_zS_y \xrightarrow{(\pi/2)2I_zS_z} S_x$$

giving in phase S spin magnetization. It is now possible (but optional) to decouple the I spins during the detection period. This will collapse all multiplets to singlets in t_2, with an effective increase in resolution and sensitivity. In addition, inspection of the $+I_x$ term on the right-hand side of (H24) shows a cosinusoidal modulation $\cos \pi J_{IS}t_1$. It is thus possible (but again optional) to decouple the S spins during t_1, since this will result in $\cos \pi J_{IS}t_1 = 1$, and the $+I_x$ term will not be annihilated. To remove offset-dependent phase shifts during τ and τ', four π-pulses can be employed. These are only necessary when pure absorption mode (phase sensitive) spectra are required. It should be noted that the experiment can be 'tuned' to the magnitude of the scalar coupling by exploiting the condition $\tau = \tau' = (2J_{IS})^{-1}$ as described above. This condition arises simply from the sinusoidal dependence of the antiphase magnetization upon J_{IS}. Since the detected signal depends upon the 'amount' of in-phase magnetization, the transfer function is

H26 $$G_{IS} = \sin(\pi J_{IS}\tau)\sin(\pi J_{IS}\tau').$$

The schemes proposed above have not found great application in biological systems, since the sensitivity is very low due to the detection of rare-spin magnetization. More recently, a series of experiments has been devised which allow for the detection of abundant spins. The sensitivity of heteronuclear COSY is proportional to the **magnetogyric ratio** of the nuclear species excited, since the initial polarization is proportional to the detected signal. The sensitivity is also proportional to $\gamma^{3/2}$ of the observed nucleus, since the observed magnetization is proportional to γ, and the induced e.m.f. is proportional to a second factor γ, while noise increases with $\gamma^{\frac{1}{2}}$. Optimum sensitivity would thus be obtained in an experiment starting with proton polarization and ending with proton detection. While there is no theoretical difficulty in this approach, a considerable drawback is that in natural-abundance, proton-detected COSY experiments, proton resonances not coupled to rare spins must be suppressed by phase cycling. Since such protons are in excess, this latter requisite is difficult to meet with perfection.

The first pulse sequence designed for proton detection was introduced by Müller, and despite various subsequent modifications, the original sequence is in many respects superior. This sequence is shown in Fig. H3. The sequence works as follows. The $90°_x(^1H)-\tau-180°(^1H, ^{13}C)-\tau-$ sequence is 'tuned' by selecting τ such that, at the end of the 2τ period

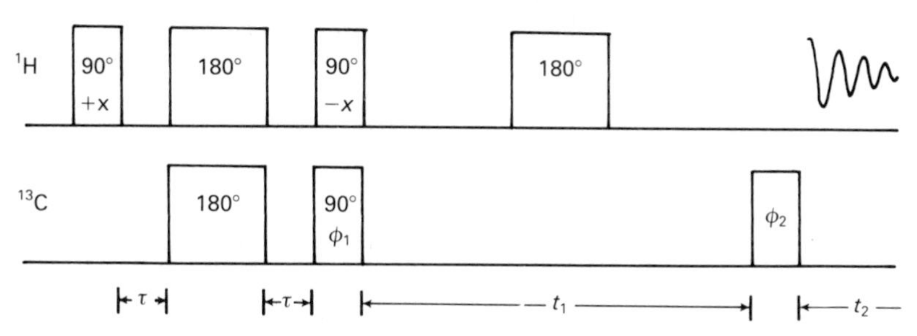

Fig. H3. Pulse sequence for acquisition of heteronuclear COSY spectra with detection of the abundant spin magnetization.

(with refocusing of chemical shifts by the 180° pulses), all protons coupled to an heteronucleus have antiphase magnetization $2I_xS_z$ with respect to J_{IS}. Since the homonuclear couplings J_{II} (assuming $I = {}^1$H) are usually at least an order of magnitude smaller than ${}^1J_{IS}$, all protons attached to ^{12}C will lie essentially along the y axis, and will give in-phase magnetization I_y, since chemical shifts are refocused and little evolution under J_{II} will occur during the relatively small 2τ period. Application of a $90°_{-x}$ pulse on the I spins thus rotates the I_y magnetization (protons attached to ^{12}C) into unobservable z magnetization. Conversely, antiphase $2I_xS_z$ magnetization (protons coupled to ^{13}C) is unaffected by the $90°_{-x}$ pulse. However, at the same time the $90°_{\phi_1}$ pulse on the S spins converts this antiphase magnetization into two-spin coherence, $2I_xS_y$, which evolves during t_1. The 180° I spin pulse in the centre of the t_1 period refocuses the I spin chemical shift evolution, such that signals are labelled with the Larmor frequency of spin S during t_1. The signals are also effectively decoupled during ω_1, since the evolution of multiple-quantum coherence is independent of the coupling J_{IS} (see **product operator formalism**). Finally, a $90°_{\phi_2}$ pulse on the S spins converts the multiple-quantum term $2I_xS_y$ into observable antiphase I spin magnetization $2I_xS_z$ (assuming $\phi_2 = +x$). This give I, S crosspeaks which are antiphase along ω_2 at the I spin frequencies, and decoupled in ω_1 at the S spin frequencies. In phase magnetization along ω_2 can be achieved with an additional refocusing period in exact analogy to the conventional heteronuclear COSY experiment described above. The sequence is repeated as usual with the relevant **phase cycling**, which is

ϕ_1	ϕ_2	R_x
$+x$	$+x$	$+$
$-x$	$+x$	$-$
$+x$	$-x$	$-$
$-x$	$-x$	$+$

In addition, the phases of all 180° pulses may be varied by 180° independently of the four-step cycle. As usual, the sequence is repeated with inclusion of **CYCLOPS**.

FURTHER READING

Bax, A. and Subramian, J. (1986). *J. Magn. Reson.* **67,** 565.
Bax, A. and Summers, M. (1986). *J. Am. Chem. Soc.* **108,** 2093.
Bodenhausen, G. and Ruben, D. J. (1980). *Chem. Phys. Lett.* **69,** 185.
Lerner, L. and Bax, A. (1986). *J. Magn. Reson.* **69,** 375.
Muller, L. (1979). *J. Am. Chem. Soc.* **101,** 4481.

Heteronuclear multiple-bond correlation (HMBC) The HMBC technique is a sensitive method for the determination of long-range (two- and three-bond) ^{1}H-heteronucleus connectivity. When applied to ^{15}N-labelled proteins, the information most frequently sought is correlations between nitrogen and the α proton of the $(i + 1)$ amino acid as well as inter- and intraresidue ^{1}H–^{15}N coupling constants. The technique is also valuable for the sequence analysis of oligosaccharides via long-range ^{1}H–^{13}C connectivities across glycosidic linkages. Two versions of the technique are in general use. The first is a modified version of the **heteronuclear multiple-quantum correlation (HMQC) experiment**, whereas the second is a modified version of the **heteronuclear single-quantum correlation (HSQC) experiment**.

The pulse scheme for the first version of the HMBC experiment is shown in Fig. H4. The first 90° (^{13}C) pulse serves as a low pass J filter, i.e. it suppresses one-bond correlations in the two-dimensional spectrum, and 'passes' long-range correlations with smaller J. This pulse creates heteronuclear **multiple-quantum coherence** for protons which are directly coupled to a ^{13}C nucleus, which is removed from the two-dimensional spectrum by alternating the **phase** of the ^{13}C pulse along the $\pm x$ axis

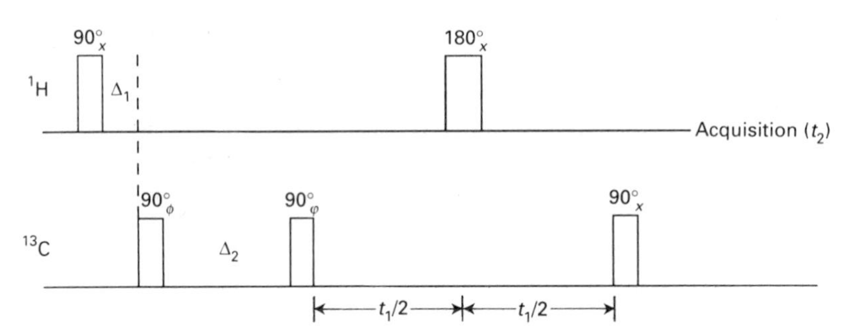

Fig. H4. Pulse scheme for the acquisition of HMBC spectra, based upon the HMQC technique. The delays $\Delta_1 = 1/(2J_{CH})$ where J_{CH} refers to the multiple bond scalar coupling constant and $\Delta_2 \sim 60$ ms. The phase cycling employed is as follows; $\varphi = 2(x), 2(-x), 2(x), 2(-x)$; ψ and receiver $= x, -x, x, -x, y, -y, y, -y$.

without changing the receiver phase. While it is not essential to remove these direct connectivities, the resulting spectrum is simplified at a very small cost in sensitivity. The second 90° (^{13}C) pulse creates ^{1}H–^{13}C multiple- (zero- and double-) quantum coherence for the long-range connectivities. The 180° proton pulse effectively removes the effect of the proton shifts from the t_1 modulation frequency by interchanging the zero- and double-quantum components. Thus, after the final 90° (^{13}C) pulse, the ^{1}H signals that originate from ^{1}H–^{13}C multiple-quantum coherence are modulated by ^{13}C chemical shifts and homonuclear proton couplings. Signals from protons which do not have a long-range coupling to ^{13}C are removed by **phase cycling** of the second 90° (^{13}C) pulse. Since the detected signal is also phase modulated (see **phase modulation**) by the homonuclear scalar coupling, absorptive two-dimensional spectra cannot be recorded and the spectra are usually presented in the **absolute value mode**.

The pulse scheme for the HSQC version of the HMBC experiment is shown in Fig. H5. In contrast to the HMQC experiment, the delay Δ need only be optimized for one-bond couplings. The HSQC version is therefore shorter than its HMQC counterpart, resulting in less attenuation of the final magnetization due to relaxation. In addition, it produces spectra that are pure phase in both dimensions, whereas the HMQC version is of mixed-mode absorption in F_1, as discussed above. Furthermore, the F_1 multiplet of a peak generated in the HSQC version of the experiment only exhibits the antiphase heteronuclear multiplet of the ^{15}N spins that give rise to it, with respect to the couplings active in both heteronuclear coherence-transfer processes. It is thus easier to extract long-range heteronuclear coupling constants. Another significant advantage of the HSQC regime is that solvent presaturation can be used for studies on proteins in H_2O. Whereas all magnetization observed in the HSQC experiment originates from the amide protons, all long-range

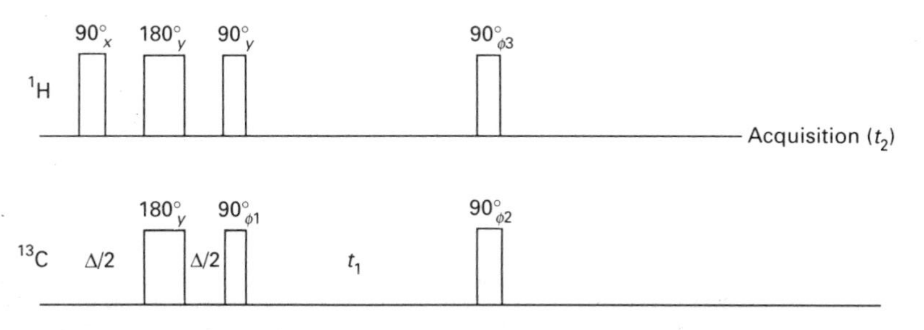

Fig. H5. Pulse scheme for the acquisition of HMBC spectra, based upon the HSQC technique. The delay $\Delta = 1/(2J_{CH})$, where J_{CH} refers to the single-bond scalar-coupling constant. The phase cycling employed is as follows; $\varphi_1 = x, -x$; φ_2 and $\varphi_3 = 8(x), 8(-x)$; receiver $= x, -x, -x, x$.

correlations to α protons observed in the HMQC experiment originate from the α protons themselves, so if these spins are saturated due to their proximity to the water resonance, correlations will not be observed.

FURTHER READING

The HMQC-derived version of the experiment is described in

Bax, A. and Summers, M. F. (1986). *J. Am. Chem. Soc.* **108,** 2093.

A good description of the HSQC-derived version of the experiment is described in

Norwood, T. J., Boyd, J., Heritage, J. E., Soffe, N., and Campbell, I. D. (1990). *J. Magn. Reson.* **87,** 488.

Heteronuclear multiple-quantum correlation (HMQC) HMQC or 'forbidden echo' experiments represent a class of pulse sequences for 'reverse correlation', i.e. heteronuclear correlation with detection of protons. These are all derivatives of experiments proposed originally by Muller (see **Heteronuclear correlation spectroscopy**). A simple but effective version of this sequence is shown in Fig. H6, and the inner workings of this experiment can conveniently be described by use of the **product operator formalism**. For clarity, only terms that contribute to the final spectrum will be discussed. For a heteronuclear **spin system** IS, ($I = {}^1$H, S = heteronucleus), the scheme in Fig. H6 can be described by

$$I_z \xrightarrow{A} -2I_xS_y \xrightarrow{t_1} -2I_xS_y \cos \omega_s t_1 \xrightarrow{B} -I_y \cos \omega_s t_1 \qquad \text{(H27)}$$

where A and B are **operators** representing the effect of the pulse sequence before and after the t_1 period respectively, and the pulse phases are all $+x$. (H27) indicates that the detected in-phase proton signal (I_y) is modulated in amplitude (see **amplitude modulation**) by ω_s, giving rise to a single absorption line in the two-dimensional spectrum.

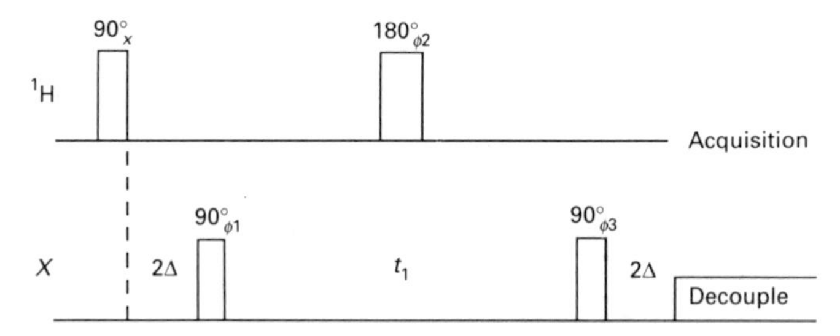

Fig. H6. Scheme for HMQC which requires presaturation of solvent when spectra are recorded in H_2O solution. To minimize relaxation effects, for proteins the delay Δ is usually set to a value ~20% shorter than $1/4(J_{IS})$. The phase cycling is as follows: $\varphi_1 = x, -x$; $\varphi_2 = x, x, y, y, -x, -x, -y, -y$; receiver $= 2(x, -x, -x, x)$. To suppress incomplete steady-state effects, φ_3 is inverted from x to $-x$ after 8 scans, together with the receiver phase. The phase ψ_1 is incremented by 90° in the normal manner to obtain pure phase absorption spectra (see **phase-sensitive experiments**).

In most circumstances of practical interest, the spin system will typically comprise more than one proton. For example, the ^{15}NH–αCH spin subsystem of amino acid residues in ^{15}N-labelled proteins consists of two coupled protons, or three in the case of glycine. It is thus instructive to consider the effect of a second proton M, from which extension to a larger number of protons is then straightforward. The effect of the relatively small homonuclear coupling J_{IM} during the short delays Δ may be neglected. During t_1, dephasing caused by any J_{SM} coupling is refocused by the 180° proton pulse. However, the effect of any J_{IM} coupling is not refocussed, since both coupled nuclei are influenced by the 180° pulse. Thus, the effect of the pulse sequence can be summarized by

H28
$$I_z \xrightarrow{At_1B} -I_y \cos \pi J_{IM} t_1 \cos \omega_s t_1 + 2I_x M_z \sin \pi J_{IM} t_1 \cos \omega_s t_1.$$

The detected signal will thus consist of four multiplet components at $\omega_s \pm \pi J_{IM}$ and $\omega_I \pm \pi J_{IM}$, and will contain both in-phase absorptive (I_y) and antiphase dispersive ($2I_x M_z$) components.

A jump-and-return version (see **solvent suppression**) of the HMQC sequence has been described by Roy *et al.* (Fig. H7) for use in ^{15}N–^{1}H correlation experiments of proteins. At first sight, the only difference from the sequence described above is that no presaturation of the H_2O resonance is required, and that the jump-and-return type pulses introduce a $\sin^3(2\pi\delta T)$ intensity dependence in the F_2 dimension, where δ is the offset from the H_2O frequency and T is the delay in the jump-and-return sequence. However, the situation is more complicated because CαH protons, which typically resonate in the vicinity of the H_2O resonance, are not inverted by the 90°_φ–2τ–$90^\circ_{-\varphi}$ sequence at the

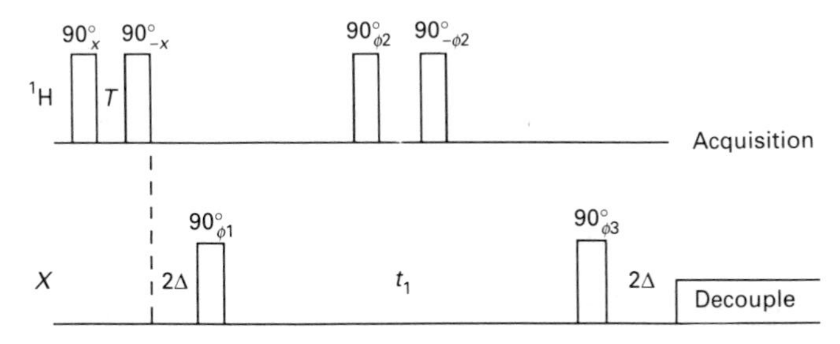

Fig. H7. Scheme for HMQC incorporating jump-and-return sequences for solvent suppression. To minimize relaxation effects, for proteins the delay Δ is usually set to a value ~20% shorter than $1/4(J_{IS})$. The phase cycling is as follows: $\varphi_1 = x, -x$; $\varphi_2 = x, x, y, y, -x, -x, -y, -y$; receiver $= 2(x, -x, -x, x)$. To suppress incomplete steady-state effects, φ_3 is inverted from x to $-x$ after 8 scans, together with the receiver phase. The phase ψ_1 is incremented by 90° in the normal manner to obtain pure phase absorption spectra (see **phase-sensitive experiments**).

midpoint of t_1. Hence the effect of homonuclear coupling with the NH protons is refocused and no homonuclear splittings appear in F_1. However, long-range heteronuclear couplings between ^{15}N and CαH and CβH protons which are not inverted by the $90^\circ_\varphi - 2\tau - 90^\circ_{-\varphi}$ sequence, remain. The relevant terms during the magnetization transfer process are summarized by

H29 $$I_z \xrightarrow{At_1} -2I_x S_y \cos \omega_s t_1 \cos \pi J_{NM} t_1 \xrightarrow{B} -I_y \cos \omega_s t_1 \cos \pi J_{NM} t_1.$$

This expression indicates that a purely absorptive signal (I_y) is obtained, with J couplings J_{NM} between ^{15}N and the CαH (and CβH) protons which resonate in the vicinity of the H_2O frequency.

The available resolution in the F_1 dimension for each of these experiments is poorer than that available using **heteronuclear single-quantum correlation** (HSQC) methods. The primary reason for this difference lies in the homonuclear splittings and mixed-mode lineshapes in F_1 obtained using the sequence in Fig. H6, and the presence of often unresolved long-range splittings in F_1 obtained using the sequence in Fig. H7. None of these splittings is found in F_1 with HSQC methods. However, the available resolution is also limited by the inherent resonance linewidths, which are greater in the HMQC experiment due to the different relaxation properties of the multiple-quantum coherence. For proteins at field strengths above $10T$, and neglecting S–M **dipolar coupling, cross-correlation**, and **chemical shift anisotropy**, the transverse relaxation (see **spin–spin relaxation**) of the I spin (^1H), S spin (heteronucleus) and multiple-quantum coherence are given by

H30 $$\begin{aligned} 1/T_{2I} &= (1/10)D_{IS}^2[2J(0) + 3J(\omega_S)] + (1/4)J(0)\sum_M D_{IM}^2 \\ 1/T_{2S} &= (1/20)D_{IS}^2[4J(0) + 3J(\omega_S)] \\ 1/T_{2MQ} &= (1/4)J(0)\sum_M D_{IM}^2 + (3/20)J(\omega_S)D_{IS}^2 \end{aligned}$$

where the spectral density functions (see **relaxation**) $J(\omega) = \tau_c/(1 + \omega^2\tau_c^2)$, and τ_c is the **correlation time**. The constant $D_{IS} = h\gamma_I\gamma_S/(2\pi r_{IS}^3)$, h is Planck's constant, γ_I and γ_S are the magnetogyric ratios of spins I and S respectively, and r_{IS} is the I–S internuclear distance. The constant $D_{IM} = h\gamma_I^2/(2\pi r_{IM}^3)$ represents the homonuclear dipolar interaction between spin I and spin M.

The ^1H–^1H dipolar broadening (D_{IM}) of the multiple-quantum coherence is stronger than the heteronuclear dipolar broadening (D_{IS}) of ^{15}N, and hence the transverse relaxation rate, and thus linewidths of the resonances, will be greater in F_1 for the HMQC experiment. In the case of ^{13}C, the heteronuclear dipolar interaction is much larger, and the ^1H–^{13}C multiple-quantum relaxation is slower than the ^{13}C relaxation, suggesting that ^{13}C–^{1}H HMQC experiments should give better F_1 resolution than their HSQC counterparts. However, the presence of ^{1}H–^{1}H J couplings in F_1 destroy this advantage, and ^{13}C–^{1}H HSQC experiments may still show a resolution advantage in comparison with HMQC methods.

FURTHER READING

The reader is referred to two very useful articles which compare HMQC methods with their HSQC counterparts:

Bax, A., Ikura, M., Kay, L. E., Torchia, D. A., and Tschudin, R. (1990). *J. Magn. Reson.* **86,** 304.

Norwood, T. J., Boyd, J., Heritage, J. E., Soffe, N., and Campbell, I. D. (1990). *J. Magn. Reson.* **87,** 488.

The 'jump-and-return' version of HMQC is described in

Roy, S., Papastavros, M. Z., Sanchez, V., and Redfield, A. G. (1984). *Biochem.* **23,** 4395.

Heteronuclear NMR Homonuclear NMR experiments, i.e. those concerned with the perturbation and observation of a single nucleus type, can provide a great deal of information on structure and dynamics in biomolecules. However, a class of experiments generally called heteronuclear NMR can provide additional information which is difficult to achieve from homonuclear methods. Essentially, a heteronuclear NMR experiment involves the perturbation of more than one nuclear type in a single experiment. Thus a simple heteronuclear experiment consists of the detection of ^{13}C NMR signals in the presence of broadband proton decoupling. More specifically we can define a series of two-dimensional heteronuclear NMR experiments in analogy to their homonuclear counterparts. Before describing these, it is important to distinguish a class of experiments which have evolved from two-dimensional NMR techniques but which are strictly one-dimensional experiments. These are the spectral editing techniques, such as **INEPT** and **DEPT**, which are very successful in distinguishing between, for example, carbon nuclei coupled to a variable number of protons. These are described under the relevant headings.

In essence, the theoretical aspects of heteronuclear two-dimensional experiments are equivalent to their homonuclear counterparts (see e.g. **heteronuclear correlation spectroscopy**). The only difference lies in the fact that the chemical shift separation between heteronuclei is much greater than that for homonuclei. Thus, whilst the concept of the correlation of ^{13}C with ^{1}H chemical shifts in a two-dimensional experiment is at first sight somewhat daunting, there is no inherent difference between this and a ^{1}H–^{1}H COSY experiment. Indeed, the large chemical shift separation precludes the occurrence of strong coupling between correlated spin pairs, and thus the weak coupling approximation is always valid between heteronuclei. Another useful aspect is that it is possible to achieve broadband decoupling of a given nuclear type without perturbation of the other. Thus, a ^{13}C–^{1}H correlation spectrum with broadband proton decoupling is perfectly feasible.

The presence of two nuclear types raises the question as to which should be detected. In the past this has invariably been the rare nucleus, due to the difficulty in suppressing unwanted signals from the abundant nuclei, which in the case of ^{13}C–^{1}H spectroscopy are many times stronger. However, this approach does limit the sensitivity of the experiment. In the case of biological NMR, this limitation has prevented the application of the majority of heteronuclear experiments unless selective enrichment is employed. For this reason a new class of experiments has been devised whereby the abundant spin is detected. This has allowed heteronuclear correlation experiments to be performed at natural abundance upon macromolecules at reasonable sample concentration.

FURTHER READING

See references under heteronuclear correlation spectroscopy (p. 144).

Heteronuclear single-quantum correlation (HSQC) The large number of different pulse sequences proposed for 'reverse correlation' (i.e. heteronuclear correlation with detection of protons, see **heteronuclear correlation spectroscopy**) can essentially be divided into two types: those which utilize **heteronuclear multiple-quantum coherence** (HMQC) during the evolution period t_1, and those which rely upon transverse magnetization of the low **magnetogyric ratio** nucleus during t_1. The latter class of experiments are sometimes called heteronuclear single-quantum correlation experiments (HSQC).

Most of the HSQC experiments are variations on an experiment first proposed by Bodenhausen and Ruben. This experiment employs two INEPT-type transfers (see **insensitive nuclei enhanced by polarization transfer**) to transfer magnetization from the protons to the low-γ nucleus and back to the protons. The enhancement in sensitivity over conventional **heteronuclear correlation spectroscopy** which is made possible with this scheme is much greater than that obtainable by exploitation of the nuclear Overhauser effect, and therefore it has been referred to as the Overbodenhausen experiment.

The HSQC pulse scheme (Fig. H8) employs an INEPT sequence to transfer ^{1}H magnetization I_z into antiphase ^{15}N magnetization. ^{1}H decoupling during t_1 is accomplished in the standard manner by the application of a 180° pulse at the midpoint of t_1. A subsequent INEPT

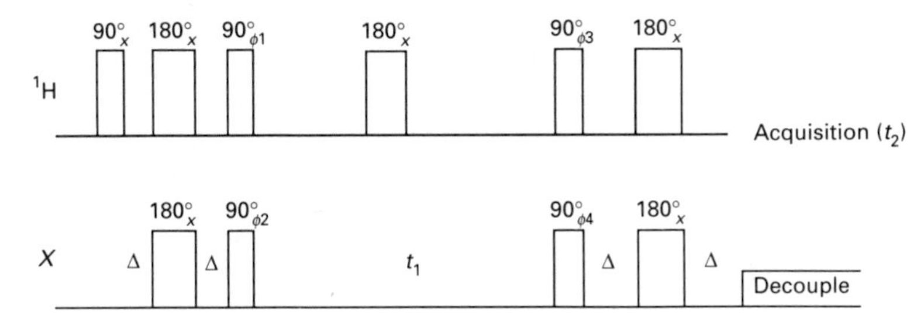

Fig. H8. Pulse scheme for HSQC utilizing single-quantum X-nucleus coherence during t_1. The phase cycling is as follows; $\varphi_1 = y, -y$; $\varphi_2 = 2(x), 2(-x)$; $\varphi_3 = 4(x), 4(-x)$; receiver $= x, -x, -x, x, 2(-x, x, x, -x), x, -x, -x, x$; $\varphi_4 = 8(x), 8(-x)$. To minimize relaxation effects, for proteins the delay Δ is usually set to a value ~20% shorter than $1/(4J_{IS})$. The phase φ_2 is incremented by 90° in the normal manner to obtain pure phase absorption spectra (see **phase-sensitive experiments**).

transfer reconverts the transverse ^{15}N magnetization into observable ^{1}H magnetization. The complete process can be analysed for a two **spin system** IS ($I = {}^1$H, $S =$ heteronucleus) by use of the **product operator formalism**:

$$I_z \xrightarrow{\text{INEPT}} -2I_zS_y \xrightarrow{t_1} -2I_zS_y \cos \omega_S t_1 \xrightarrow{\text{reverse INEPT}} -I_x \cos \omega_S t_1 \quad \text{(H31)}$$

where for clarity only those terms that contribute to the final spectrum are retained, and pulse phases corresponding to the first step of the phase cycle (Fig. H8) are assumed. Equation H31 indicates that pure absorptive lineshapes can be obtained. The F_1 linewidth is significantly narrower in comparison with **heteronuclear multiple-quantum correlation** (HMQC) type experiments, since it is not affected by ^{1}H–^{1}H or ^{1}H-heteronuclear J couplings, and neglecting static field inhomogeneity, it is solely determined by the average relaxation rate of S_x and I_zS_y. The **spin–spin**

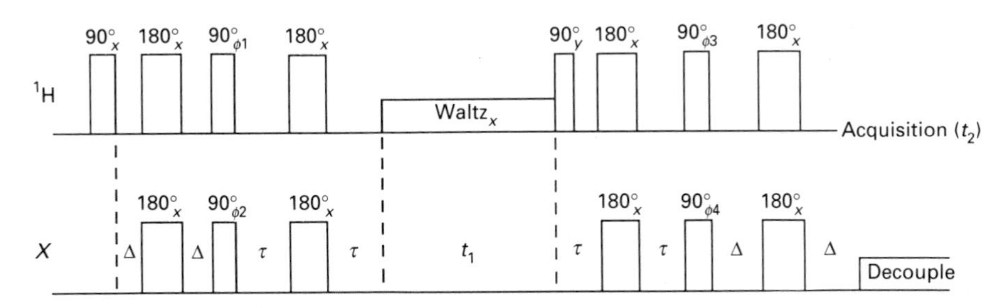

Fig. H9. Pulse scheme for HSQC incorporating a composite pulse decoupling scheme preceded by a refocussing interval $2\tau = 1/(2J_{IS})$, and followed by a defocussing period of duration 2τ. The phase cycling is as follows; $\varphi_1 = y, -y$; $\varphi_2 = 2(x), 2(-x)$; $\varphi_3 = 4(x), 4(-x)$; receiver $= x, -x, -x, x, 2(-x, x, x, -x), x, -x, -x, x$; $\varphi_4 = 8(x), 8(-x)$. After 16 scans, the phase of the first 180° (x) pulse following t_1 is inverted, without changing the receiver phase. To minimize relaxation effects, for proteins the delay Δ is usually set to a value ~20% shorter than $1/(4J_{IS})$.

relaxation rate of I_zS_y corresponds to the sum of the rate of decay of S_y (the reciprocal of the spin–spin relaxation time of the heteronucleus) and the **spin–lattice relaxation** rate of I_z. The latter contribution is essentially scalar relaxation of the second kind (see **scalar coupling relaxation**). Whenever I_z changes its spin state, the heteronuclear doublet component changes its frequency by J_{IS}. Thus the F_1 linewidth corresponds to the linewidth of a ^1H coupled heteronucleus. Narrower lines without the scalar relaxation broadening can be obtained by decoupling the protons during t_1 using the modified pulse sequence of Fig. H9. For a more detailed comparison of HMQC with HSQC methods, see **heteronuclear multiple-quantum correlation**.

FURTHER READING

Bodenhausen, G. and Reuben, D. J., (1980). *Chem. Phys. Lett.* **69,** 185.

The reader is also referred to two very useful articles which compare HSQC methods with their HMQC counterparts:

Bax, A., Ikura, M., Kay, L. E., Torchia, D. A., and Tschudin, R. (1990). *J. Magn. Reson.* **86,** 304.

Norwood, T. J., Boyd, J., Heritage, J. E., Soffe, N., and Campbell, I. D. (1990). *J. Magn. Reson.* **87,** 488.

High-field approximation Consider two scalar coupled nuclei IS in a static magnetic field. The **Hamiltonian** for this system can be written as the sum of the Zeeman Hamiltonian $\mathcal{H}_Z$, which represents the interaction of the spins with the magnetic field, and the scalar (J) coupling Hamiltonian $\mathcal{H}_J$, representing the interaction of the spins with each other indirectly via bonding electrons:

H32 $$\mathcal{H} = \mathcal{H}_Z + \mathcal{H}_J = \omega_I I_z + \omega_S S_z + 2\pi J_{IS}\mathbf{I}\cdot\mathbf{S}$$

where ω_I and ω_S are the **Larmor precession** frequencies of the nuclei I and S respectively, I_z and S_z are the z-component spin **angular momentum** operators, J_{IS} is the spin-coupling constant, and $\mathbf{I}$, $\mathbf{S}$ are the total angular momentum operators for spins I and S, respectively. Given that

$$\mathbf{I} = (I_x \quad I_y \quad I_z) \text{ is a row vector,}$$

and

H33 $$\mathbf{S} = \begin{bmatrix} S_x \\ S_y \\ S_z \end{bmatrix} \text{ is a column vector,}$$

(H32) can be expanded:

H34 $$\mathcal{H} = \omega_I I_z + \omega_S S_z + 2\pi J(I_xS_x + I_yS_y + I_zS_z).$$

If we form the **matrix representation** of (H34), using as **basis states** the

1 $|\alpha\alpha>$

3 $|\beta\alpha>$ $|\alpha\beta>$ 2

4 $|\beta\beta>$

Fig. H10. The basis states of two weakly coupled protons *IS*.

wavefunctions for a two-spin system (where we use the **bra-ket notation** Fig. H10) we obtain the following result:

$$\begin{bmatrix} \frac{1}{2}(\omega_I+\omega_S)+\frac{1}{4}J & 0 & 0 & 0 \\ 0 & \frac{1}{2}(\omega_I-\omega_S)-\frac{1}{4}J & \frac{1}{2}J & 0 \\ 0 & \frac{1}{2}J & \frac{1}{2}(-\omega_I+\omega_S)-\frac{1}{4}J & 0 \\ 0 & 0 & 0 & \frac{1}{2}(-\omega_I-\omega_S)+\frac{1}{4}J \end{bmatrix}. \tag{H35}$$

In high magnetic fields, the off-diagonal elements of matrix (H35) become much smaller than the diagonal elements, $(\omega_I-\omega_S)\gg J_{IS}$, and can be neglected. In terms of the Hamiltonian (H34), this is equivalent to neglecting the terms I_xS_x and I_yS_y, and the truncated (sometimes called **weak coupling**) Hamiltonian in this high-field approximation is therefore

$$\mathcal{H}=\omega_I I_z+\omega_S S_z+2\pi J I_z S_z. \tag{H36}$$

The high-field approximation is equivalent to the weak coupling approximation, since the σ_{23} and σ_{32} elements of (H35), which are responsible for the mixing of states $|\alpha\beta\rangle$ and $|\beta\alpha\rangle$ in the **strong coupling** case, are neglected. Note that under this approximation, the matrix of the Hamiltonian is diagonal, and thus the product functions in Fig. H10 correspond to the **eigenbasis** in the limit of weak coupling. Of course, this approach is only an approximation and we may ask what are the consequences of neglecting the off-diagonal elements of (H35) in practical calculations. If, for example, we were to calculate the signal intensities and transition frequencies for a weakly coupled two-spin system *IS*, assuming the high-field approximation, we might obtain the result in Fig. H11. In the practical case, however, we find that the intensities of the lines are not exactly equal (see Fig. H12). The degree of inequality becomes progressively worse as ω_I approaches ω_S, since the

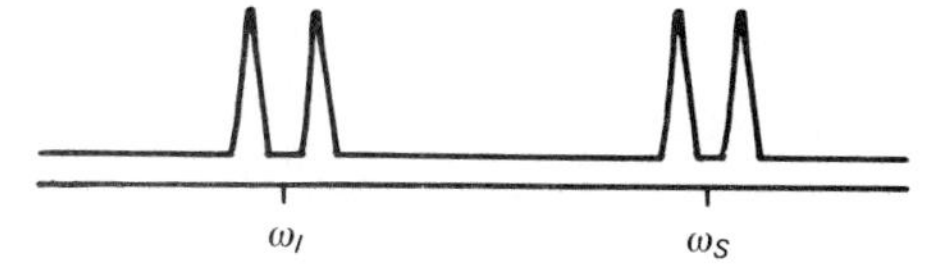

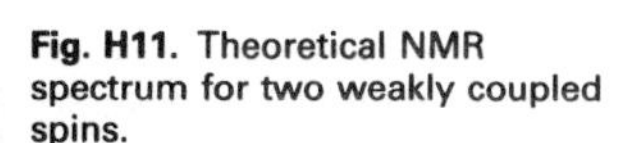
Fig. H11. Theoretical NMR spectrum for two weakly coupled spins.

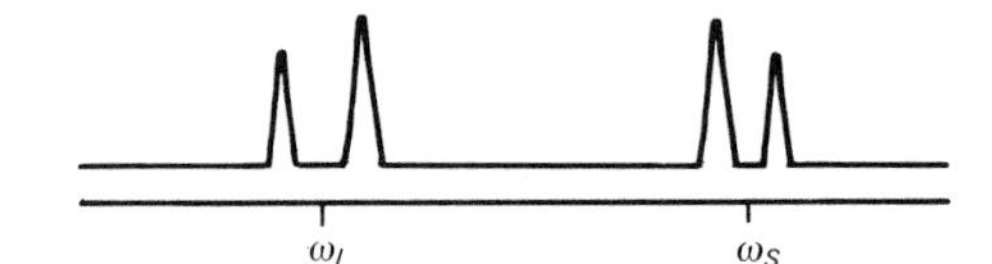

Fig. H12. Diagrammatic representation of experimental spectrum corresponding to Fig. H11, illustrating the effect of the high-field approximation.

spins become more strongly coupled, and the approximation becomes invalid. In addition, we find different transition frequencies as ω_I approaches ω_S. However, in those cases where $(\omega_I - \omega_S) > \sim 10\, J_{IS}$, the approximation is a good one.

Hilbert space Consider a vector plotted with respect to three orthogonal axes, x, y, z (see Fig. H13). We can define the direction of the vector in the cartesian coordinate system with respect to the three axes x, y, z; $x = 2$, $y = 1$, $z = 3$. We can simplify this even further by writing the coordinates in a linear fashion

H37 $$(2 \quad 1 \quad 3)$$

where the labels x, y, z are implied. In fact, we can define the position of any vector using the generalized notation

H38 $$(x \quad y \quad z).$$

This somewhat trivial explanation allows us to define (H38) as a vector mapped in three-dimensional space. If we now define another vector, such as

H39 $$(v \quad w \quad x \quad y \quad z)$$

then (H39) describes another vector, but in five-dimensional space. This is obviously impossible to visualize, but it does allow us to define a generalized n-dimensional space, often termed **Hilbert space**, within which we can 'visualize' in mathematical terms the relationships between vectors. For example, the orthogonality of a basis set (see **basis state**) of n wavefunctions can be 'visualized' in terms of the n-dimensional Hilbert space which they span.

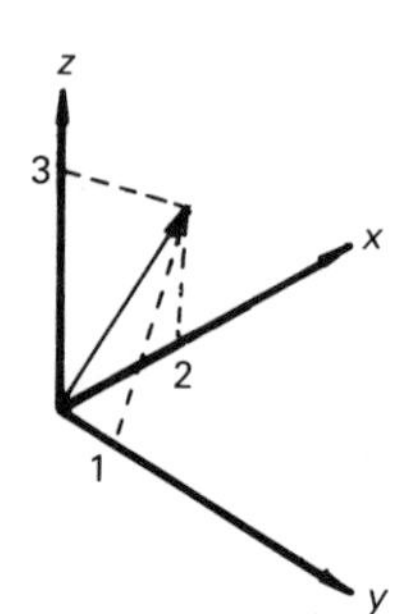

Fig. H13. An arbitrary vector in cartesian space can be specified with respect to three orthogonal axes *x*, *y*, and *z*.

Hilbert transform The Hilbert transform of a function $f(x)$ can be described as the **convolution** of $f(x)$ by the function $(\pi x)^{-1}$:

H40 $$F_{\mathrm{Hi}}(x) = \frac{-1}{\pi x} * f(x).$$

The Fourier transform of $(-\pi x)^{-1}$ is a signum function, $i \,.\, \mathrm{sgn} \,.\, s$, where s is the co-domain function of x; sgn has the value -1 for $x < 0$, and $+1$ for $x > 0$, see Fig. H14. Thus if we multiply the **Fourier transform** of $g(x)$ by $i \,.\, \mathrm{sgn} \,.\, s$, and Fourier transform the result, the convolution theorem dictates that the result will be $F_{\mathrm{Hi}}(x)$. The Hilbert transform is of importance in NMR in that the real and imaginary parts (see **complex number**) of the NMR spectrum are Hilbert transform pairs. Consider a real function $f(t)$. This has an associated complex function

H41 $$f(t) - iF_{\mathrm{Hi}}(t),$$

whose real part is $f(t)$. This complex function is known as the analytical signal, and the Hilbert transform is known as the quadrature function of $f(t)$. In NMR, the quadrature function of $\cos \omega t$ is $-\sin \omega t$, and the corresponding analytical signal is $\exp(\mathrm{i}\omega t)$. This function is a component of the complex free induction decay obtained from **quadrature detection**.

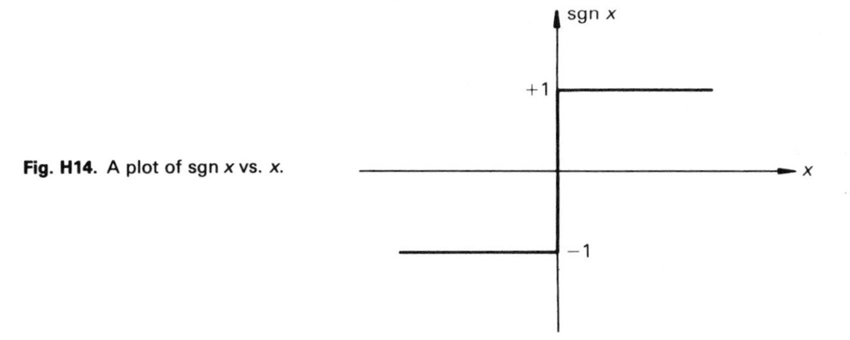

Fig. H14. A plot of sgn x vs. x.

FURTHER READING

Bracewell, R. M. (1965). *The Fourier transform and its applications.* McGraw-Hill, New York.

HMQC–COSY The HMQC–COSY experiment is a combination of a **heteronuclear multiple-quantum correlation** (HMQC) experiment and **correlated spectroscopy** (COSY). The pulse scheme is shown in Fig. H15. In addition to the single-bond ^{1}H-heteronucleus crosspeaks of the basic experiment, HMQC–COSY spectra exhibit homonuclear proton correlation peaks from heteronucleus-bonded protons. For example, in the case of a ^{15}N-labelled protein, each amino acid residue (except proline) would

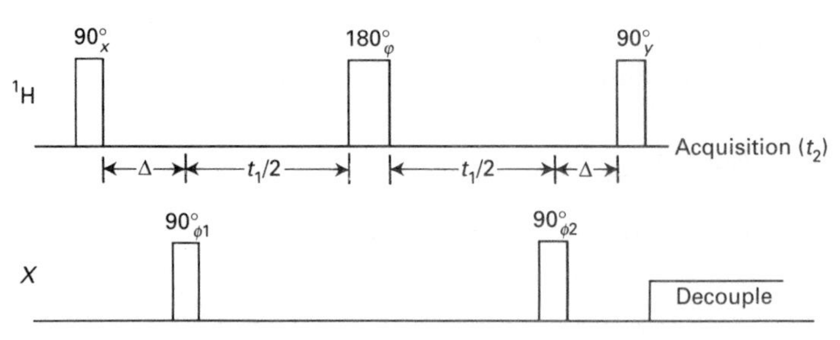

Fig. H15. Pulse scheme for HMQC–COSY. In order to minimize relaxation effects, the delay Δ is set to a value slightly shorter than $1/(2J_{XH})$, where J_{XH} is the single-bond heteronuclear scalar coupling constant. The phase cycling employed is as follows: $\psi = 2(x)$, $2(-x)$; $\varphi_1 = x, -x$; $\varphi_2 = 4(x), 4(-x)$; receiver $= 2(x, -x), 2(-x, x)$. To obtain a pure phase absorption spectrum in F_1, the phase φ_1 is incremented by 90° in the manner common to all **phase-sensitive experiments**.

give rise to a peak between the amide proton and its bonded nitrogen and, at the same nitrogen frequency, a correlation to the α proton in antiphase with respect to the active proton coupling in F_2. As with a COSY spectrum these two types of peak will be 90° out of phase in F_2. Homonuclear coherence transfer is brought about by the final 90° proton pulse, and this will only be effective if a substantial amount of homonuclear proton scalar coupling evolution has occurred prior to the pulse. As in a conventional COSY experiment, this occurs during the t_1 evolution period, which thus gives rise to F_1 multiplet structure. To minimize spectral crowding and to maximize sensitivity it is essential to remove the heteronuclear coupling in both frequency dimensions. In F_2 this can be achieved by irradiation of the ^{15}N nuclei with an efficient **broadband decoupling** sequence. In F_1, ^1H-heteronuclear zero- and double-quantum coherence (see **multiple-quantum coherence**) is present. The 180° proton pulse at the centre of t_1 interchanges zero- and double-quantum coherence, resulting in observed resonances which appear only to be modulated by the heteronuclear shift. In the case of NH_2 groups in ^{15}N-labelled proteins, the zero- and double-quantum coherences are modulated by the passive J coupling to the second proton. Ideally, the effect of this coupling is also removed by the 180° proton pulse. However, r.f. inhomogeneity prevents perfect inversion of the passive proton, and consequently a low-intensity doublet superimposed on the decoupled singlet resonance is often observed for NH_2 correlations.

FURTHER READING

The HMQC–COSY experiment is described in

Clore, G. M., Bax, A., Wingfield, P., and Gronenborn, A. M. (1988). *FEBS Lett.* **238,** 17.

HMQC–HOHAHA The HMQC–HOHAHA experiment is a combination of a **heteronuclear multiple-quantum correlation** (HMQC) experiment and **homonuclear Hartmann–Hahn spectroscopy** (HOHAHA). The pulse scheme is shown in Fig. H16. In addition to the single-bond ^{1}H-heteronucleus crosspeaks of the basic experiment, HMQC–HOHAHA spectra exhibit homonuclear proton correlation peaks from heteronucleus-bonded protons. For example, in the case of a ^{15}N labelled protein, each amino acid residue (except proline) would give rise to a peak between the amide proton and its bonded nitrogen and, at the same nitrogen frequency, a correlation to the α proton, and to other protons depending upon the length of the spin-lock time. In common with conventional HOHAHA, all peaks are approximately in phase. To minimize spectral crowding and to maximize sensitivity it is essential to remove the heteronuclear coupling in both frequency dimensions. In F_2 this can be achieved by irradiation of the ^{15}N nuclei with an efficient **broadband decoupling** sequence. In F_1, ^{1}H-heteronuclear zero- and double-quantum coherence (see **multiple-quantum coherence**) is present. The 180° proton pulse at the centre of t_1 interchanges zero- and double-quantum coherence, resulting in observed resonances which appear only to be modulated by the heteronuclear shift. In the case of NH_2 groups in ^{15}N-labelled proteins, the zero- and double-quantum coherences are modulated by the passive J coupling to the second proton. Ideally, the effect of this coupling is also removed by the 180° proton pulse. However, r.f. inhomogeneity prevents perfect inversion of the passive proton, and consequently a low-intensity doublet superimposed on the decoupled singlet resonance is often observed for NH_2 correlations.

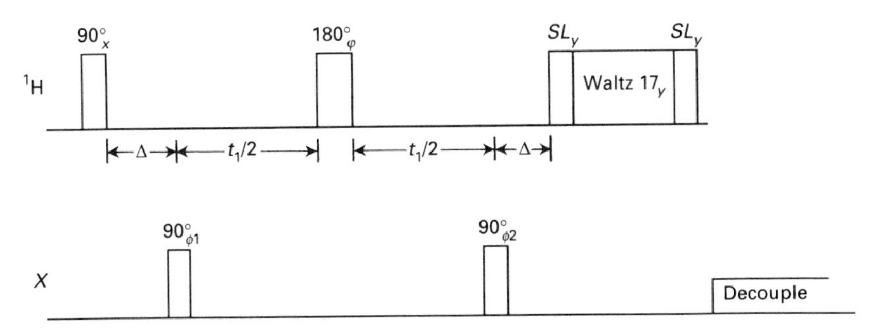

Fig. H16. Pulse scheme for HMQC–HOHAHA. In order to minimize relaxation effects, the delay Δ is set to a value slightly shorter than $1/(2J_{XH})$, where J_{XH} is the single bond heteronuclear scalar coupling constant. The phase cycling employed is as follows; $\psi = 2(x), 2(-x)$; $\varphi_1 = x, -x$; $\varphi_2 = 4(x), 4(-x)$; receiver $= 2(x, -x), 2(-x, x)$. To obtain a pure phase absorption spectrum in F_1, the phase φ_1 is incremented by 90° in the manner common to all **phase-sensitive experiments**.

FURTHER READING

The HMQC–HOHAHA experiment is described in

Gronenborn, A. M., Bax, A., Wingfield, P. T., and Clore, G. M. (1988). *FEBS Lett.* **243,** 93.

HMQC–NOESY The HMQC–NOESY experiment is a combination of a **heteronuclear multiple-quantum correlation** (HMQC) experiment and **nuclear Overhauser effect spectroscopy** (NOESY). The pulse scheme is shown in Fig. H17. In addition to the crosspeaks correlating ^1H shifts to the directly-bonded heteronucleus, HMQC–NOESY spectra display homonuclear ^1H proton **nuclear Overhauser effect** (NOE) peaks. This technique has found its primary application in the assignment of ^{15}N-labelled proteins. In these cases, an NOE peak will occur at the nitrogen frequency in F_1 of the crosspeak of the amide proton from which it originates, but at the proton frequency in F_2 of the spin magnetization to which it is transferred. A correlation between two amide protons is thus characterized by four peaks located at the corners of a rectangle. The conventional HMQC peaks and the two NOE peaks each occur at opposite corners of the rectangle. The spectrum thus lacks the plane of symmetry found in conventional homonuclear NOESY spectra. This is advantageous since the probability that a given correlation between two amide protons will be observed is increased: if one correlation is obscured by overlap, the other may still be observable. However, a correlation between two amide protons will always be unresolved if either the nitrogen or the proton frequencies of the two corresponding conventional HMQC peaks are degenerate. Significantly greater resolution can be obtained by extending the experiment into three dimensions (see **three-dimensional NMR**), giving **three-dimensional NOESY–HMQC.** To minimize spectral crowding and to maximize sensitivity it is essential

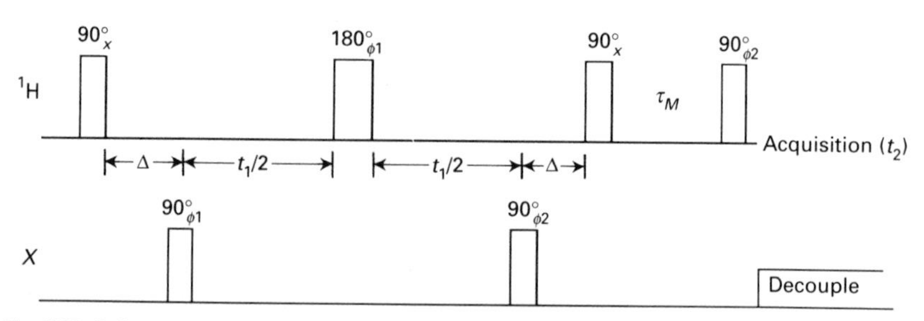

Fig. H17. Pulse scheme for HMQC–NOESY. The optimal value of Δ is $1/(2J_{HX})$, where J_{HX} is the single-bond heteronuclear scalar coupling. The phase cycling employed is: $\varphi_1 = 2(x), 2(-x)$; $\varphi_2 = 4(x), 4(y), 4(-x), 4(-y)$; $\psi_1 = x, -x$; $\psi_2 = x$ (and may be inverted together with the receiver phase after the basic phase cycle is completed); receiver $= 2(x, -x), 2(y, -y), 2(-x, x), 2(-y, y)$. To avoid effects of an incomplete steady state, the phase ψ_2 and the receiver phase may be inverted after completion of the above cycle. The phase ψ_1 is incremented by 90° in the normal manner to obtain pure phase absorption spectra (see **phase-sensitive experiments**).

to remove the heteronuclear coupling in both frequency dimensions. In F_2 this can be achieved by irradiation of the ^{15}N nuclei with an efficient **broadband decoupling** sequence. In F_1, ^1H-heteronuclear zero and double-quantum coherence is present. The 180° proton pulse at the centre of t_1 interchanges zero- and double-quantum coherence, resulting in observed resonances which appear only to be modulated by the heteronuclear shift. In the case of NH_2 groups in ^{15}N-labelled proteins, the zero- and double-quantum coherences are modulated by the passive J coupling to the second proton. Ideally, the effect of this coupling is also removed by the 180° proton pulse. However, **radio frequency** field inhomogeneity prevents perfect inversion of the passive proton, and consequently a low-intensity doublet superimposed on the decoupled singlet resonance is often observed for NH_2 correlations.

FURTHER READING

The HMQC–NOESY experiment is described by

Gronenborn, A. M., Bax, A., Wingfield, P. T., and Clore, G. M. (1989). *FEBS Lett.* **243,** 93.

HOHAHA See **homonuclear Hartmann–Hahn spectroscopy**.

Homonuclear Hartmann–Hahn spectroscopy (HOHAHA) Homonuclear Hartmann–Hahn spectroscopy (HOHAHA) can be thought of as an alternative version of **correlated spectroscopy** (COSY). However, the method has important additional advantages over COSY. These result from the fact that the mechanism of **coherence transfer** in HOHAHA and in COSY is fundamentally different. The method relies on the principle of **cross-polarization**. In the simplest case cross-polarization can be obtained using a single coherent r.f. field. If the effective r.f. fields experienced by two spins are identical, the **Hartmann–Hahn condition** is established, giving rise to oscillatory exchange of spin-locked magnetization between spins. For a simple two-spin AX system, complete exchange is obtained for a spin-lock time equal to $(2J_{AX})^{-1}$. This is analogous to the closely related **total correlation spectroscopy** (TOCSY) experiment. For large spin systems the time dependence of exchange is very complicated and there is no simple analytical solution. The simplest pulse scheme for this experiment is shown in Fig. H18. It is convenient to perform this experiment in the phase-sensitive mode (see **phase-sensitive**

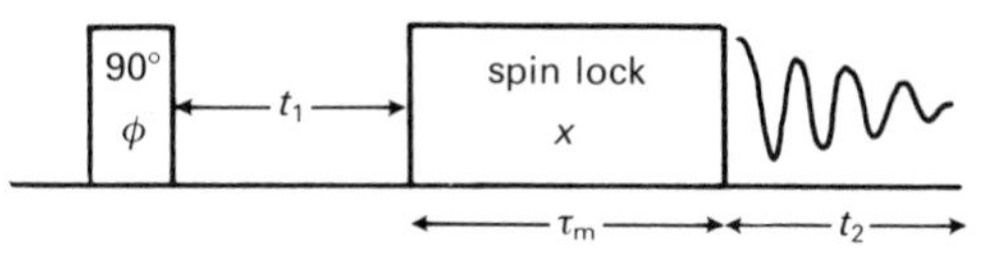

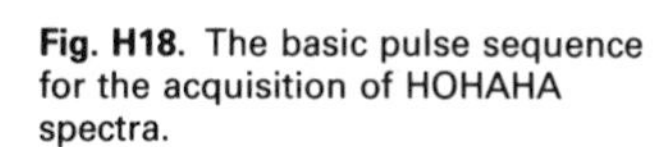

Fig. H18. The basic pulse sequence for the acquisition of HOHAHA spectra.

experiments), in which case the phase cycling scheme is

ϕ	receiver	
$+x$	+	location 1
$-x$	+	
$+y$	+	location 2
$-y$	+	

As usual, this sequence is repeated four times with phase incrementation for **CYCLOPS** phase cycling, resulting in a total of 16 n scans per t_1 increment.

An advantage of cross-polarization coherence transfer is that net magnetization transfer occurs, by analogy with the TOCSY experiment. In principle, therefore, all peaks in the spectrum can be obtained in near-absorption mode. This situation is different from that observed in COSY experiments, where crosspeak multiplets are 180° out of phase since no net coherence transfer is achieved. Therefore the undesirable cancellations which may occur in crosspeak multiplets in COSY under certain conditions (see **correlated spectroscopy**) do not occur in HOHAHA, and it is possible, for example, to find detectable crosspeaks from resonances which are J coupled with a magnitude much less than the linewidths. Another consequence of net coherence transfer is the appearance of relay and multiple relay peaks in the spectrum. The number of relay peaks is related to the spin-lock time. Although multiple-relay can be achieved using conventional coherence transfer methods (see **relayed correlation spectroscopy**), HOHAHA yields the important advantage that the efficiency of relayed transfer is not particularly sensitive to spin coupling topography. For example, it is possible to relay magnetization through strongly coupled systems using HOHAHA, a procedure which is difficult using conventional relayed correlation spectroscopy.

On a practical level, the simple scheme in Fig. H18 is unlikely to give good results since the r.f. field generated by a single coherent field of fixed phase has a severe offset dependence. As shown by Bax *et al.* (1985), this can be alleviated by switching the phase of the spin-lock field by 180° periodically (see Fig. H19). The total number of $+x$ vs. $-x$ periods differ to prevent the formation of **rotary echoes**, which would introduce undesirable lineshape distortions since the r.f. field inhomogeneity effects would be refocused (see **total correlation spectroscopy**). A still more efficient spin-lock sequence involves the application of the WALTZ or MLEV decoupling sequence (see **broadband decoupling**). In each of these modifications, the desired effect is to achieve efficient spin-locking of resonances which are far off-

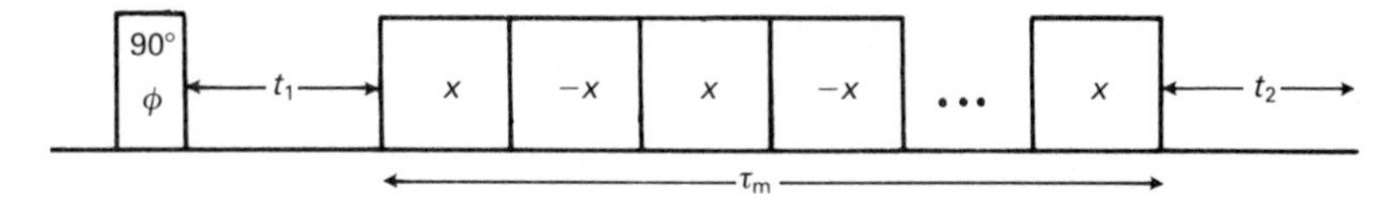

Fig. H19. Pulse sequence with modified spin-lock period to increase the bandwidth and to prevent the formation of rotary echoes.

resonance, and which do not have equal (but opposite) offsets from the transmitter carrier, a situation which will generally be found in practical experiments on macromolecules.

The HOHAHA sequence is essentially identical to that used for **rotating frame Overhauser effect spectroscopy** (ROESY). However, for the small spin-lock times usually employed in HOHAHA, ROESY crosspeaks are small. In addition, the latter appear with opposite phase to HOHAHA crosspeaks and can therefore be distinguished easily.

FURTHER READING

Bax, A., Davies, D. G., and Sarkar, S. K. (1985). *J. Magn. Reson.* **63,** 230.

Hypercomplex Fourier transformation See **phase-sensitive experiments**.

I

Identity operator The identity operator, often abbreviated **1** or E, is an operator which leaves the wavefunction upon which it operates unaffected:

I1 $$\mathbf{1}\,|\psi\rangle = |\psi\rangle.$$

The **matrix representation** of the identity operator is, not surprisingly, equal to the unit matrix:

I2 $$\begin{bmatrix} 1 & 0 \\ 0 & 1 \end{bmatrix}.$$

The identity operator is important in the computation of matrix elements (see **matrix representation**). Since the identity operator commutes with all operators (see **commutator**), it is unchanged under evolution, and can never correspond to observable magnetization (see also **partition function**.)

Image response Image responses can result under certain circumstances in systems equipped with quadrature detection. In order to achieve 'frequency discrimination' between magnetization components with offsets $\pm\delta\omega$ from the transmitter **carrier**, ω, modern spectrometers use quadrature detection, resulting in two signals in phase quadrature which are fed into the analogue-to-digital converters. The resulting complex **free induction decay** is described by

I3 $$f(t) = \exp\{\mathrm{i}\,\Delta\omega t\}\,\exp\{-t/T_2\}.$$

This function generates absorption and dispersion signals at $+\Delta\omega$ on **Fourier transformation**:

I4 $$FT\{\exp\{\mathrm{i}\,\Delta\omega t\}\,\exp\{-t/T_2\}\} = \mathrm{Abs}(+\Delta\omega) + \mathrm{i}\,\mathrm{Dis}(+\Delta\omega).$$

If the two channels are not exactly 90° out of phase with each other and/or the respective gains are not equal, then the function in (I3) is contaminated with an additional term as follows:

I5 $$f(t) = \exp\{\mathrm{i}\,\Delta\omega t\}\,\exp\{-t/T_2\} + K(\exp\{-\mathrm{i}\,\Delta\omega t\}\,\exp\{-t/T_2\})$$

where K is a constant which is a measure of the degree of phase/gain mismatch of the two channels. The resulting signal after Fourier transformation is

I6
$$\mathrm{FT}[\exp\{\mathrm{i}\,\Delta\omega t\}\exp\{-t/T_2\} + \exp\{-\mathrm{i}\,\Delta\omega t\}\exp\{-t/T_2\}]$$
$$= \mathrm{Abs}(+\Delta\omega) + \mathrm{i}\,\mathrm{Dis}(+\Delta\omega) + K[\mathrm{Abs}(-\Delta\omega) + \mathrm{i}\,\mathrm{Dis}(-\Delta\omega)],$$

which gives a small 'ghost' or quadrature image of the resonance line at $-\Delta\omega$. This response can be attenuated by employing a **cyclically ordered phase sequence** (CYCLOPS) to the phase of the r.f. excitation together with appropriate data routing in the receiver.

Imaginary part See **complex number**.

Imaging (magnetic resonance imaging) Simple NMR theory shows that a system of nuclei of a given type (e.g. protons) will precess with identical Larmor frequency (ω), if the effective field B_0 experienced by all nuclei is the same:

I7
$$\omega = \gamma B_0,$$

where γ is the **magnetogyric ratio** for the nuclei. Of course, in a high-resolution NMR experiment, we detect the sensitivity of each nucleus to small changes in B_0 dictated by the microenvironment. Since these changes are very small, it is necessary to employ a magnetic field which is spatially homogeneous to a very high degree across the sample volume. A corollary of this requirement is that spatial information might be available if we impose deliberate magnetic field inhomogeneity across the sample volume. More specifically, a linear magnetic field gradient will impose corresponding linear shifts in the Larmor frequencies ($\delta\omega$) of nuclei across the sample volume since each will experience an effective field which is different from B_0:

I8
$$\delta\omega = \gamma\delta B_0.$$

This principle is the basis of magnetic resonance imaging. Consider for example two tubes of water placed in a linear field gradient (Fig. I1). Nuclei at location A will experience a static field $B_0 + \delta B_0$ and will therefore possess a chemical shift $\omega + \delta\omega$. Similarly, nuclei at location B will possess a chemical shift $\omega - \delta\omega$. Nuclei which lie between these extremities will experience a chemical shift somewhere between $\omega + \delta\omega$ and $\omega - \delta\omega$. In addition, since intensity is proportional to the number of spins per unit volume, the NMR spectrum of the tubes of water will map a cross-section through the tubes (Fig. I1). This section is, however, only a two-dimensional image. We can obtain information in three dimensions by changing the direction of the field gradient or by rotating the sample. From a series of projections, the object can be reconstructed using image

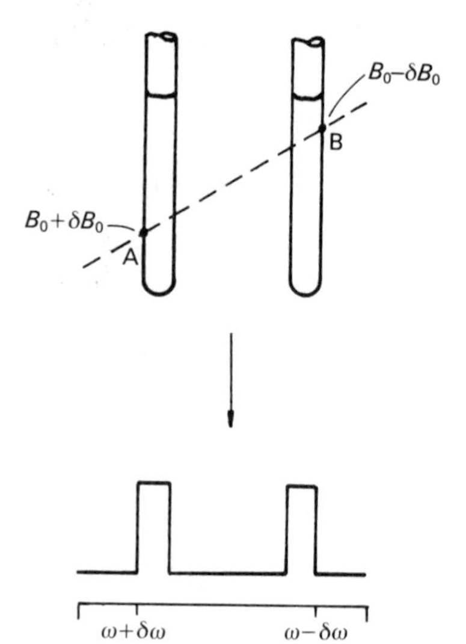

Fig. I1. Simple illustration of magnetic resonance imaging of two tubes of water in a linear field gradient. See text for details.

reconstruction. This is known as the projection–reconstruction technique.

In the context of multidimensional Fourier transform NMR, a second technique exists, which is known as Fourier imaging. In the manner of two-dimensional NMR, the two (or three) frequency coordinates which correspond to a given volume element are measured sequentially in an experiment with one (or two) evolution periods together with a detection period. For example, a two-dimensional version of the experiment is shown in Fig. I2. Firstly, a selective pulse is applied in a presence of a static magnetic field gradient (e.g. g_x). This results in the excitation of only those nuclei which are located in the sample volume where the value of the static magnetic field gradient gives rise to the resonance condition at the frequency of the selective pulse. If the field gradient is along the x direction, then a plane will be selected parallel to the y–z plane. Evolution takes place under a g_y gradient, and detection is achieved under a g_z gradient. In the manner of two-dimensional spectroscopy (see **two-dimensional NMR**), the experiment is repeated for a series of increments in the evolution period. In a two-dimensional version of the experiment, g_x and g_y form two evolution periods, and the lengths of both must be varied between experiments.

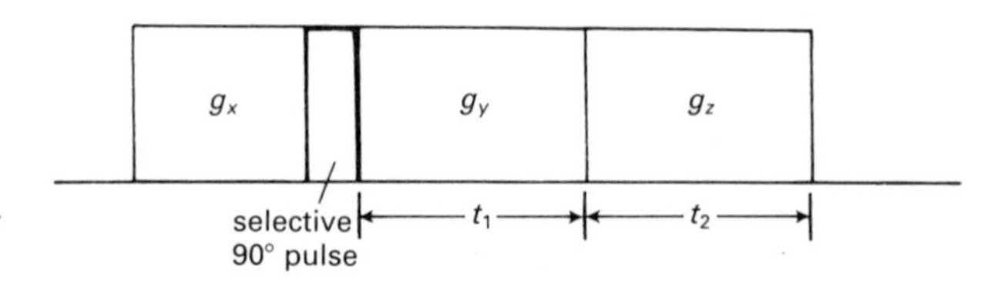

Fig. I2. Pulse sequence for Fourier imaging.

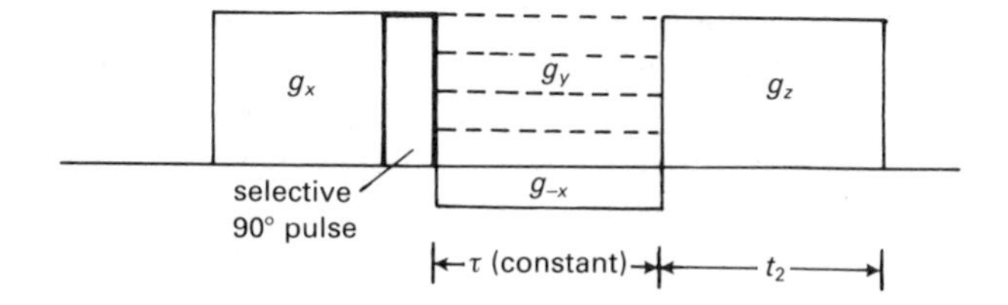

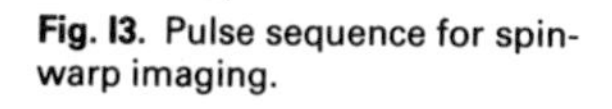
Fig. I3. Pulse sequence for spin-warp imaging.

The time-domain data represent a grid of sampling points of the two- (or three-) dimensional **Fourier transform** of the object. The desired image can be obtained from a two- (or three-) dimensional Fourier transform of the data.

Present-day imaging methodology employs a modified form of the Fourier technique. Known as spin-warp imaging, it is the most frequently applied method. Spin-warp imaging differs from conventional Fourier imaging in the fixed length of the evolution period. Instead, the amplitude of the applied field gradients is incremented between experiments. The fixed evolution period is reminiscent of that used in other so called **'constant-time' experiments**, and the achievable resolution is in fact independent of **relaxation**. The experimental scheme of spin-warp imaging is shown in Fig. I3. Excitation is effected by a selective pulse in the presence of a gradient (e.g. g_x). During evolution, it is useful to apply a reversed gradient $-g_x$ to refocus excited magnetization. At the same time a gradient g_y allows the volume elements in the y direction to be separated. The variable amplitude in g_y between experiments introduces a **phase modulation** of free precession at the end of the evolution period. Finally, a g_z gradient during detection serves to disperse the volume elements in the z direction. Extension to three dimensions is obviously straightforward.

Another variant of Fourier imaging is the technique known as rotating frame imaging. In this method, the preparation and evolution periods are combined into one single interval (Fig. I4). Transverse magnetization is excited by a linearly inhomogeneous r.f. field. With an r.f. field gradient such as g_x, the effective rotation angle of the r.f. pulse will be dependent upon the spatial location of the nucleus in the x direction. If the width of the pulse is now varied systematically between experiments, an amplitude modulation of the resulting signal occurs, which carries the x coordinate

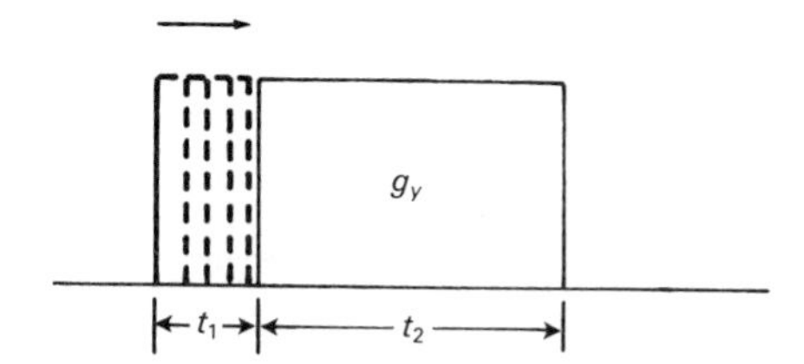

Fig. I4. Pulse sequence for rotating frame imaging.

information. If detection takes place under a static g_y field gradient, two-dimensional time-domain data are obtained in a manner entirely equivalent to conventional Fourier imaging. Identical data-processing procedures are used. The advantage of rotating-frame imaging is that no switched static field gradients are required. However, it is difficult to create a clean linear r.f. field gradient.

A variant of rotating-frame imaging can be obtained if no static field gradient is employed during detection. In this case, under high-resolution conditions, the time-domain data after two-dimensional Fourier transformation display the conventional NMR spectrum along one axis, with spatial information regarding the x coordinates of the nuclei along the orthogonal axis.

FURTHER READING

Several good texts exist in this field. See for example:

Kaufman, L., Crooks, L. E., and Margulis, A. R. (1981) *NMR imaging in medicine*. Igakun-shoin, Tokyo.

Morris, P. G. (1986). *NMR imaging in medicine and biology*. Oxford University Press, Oxford.

For a good introduction to Fourier imaging, see also:

Ernst, R. R., Bodenhausen, G., and Wokaun, A. (1987). *Principles of NMR in one and two dimensions,* Chapter 10. Clarendon Press, Oxford.

Impulse See **delta function**.

INADEQUATE See **double-quantum correlated spectroscopy**.

INEPT See **insensitive nuclei enhanced by polarization transfer**.

Insensitive nuclei enhanced by polarization transfer (INEPT) As its name suggests, the purpose of the INEPT experiment is to improve the sensitivity of NMR experiments on rare and low **magnetogyric ratio** nuclei. The simplest pulse sequence relevant to INEPT is shown in Fig. I5. As an example, consider a two-spin system IS, where S refers to a

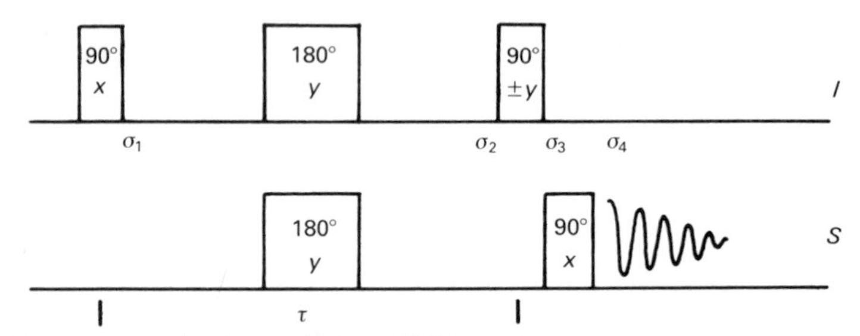

Fig. I5. Pulse sequence for the acquisition of INEPT spectra.

rare nucleus (e.g. ^{13}C). The equilibrium density operator, expressed in terms of cartesian spin operators (see **product operator formalism**) is proportional to

$$\sigma_{(0)} \approx I_z + (\gamma_S/\gamma_I)S_z. \tag{I9}$$

After the first 90° pulse, which is applied only to the I spins, we find

$$\sigma(1) \approx -I_y + (\gamma_S/\gamma_I)S_z. \tag{I10}$$

The spin system now evolves during τ, which contains a pair of π pulses applies simultaneously to I and S spins. Since the latter effectively refocus chemical shifts, the τ period is equivalent to the following transformation:

$$\begin{aligned} &-I_y + (\gamma_S/\gamma_I)S_z \xrightarrow{\pi Iy} \xrightarrow{\pi Sy} \xrightarrow{\pi J_{IS}\tau 2I_zS_z} \\ &I_y \cos \pi J_{IS}\tau - 2I_xS_z \sin \pi J_{IS}\tau - (\gamma_S/\gamma_I)S_z = \sigma(2). \end{aligned} \tag{I11}$$

After a $\pi/2$ pulse on the I spins, which will be required to have a phase of $\pm y$ in alternate experiments as explained below, we find

$$\sigma_3 \approx I_y \cos \pi J_{IS}\tau \pm 2I_zS_z \sin \pi J_{IS}\tau - (\gamma_S/\gamma_I)S_z. \tag{I12}$$

The final $\pi/2$ pulse on the S spins, of phase $+x$, gives

$$\sigma_4 \approx I_y \cos \pi J_{IS}\tau \mp 2I_zS_y \sin \pi J_{IS}\tau + (\gamma_S/\gamma_I)S_y. \tag{I13}$$

The last term on the right-hand side of (I13) results from the polarization of native spins, which is converted to observable magnetization by the final $\pi/2$ pulse. It can be cancelled by subtracting the two experiments with the different phases described above. The only term which survives is then

$$\sigma_{\text{obs}} \approx -2I_zS_y \sin \pi J_{IS}\tau. \tag{I14}$$

Now, if $\tau = 1/2J_{IS}$, $\sin \pi J_{IS}\tau = 1$, and the observed signal is maximal. Importantly, this signal will evolve during the detection period to generate antiphase magnetization which is enhanced by a factor γ_I/γ_S with respect to the native spin magnetization $(\gamma_S/\gamma_I)S_y$. Also, since the detected signal depends upon transfer of polarization (the detected signal derives from I_z), the repetition rate between experiments can be on the order of T_1 (see **spin–lattice relaxation**) for the abundant spin, which is usually significantly smaller than T_1 for the rare spin.

A modification of this experiment involves delaying acquisition of the free induction decay of the S spin so that the antiphase magnetization in (I14) is allowed to rephase. This 'refocused INEPT' experiment allows for decoupling of the I spins during acquisition. For systems containing a variety of couplings, and in three- and four-spin systems, perfect rephasing is not possible, and further modifications such as DEPT would appear to be more useful.

FURTHER READING

Morris, G. A. and Freeman, R. (1979). *J. Am. Chem. Soc.* **101,** 760.

Intensity The intensity of a resonance line is one of the five parameters which characterize it (see **chemical shift**, **spin–lattice relaxation**, **spin–spin relaxation**, **scalar coupling**). The intensity is simply proportional to the number of equivalent spins per unit volume. This is the only inherent information available from this parameter. However, the measurement of other parameters (T_1, T_2) depend directly upon the measurement of the intensities of resonance lines. In modern spectrometers, software-driven integration procedures allow intensity to be measured easily. However, it must always be remembered that under certain conditions anomalous intensities may be produced. An obvious example is the situation where partial saturation occurs. Another is the intensity distortions inherent in ^{13}C spectra under conditions where the ^{1}H–^{13}C **nuclear Overhauser effect** is being exploited to enhance sensitivity. Indeed, in any NMR experiment in which the spin system is prepared in an arbitrary non-equilibrium state, theoretical considerations should be clearly understood before intensity measurements are used. This of course includes all two-dimensional experiments.

Further difficulties can arise in intensity measurements when the **free induction decay** is weighted (see **convolution**) prior to **Fourier transformation**. Most weighting functions distort lineshapes and also intensities. However, a simple exponential weighting function preserves the correct intensities at least for Lorentzian **lineshapes**. This may be rationalized by noting that the first point in the free induction decay is proportional to the total integrated intensity of the spectrum. This point is multiplied by unity on application of a decaying exponential of arbitrary time constant.

Interaction representation See **average Hamiltonian theory**.

Interferogram See **free induction decay**.

Intermediate exchange See **chemical exchange**.

Intermediate frequency Modern r.f. receivers, which includes the NMR receiver, generally operate on the superheterodyne ('superhet') principle. This involves the conversion of the input signal, which has a variable frequency, to a constant intermediate frequency. The conversion is achieved using a **phase sensitive detector** or mixer. For the case of a

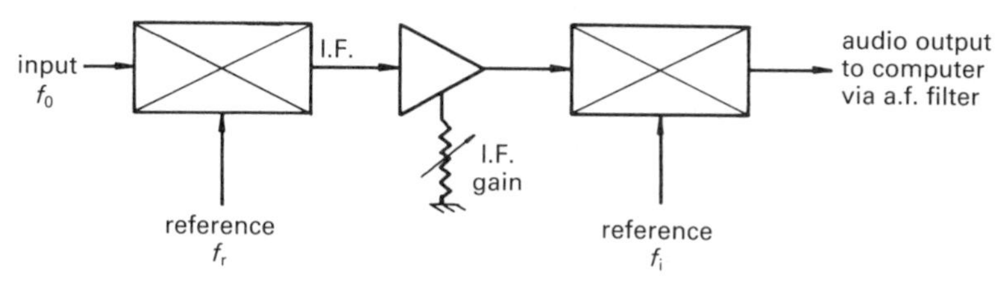

Fig. I6. Block diagram of the IF stage of a typical NMR receiver.

simple single channel (i.e. non-quadrature) detection system, the building blocks are very simple (Fig. I6). The rationale behind this design is that a variable-frequency input is converted to a fixed intermediate frequency. The gain-determining stages of the spectrometer can therefore be conveniently run at the intermediate frequency, and any necessary r.f. filtration can be placed here also. A disadvantage of the 'superhet' principle is the response of the mixers to the input frequency. With regard to the first mixer in Fig. I6 for a given value of f_r, two input frequencies are capable of generating a given intermediate frequency. This is because a mixer generates output signals which, amongst others, are equal to the sum and difference of the input and reference, i.e. $f_0 \pm f_r$. Assuming a reference frequency of 500 MHz, for example, and an intermediate frequency of 50 MHz, input signals of 450 MHz and 550 MHz will be detected with equal strength. To avoid this problem, the preamplifier (see **amplifier**) is designed with a bandwidth which is narrow enough to pass the desired frequency at the expense of the other. In addition, it is obviously advantageous to work with an intermediate frequency (i.f.) as high as possible, such that the wanted and unwanted signals, which are separated by $2 \times$ i.f., are as far apart as practicable. In practice, the i.f. cannot be chosen to be arbitrarily high, since in a multinuclear spectrometer, there exists the possibility of choosing an i.f. which matches the Larmor frequency of a relevant nucleus, which is highly undesirable.

Inversion recovery sequence The inversion recovery pulse sequence is typically used to measure **spin–lattice relaxation** (T_1) rates. It consists of two non-selective r.f. pulses and a variable delay, τ (Fig. I7). Consider the effect of this sequence upon a group of equivalent spins at thermal equilibrium. The vector representing spin magnetization (see **classical formalism**) will lie along the $+z$ axis. After application of a perfect 180° pulse, it will lie along the $-z$ axis (Fig. I8). If now, $\tau = 0$, a 90° pulse

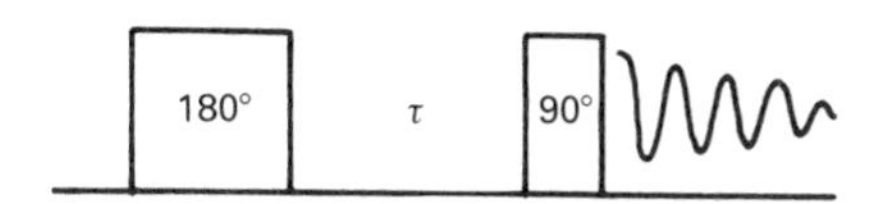

Fig. I7. Inversion recovery sequence for the measurement of T_1.

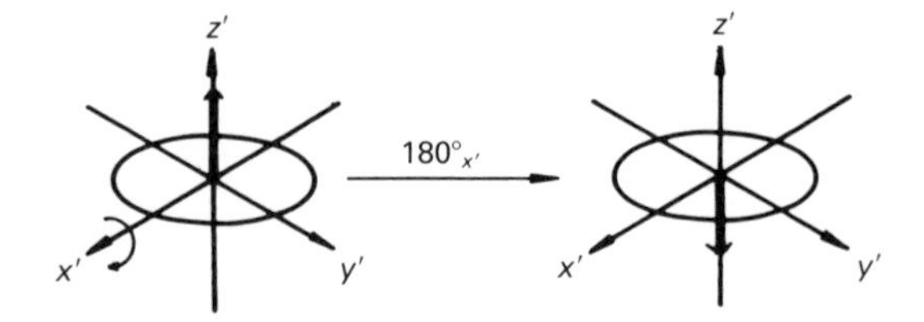

Fig. I8. Effect of 180° x pulse on equilibrium z magnetization.

along the x axis will rotate the magnetization along the $-y$ axis (Fig. I9). If the magnetization is now allowed to precess freely during the acquisition period with the receiver phase along the $+y$ axis, after **Fourier transformation** the spectrum will appear inverted. If, now, the experiment is repeated with increasing values of τ, then after the 180° pulse (Fig. I8), the vector will gradually decay along the $+z$ axis with

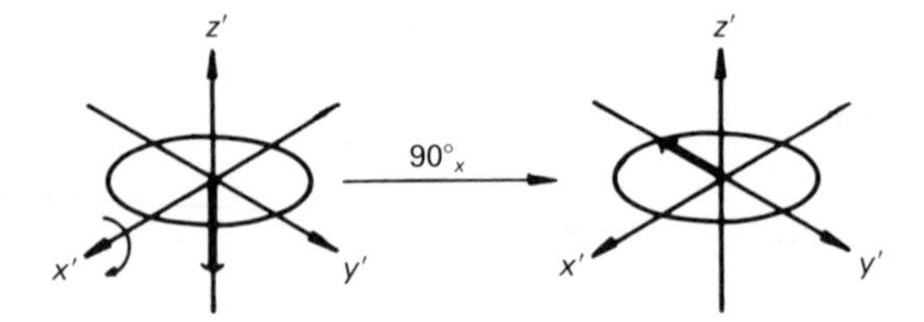

Fig. I9. Effect of 90° x pulse on $-z$ magnetization.

increasing τ due to spin–lattice (longitudinal) relaxation. This is 'read' by the 90° pulse to generate a series of spectra, one for each τ value. If the intensities A of these resonances are now plotted against τ, we obtain a graph such as that shown in Fig. I10. In this example, T_1 relaxation has an exponential decay $M_z(\tau) = M_0[1 - 2\exp(-\tau/\tau_1)]$. Therefore if we plot $\ln(A_\infty - A_\tau)$ against τ then we obtain a straight line of slope T_1. An alternative but less accurate measure of T_1 is obtained from the 'null-point' (p) in Fig. I10 which equals $0.693T_1$.

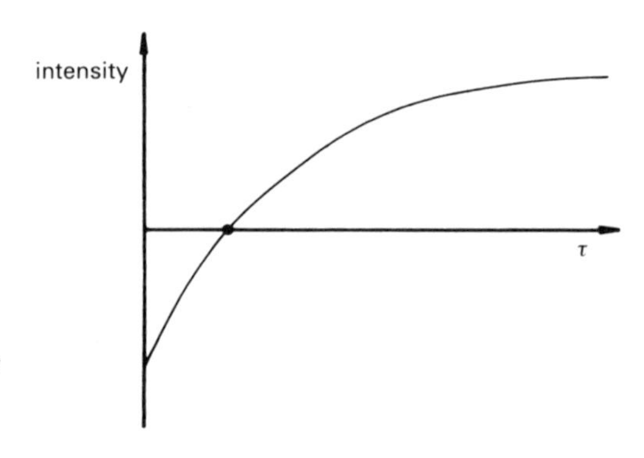

Fig. I10. Plot of intensity (A_τ) *vs.* τ for a typical inversion recovery experiment.

In common with every NMR experiment involving spin systems prepared in a non-equilibrium state, the inversion-recovery experiment is susceptible to artefacts which can cause systematic errors. An obvious requirement is to wait at least five times T_1 between scans if signal averaging is employed. This presents an apparent paradox, since the purpose of the experiment is to measure T_1. However, with experience an approximate value for T_1 can always be estimated.

A second source of artefacts is imperfection in the 180° pulse. If the magnetization is not perfectly inverted by this pulse, then transverse magnetization will be present during τ. However, this can simply be removed by alternating the phase of the 180° pulse by π radians at each transient. Residual transverse magnetization is then cancelled. Finally, a more subtle class of artefacts arises from the fact that the 90° pulse acts upon the spin system in a non-equilibrium state. This can result in the creation of multiple-quantum coherences, which interfere with the measured intensities in a systematic manner. These can be removed by phase cycling the 90° pulse.

FURTHER READING

Farrar, T. C. and Becker, E. D. (1971). *Pulse and Fourier transform NMR.* Academic Press, New York.

For a discussion of systematic errors in the inversion recovery sequence due to multiple-quantum interference, see:
Bodenhausen, G. (1981). *Progr. NMR Spectr.* **14,** 137.

Isotropic Hamiltonian See **Hamiltonian**.

J

J-modulation See ***J*-spectroscopy**.

***J*-spectroscopy** J-spectroscopy is one of the simplest **two-dimensional NMR** experiments. Its purpose is to allow the multiplet patterns of overlapping lines to be detected, and the measurement of the respective spin-coupling (J) values to high accuracy. Under the correct conditions it is also possible, by software manipulations, to obtain a 'proton-decoupled' proton spectrum for the sample of interest.

Two-dimensional J-spectroscopy (2D-J) involves a pulse sequence (Fig. J1) which consists essentially of a 90° pulse to generate transverse magnetization, followed by a **spin echo** evolution period, where the 180° pulse serves to refocus chemical shifts. The two-dimensional sequence differs from conventional spin echo spectroscopy in that the evolution period τ becomes the t_1 period, and is incremented sequentially from experiment to experiment in the normal manner (see **two-dimensional NMR**). The key principle to the workings of 2D-J spectroscopy lies in the concept of J-modulation. This can most easily be explained using the ubiquitous **product operator formalism**. Assuming the spin system is at thermal equilibrium, the initial longitudinal magnetization just before the 90° pulse (σ_0) for a weakly coupled two-spin system may be described by;

$$\sigma_{(0)} = I_z + S_z. \tag{J1}$$

A 90° pulse along the x axis then creates transverse magnetization:

$$I_z + S_z \xrightarrow{\pi/2(I_x)+\pi/2(S_x)} -I_y - S_y. \tag{J2}$$

During the subsequent evolution period, it is necessary only to consider the effect of the spin-coupling **Hamiltonian**, since chemical shift terms are refocused by the 180° pulse (**weak coupling** only!). At the end of the t_1 period, we find therefore

$$\begin{aligned} -I_y - S_y \xrightarrow{\pi J t_1 2I_zS_z} & -I_y \cos \pi J_{IS}t_1 + 2I_xS_z \sin \pi J_{IS}t_1 \\ & - S_y \cos \pi J_{IS}t_1 + 2S_xI_z \sin \pi J_{IS}t_1. \end{aligned} \tag{J3}$$

At this point we find two 'observable' terms $-I_y$ and $-S_y$ which possess a cosinusoidal modulation in J during the t_1 period. This is commonly known as J-modulation in conventional spin-echo spectra. The second

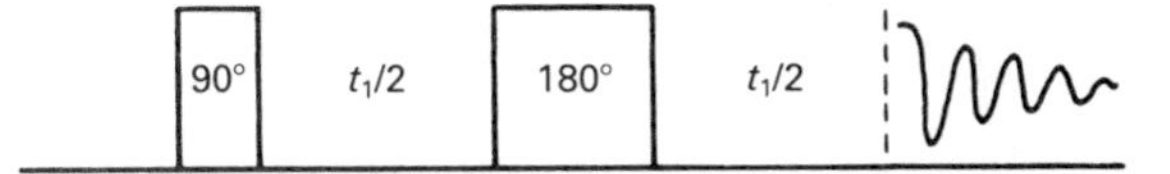

Fig. J1. Pulse sequence for the acquisition of *J* spectra.

pair of terms on the right-hand side of (J3) do not formally constitute observables, but they will evolve into observables in S_y during the t_2 period, with a sinusoidal dependence on J during t_1. After two-dimensional Fourier transformation, there is no chemical shift information in the ω_1 dimension, and the spectrum is composed of individual multiplets for each resonance. However, each multiplet is composed of two terms, one with a cosinusoidal J-modulation during t_1 and a second with sinusoidal modulation, as described above. This imparts an admixture of absorption- and dispersion-mode contributions to each resonance line, resulting in the well-known phase-twist lineshape. It is therefore not possible to obtain pure absorption-mode lineshapes in this particular experiment. The form of the spectrum in the ω_2 dimension will contain both chemical shift and spin coupling information, and thus resembles the conventional one-dimensional spectrum in cross-section.

To illustrate some interesting features of 2D-J spectra, the result of this experiment applied to a solution of tryptophan is shown in Fig. J2. In this contour plot (see **correlated spectroscopy**) of the spectrum, the lack of chemical shift information in the ω_1 dimension is clearly seen. In the case of proton 2D-J spectroscopy, the sweep width in the ω_1 dimension need only be of the order of ± 15 Hz maximum. The digital resolution in Hz/point in ω_1 can therefore be made small, thus allowing the J values to be measured accurately after tilting the spectrum (see below). However, it must be borne in mind that the lineshapes are not in pure absorption mode, and for small values of J, can give misleading values, which detracts somewhat from the usefulness of the technique. A second point of note in Fig. J2 is that the individual multiplets lie along a line which is tilted with respect to the ω_2 axis. For this reason the multiplet patterns are preserved in ω_2. However, if we were to observe the spectrum along the plane at 45° to the ω_2 axis, then the multiplets would collapse to singlets—in other words, would we observe an effective 'proton-decoupled' proton spectrum. This can readily be achieved using modern software 'tilting' manipulations, Unfortunately, this procedure does not work in the case of strongly coupled systems (see **strong coupling**), since chemical shift information is not completely refocused by the 180° pulse. Spurious lines therefore result, and the spectrum becomes difficult to interpret. In addition, the procedure will only work on spectra presented in the absolute value mode, which is a consequence of the cross-section projection theorem (see *Further reading*).

As usual with two-dimensional experiments, it is desirable to employ phase cycling procedures to remove unwanted artefacts in the two-

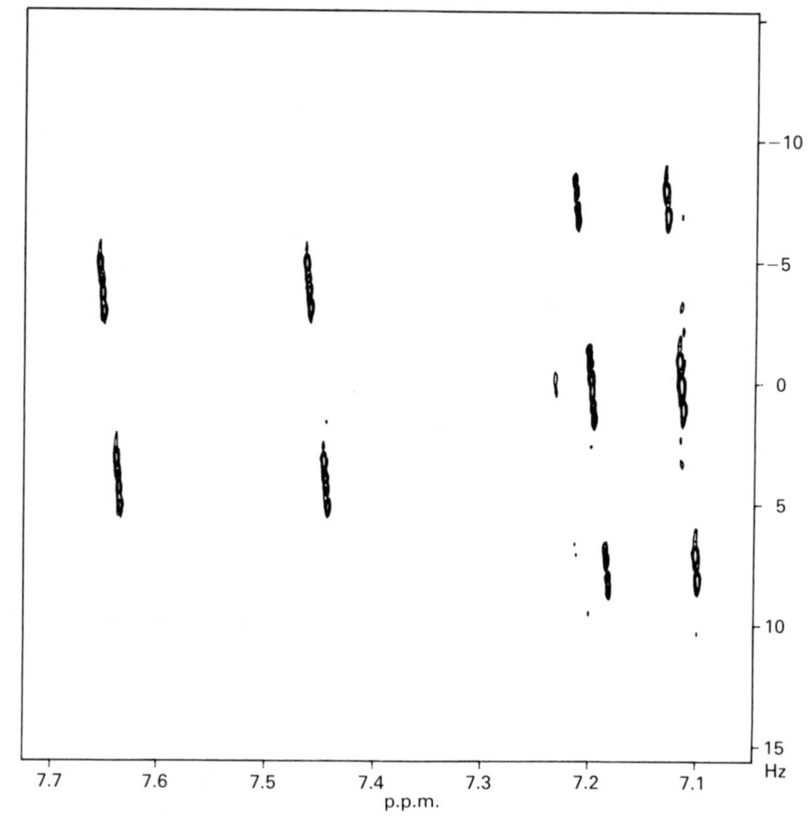

Fig. J2. Contour plot of the aromatic region of a *J* spectrum of tryptophan in D_2O.

dimensional spectrum. In the case of 2D-J spectroscopy, the desired phase cycling has been termed EXORCYCLE.

FURTHER READING

Bax, A. (1982). *Two-dimensional NMR in liquids*. Delft University Press, Dordrecht.

The cross-section projection theorem is nicely described in:

Ernst, R. R., Bodenhausen, G. and Wokaun, A. (1987). *Principles of NMR in one and two dimensions*, pp. 304–6. Clarendon Press, Oxford.

Jump-and-return sequence See **solvent suppression**.

K

Karplus equation In principle, scalar spin coupling constants (J values) can yield detailed geometric information in view of their orientational dependence. The theoretical prediction of J values is however complicated by the large numbers of electrons and orientation states. One situation commonly found in biological systems, which is amenable to analysis by empirical means, is the vicinal coupling between hydrogens attached to two carbon atoms (Fig. K1). The value of this coupling is given by the Karplus equation

K1 $$J(\theta) = A \cos^2 \theta + B \cos \theta + C$$

where θ is the dihedral angle between protons (see Fig. K1). The values A, B, C depend upon the precise system under investigation, and in particular are sensitive to the electronegativity of the substituents on the carbons. For tetrahedral carbons substituted with hydrogen, $A = 4.22$, $B = -0.5$, and $C = 4.5$. Due to its empirical nature, care should be taken in generalizing any parametrization to an unknown system. A qualitative interpretation of the Karplus equation is useful in the determination of the state of ring puckering in carbohydrates.

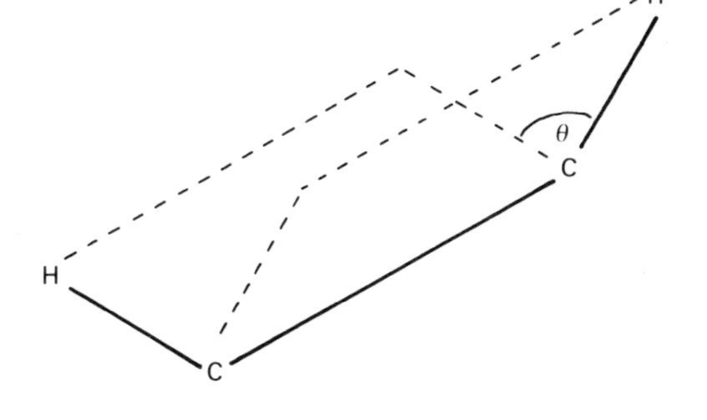

Fig. K1. Definition of the dihedral angle θ in the Karplus equation.

FURTHER READING

Karplus, M. (1963). *J. Am. Chem. Soc.* **85,** 2870.

A useful modification of the Karplus equation which includes electronegativity is described by

Haasnoot, C. A. G., De Leeuw, F. A. A. M., and Altona, C. (1980). *Tetrahedron* **36,** 2783.

L

Larmor precession All NMR active nuclei possess a **magnetic moment** (μ), the generation of which can be thought of as a rotation of charge. If a nucleus is placed in a magnetic field B_0, the magnetic moment will experience a torque given by $\mu \times B_0$. For example, a bar magnet (or compass needle) will align along the direction of B_0. However, since the rotation confers the property of **angular momentum** upon the nucleus, the situation is modified, and the nucleus behaves like a gyroscope. The net effect, in classical terms, is precession of the magnetic moments about B_0. The frequency of this precession is found from the equation

L1 $$\omega = \gamma B_0$$

where ω is the Larmor precession frequency, γ is the **magnetogyric ratio**, and B_0 is the magnetic field strength. A quantum mechanical description of Larmor precession defines a Zeeman **Hamiltonian** for the description of the interaction of the nucleus with the applied field:

L2 $$\mathscr{H}_Z = \omega I_z.$$

We can form the **matrix representation** of this Hamiltonian for a one-spin system (Fig. L1) by operating on each eigenstate (see **eigenfunction**) individually. We find, using the rules formulated for the z component angular momentum operator I_z,

L3 $$I_z\,|\alpha\rangle = +\tfrac{1}{2}\,|\alpha\rangle,$$
$$I_z\,|\beta\rangle = -\tfrac{1}{2}\,|\beta\rangle.$$

These can be recognized as **eigenvalue** equations, and the matrix representation of $\mathscr{H}_Z$ is therefore diagonal:

L4 $$\begin{array}{c} \\ |\alpha\rangle \\ |\beta\rangle \end{array}\begin{array}{c} \begin{array}{cc} |\alpha\rangle & |\beta\rangle \end{array} \\ \begin{bmatrix} +\tfrac{1}{2}\omega & 0 \\ 0 & -\tfrac{1}{2}\omega \end{bmatrix} \end{array}.$$

Consequently, the diagonal elements are the eigenvalues or energies of the states $|\alpha\rangle$ and $|\beta\rangle$. We find therefore that a transition between states is associated with a frequency $\omega = \gamma B_0$. The precession frequency is thus identical in magnitude with the frequency needed for magnetic resonance absorption.

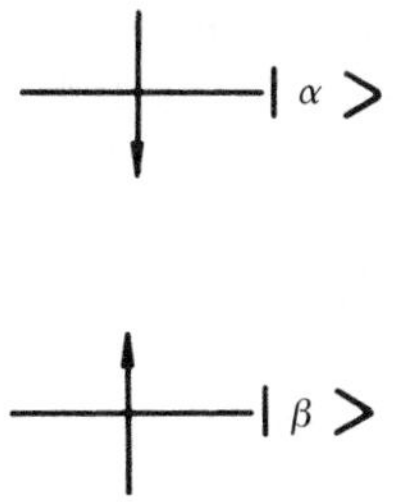

Fig. L1. The spin states of a single spin $\frac{1}{2}$.

Lifetime broadening See **chemical exchange**.

Linear amplifier As its name suggests, a linear amplifier operates within the linear approximation of the amplifying devices. The output signal is therefore in principle a faithful reproduction of the input. Most present-day commercial spectrometers are actually not equipped with linear amplifiers in the final stage of the transmitter. However, under normal circumstances this is of no consequence since the amplification of a pulsed waveform need not be linear. Indeed, there are advantages in avoiding linearity in this case since a non-linear amplifier is inherently less noisy. On the other hand an increasing number of experiments involving 'tailored' r.f. pulses are becoming popular. An example is the **Gaussian pulse** designed for its frequency-domain selectivity. If amplification of a gaussian pulse is attempted in a non-linear amplifier, the output will certainly not be a Gaussian pulse. In this situation a linear amplifier is required, unless it is proposed to modulate a final non-linear stage, operating under continuous-wave conditions, with a gaussian envelope. The design of a linear amplifier involves careful choice of operating voltages and driving-circuit considerations. The overall aim is to adjust operation in such a way that the power output is proportional to the square of the r.f. exciting voltage.

Linearity (linear response theory) A system which may be represented by an operator ϕ is said to be linear if it obeys the superposition principle:

$$\phi\{x_1(t)+x_2(t)\} = \phi\{x_1(t)\} + \phi\{x_2(t)\} = y_1(t) + y_2(t). \tag{L5}$$

Thus, any input signal can be represented by a linear combination of base functions $g_k(t)$,

$$x(t) = \sum_k X_k g_k(t) \tag{L6}$$

and it is possible to consider the response of each constituent function separately:

$$y(t) = \phi\{x(t)\} = \sum_k X_k \phi\{g_k(t)\}. \tag{L7}$$

Of particular interest in response theory is the impulse response $h(t)$ of the system, which is the response to a **delta function** input signal:

L8 $$h(t) = \phi\{\delta(t)\}.$$

The value of the impulse response is that the response for an arbitrary input signal is equal to the **convolution** of the input signal ($x(t)$) with the impulse response ($h(t)$) of the system:

L9 $$y(t) = h(t) * x(t).$$

The impulse response therefore characterizes completely a linear, time-independent system.

If the input signal is an exponential function, $\exp\{pt\}$, then it can be shown that $\exp\{pt\}$ is reproduced at the output, multiplied by the complex phase and amplitude factors $H'(p)$ introduced by the system. Since $\exp\{pt\}$ is unchanged the $H'(p)$ are **eigenvalues** of the system. $H'(p)$ can be considered to be a linear function of p and is called the transfer function of the system.

If p is specially chosen to be an harmonic function, $p = \exp\{i\omega t\}$, the frequency response function is obtained:

L10 $$H(\omega) = H'(i\omega),$$

and the impulse response $h(t)$ and the frequency response $H(\omega)$ form a **Fourier transform** pair. In Fourier spectroscopy, the **free-induction decay** can be identified with the impulse response, and the complex spectrum is equivalent to the frequency response function.

The nuclear spin system is actually a non-linear system. Thus, (L5) does not generally apply. Nevertheless, linear response theory is still applicable following the application of an r.f. pulse. This is because the non-linear effect of the r.f. pulse defines the initial conditions. Subsequent evolution occurs in the absence of r.f. fields and the system can be treated in a linear manner. In multiple-pulse experiments, this situation does not hold, and non-linearity has to be taken into consideration.

FURTHER READING

Ernst, R. R., Bodenhausen, G. and Wokaun, A. (1987). *Principles of NMR in one and two dimensions*, p. 93ff. Clarendon Press, Oxford.

Lineshape The NMR spectrum represents the frequency-domain response of the spin system to a r.f. pulse. This response is obtained from data in the time domain (the **free induction decay**) by **Fourier transformation**. In the mathematical sense, the resulting spectrum is complex, i.e. it has a real part together with an imaginary part:

L11 $$M = A + iD.$$

The dispersive component, D, is the component which is in phase with the exciting r.f. energy. The absorptive component A (the real part) is the component which is 90° out of phase with the exciting r.f. field. If, therefore, we were to construct a **probe** consisting of two pairs of coils at right angles, we would expect to observe both components. In fact we can achieve this with a single-coil arrangement using a procedure known as **quadrature detection**, and both components are indeed detected by the spectrometer. In liquids, the solution of the **Bloch equations** gives us expressions for the magnetization along both the x and y axes:

$$D = \frac{M_0 \gamma B_1 T_2^2(\omega_0 - \omega)}{1 + 4\pi^2 T_2^2(\omega_0 - \omega)^2}, \tag{L12}$$

$$A = \frac{M_0 \gamma B_1 T_2}{1 + 4\pi^2 T_2^2(\omega_0 - \omega)^2}. \tag{L13}$$

These equations predict two quite different responses, which are collectively known as a Lorentzian lineshape. This lineshape is characteristic of damped oscillatory motion (see **damped oscillator**). If we plot the absorptive and dispersive components as a function of frequency, we obtain lineshapes similar to those in Fig. L2.

The absorption lineshape is characterized by positive **intensity** for all frequancies, and is the mode which is normally plotted in NMR. The dispersion component has undesirable broad 'wings', and its integrated intensity is zero. Actually, the association of the absorption lineshape with the x or y component is rather academic, since in any practical case involving one-dimensional NMR we can phase the response from either component to pure adsorption see **phase correction**. Note, however, that this is not the case in certain two-dimensional NMR experiments, Despite their different appearance, the absorption and dispersion lineshapes are inextricably linked: given the form of one component, the other can be calculated. They are in fact related by the **Hilbert transform**.

Since (L12) and (L13) contain terms in T_2, it is clear that **relaxation** processes contribute to the linewidth of the resonance line. In addition, such processes can, under certain conditions, change the lineshape due to non-exponential relaxation (see **relaxation**).

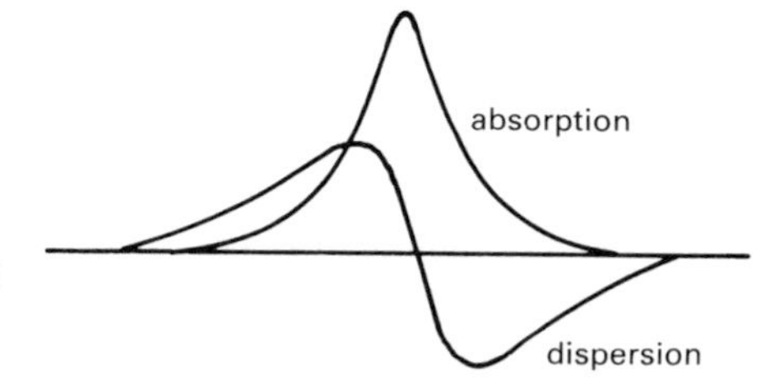

Fig. L2. The absorption-mode and dispersion-mode lineshapes inherent in NMR spectroscopy.

Another lineshape which is found in NMR of crystalline solids is the Gaussian lineshape. This is characterized by a function of the form

L14 $$M = \exp\{(-2\pi\,\Delta U)^2/a^2\}$$

which is a lineshape that drops off more rapidly towards the wings in comparison with the Lorentzian. For this reason a **convolution** function providing Lorentzian–Gaussian lineshape transformation is useful as a resolution enhancement function. The form of the (time-domain) convolution function is similar in form to (L14), since the **Fourier transform** of a Gaussian is also Gaussian. This latter property forms the basis of the **Gaussian pulse**.

Linewidth See **spin–spin relaxation**.

Liouville space See **superoperator**.

Liouville–von Neumann equation The Liouville–von Neumann (or 'density operator') equation is a differential equation expressing the time evolution of the density operator (see **density matrix**) under an **Hamiltonian** $\mathscr{H}$;

L15 $$\frac{\mathrm{d}\rho}{\mathrm{d}t} = -\mathrm{i}\hbar^{-1}[\mathscr{H}(t), \rho(t)]$$

where $[\mathscr{H}(t), \rho(t)]$ represents the **commutator** of $\mathscr{H}(t)$ and $\rho(t)$:

L16 $$[\mathscr{H}(t), \rho(t)] = \mathscr{H}(t)\rho(t) - \rho(t)\mathscr{H}(t).$$

The formal solution of (L15) is

L17 $$\rho(t) = T\exp\left[-\mathrm{i}\int_0^t \mathscr{H}(t')\,\mathrm{d}t'\right]\rho(0)\exp\left[+\mathrm{i}\int_0^t \mathscr{H}(t')\,\mathrm{d}t\right]$$

where T is the Dyson time ordering operator (see **Dyson expression**). If $\mathscr{H}$ is time independent, then the evolution of ρ can be expressed by a series of **unitary transformations**:

L18 $$\rho(t_1+t_2+t_3) = \exp\{-\mathrm{i}\mathscr{H}_3 t_3\}\exp\{-\mathrm{i}\mathscr{H}_2 t_2\}\rho_{t_1}\exp\{\mathrm{i}\mathscr{H}_2 t_2\}\exp\{\mathrm{i}\mathscr{H}_3 t_3\}.$$

Actually (L15) is not a correct expression for the time evolution of the density matrix, since we have ignored relaxation. In order to introduce relaxation terms in a manageable way, we must introduce the concept of the 'reduced density operator'. For magnetic resonance applications, it is sufficient to consider **expectation values** for a set of operators which act upon nuclear or electronic spin variables. The remaining degrees of freedom are then referred to as the lattice. Equation (L15) can then be written for the reduced density operator:

$$\frac{d\sigma(t)}{dt} = -i\hbar^{-1}[\mathcal{H}, \sigma(t)] - \hat{\hat{\Gamma}}[\sigma(t) - \sigma_0] \tag{L19}$$

where now $\hat{\hat{\Gamma}}$ is the relaxation **superoperator** which accounts for relaxation between the spin system and the lattice. It is general practice to ignore relaxation terms in most density matrix calculations, as has been done with the majority of examples in this book. The integrated form of (L19) ia actually much simpler to obtain if relaxation is ignored, and by analogy with (L18) we find

$$\sigma(t_1 + t_2 + t_3) = \exp\{-i\mathcal{H}_3 t_3\} \exp\{-i\mathcal{H}_2 t_2\} \sigma_{t_1} \exp\{i\mathcal{H}_2 t_2\} \exp\{i\mathcal{H}_e t_3\}. \tag{L20}$$

However, it must always be understood that dissipative interactions between the spin system and the lattice are constantly driving $\sigma(t)$ to its equilibrium value $\sigma(0)$. This must always be considered when assessing the worth of a complex **pulse sequence**. In addition, the exclusion of the relaxation terms in (L19) can sometimes (though rarely) fail to account for some types of peak in two-dimensional NMR spectra.

FURTHER READING

Ernst, R. R., Bodenhausen, G., and Wokaun, A. (1987). *Principles of NMR in one and two dimensions*. Clarendon Press, Oxford.

Liquid state The majority of NMR experiment on biomolecules, with the possible exception of membrane systems, are performed in the liquid state. In this manner experimental results *in vitro* can be related to those *in vivo*. In some respects the inherent simplifications upon the NMR spectrum imposed by the spin physics of liquids is an advantage, but in other respects important information is lost. In essence, the random rotational and reorientational motions of the molecules in a liquid cause an 'averaging' of the various interactions between a spin and the static magnetic field, or between spins. It is this averaging which is responsible for the high resolution of liquid state NMR spectra. Of the many interactions between spins which govern the appearance of a **solid state NMR** spectrum, only an isotropic chemical shift and scalar spin–spin coupling's (J's) survive. In addition, the rapid molecular motion results in inefficient **relaxation** between spins, resulting in narrow lines.

Lock (field-frequency lock) Although the frequencies generated in modern NMR spectrometers are stable to a very high degree, this is not true of the **Larmor precession** frequencies ($\omega = \gamma B_0$) of the nuclei under investigation. Of course, there is no inherent instability in the **magnetogyric ratio** (γ) of the nucleus, but the static field (B_0) generated by the superconducting magnet decays slowly with time and is not of sufficient stability for high-resolution NMR. In order to improve the stability, an electronic device termed a field-frequency lock is incorporated into the modern superconducting console. Its mode of operation is quite straightforward. Essentially, a second NMR experiment is performed continuously and automatically by the spectrometer at all times. This experiment invariably uses deuterium as the perturbed nucleus, since it is present at a very high concentration in the deuterated solvents commonly used in NMR. In practice, a continuous train of pulses is applied to the sample at the Larmor frequency of deuterons. Since this varies depending upon the solvent, it is necessary to bring the signal on to resonance by adjusting the field manually, or, as is becoming increasingly common, under computer control. Once the resonant frequency has been found, the lock circuit maintains the resonance condition, thus locking the field to the exciting frequency. Since all frequencies in a well-designed spectrometer are generated from a common source, the field is locked to the exciting frequency irrespective of the nucleus being studied in the actual experiment. The key principle in the operation of the lock circuit is the response of the receiver. The **phase-sensitive detector** of the receiver is set to detect the dispersion mode signal At resonance, this leads to zero signal (Fig. L3). If the resonance condition is violated, i.e. if the field drifts, then an error signal is generated. This can be amplified, and fed back to a correcting coil in the magnet to effect a shift in the magnitude of the static field in a direction which opposes the drift. Of course, such a system must be carefully designed if the system is not to oscillate about the resonance condition. The system we have described is similar to a **phase-locked loop** circuit. The irradiating frequency is the reference oscillator, the perturbed sample is the voltage-controlled oscillator (VCO), and the receiver generates the necessary error signal (Fig. L4).

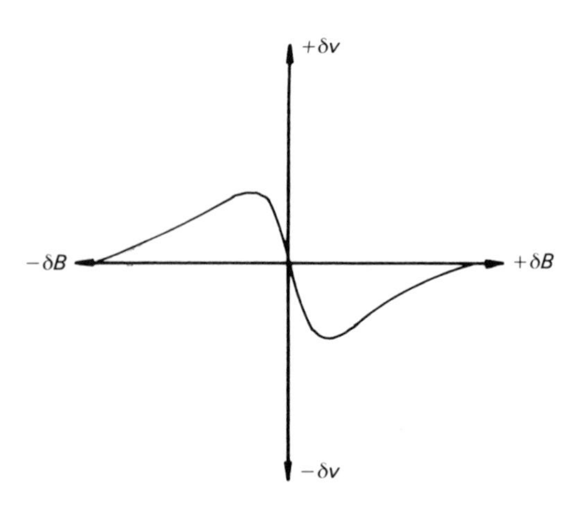

Fig. L3. Dispersion-mode signal used for field/frequency locking.

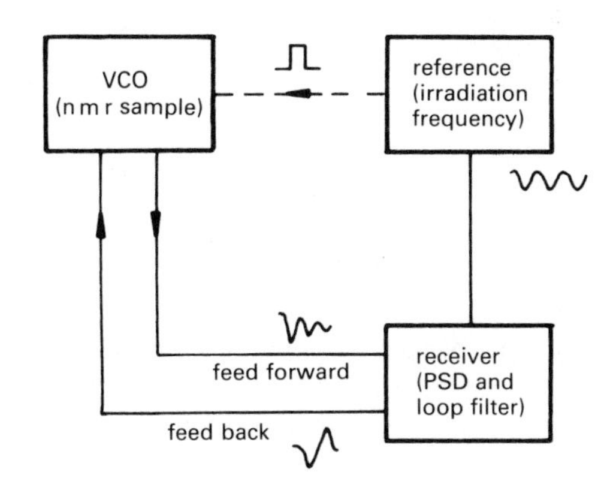

Fig. L4. The lock circuitry is essentially a phase-locked loop system with a stability which is determined by the spectrometer reference frequency.

The difference between the circuit of Fig. L4 and a classical phase-locked loop is that the VCO is not sustained and requires 'pumping' with a pulse derived from the reference generator. The system adequately maintains field/frequency stability to a high degree.

Longitudinal magnetization See **classical formalism**.

Longitudinal spin order In certain two-dimensional NMR experiments, signals may arise from the phenomenon known as longitudinal spin order. For example, in the two-dimensional ^1H–^1H **nuclear Overhauser effect** (NOESY) experiment, if the rotation angle of the second pulse $\beta \neq \pi/2$, antiphase single-quantum coherence generated during the t_1 period is converted into four terms:

$$2I_yS_z \xrightarrow{\beta(I_x+S_x)} 2I_yS_z \cos^2\beta + 2I_zS_z \sin\beta\cos\beta - 2I_yS_y \sin\beta\cos\beta - 2I_zS_y \sin^2\beta. \quad \text{L21}$$

The second term is known as longitudinal two-spin order. It can be converted into observable antiphase magnetization by a third pulse with $\beta \neq \pi/2$. Experiments such as z–z spectroscopy and **z-filtered COSY** depend for their success upon the generation of $2I_zS_z$ terms during the evolution of the spin system. In the NOESY experiment proper, or indeed in exchange spectroscopy, crosspeaks derived from spin order are often undesirable, and they can be eliminated by careful calibration of the flip angles of the pulses.

FURTHER READING

Bodenhausen, G., Wagner, G., Rance, M., Sørensen, O. W., Wuthrich, K., and Ernst, R. R. (1984). *J. Magn. Reson.* **59,** 542.

Lorentzian line See **lineshape**.

Lowering operator See **shift operator**.

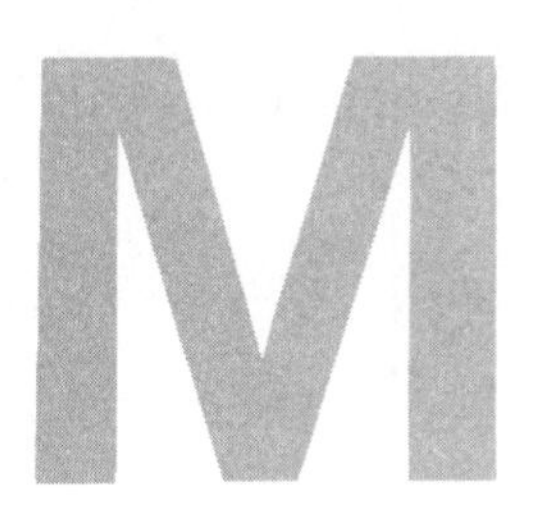

Magic-angle spinning Magic-angle spinning (MAS) is a technique which was developed by Lowe and Andrew as a means by which dipole–dipole couplings could be suppressed in **solid state NMR** spectra. MAS can be a very effective method for the suppression of such couplings, but only in cases where the magnitude of the coupling is less than the attainable spinning speeds (5 KHz). Moreover, homogeneous dipolar broadening can be removed by rotations in **spin space** using r.f. decoupling. However, MAS has notable effects upon other spin interactions, of which the most important is the chemical shift. More specifically, MAS narrows the **chemical shift** dispersion which is an inherent property of solid state NMR spectra. In an amorphous solid or crystal powder, a complicated lineshape is observed that arises from the sum of all possible chemical shifts (see **powder spectrum**). For example, in ^{13}C solid state NMR spectra, where the solid is typically composed of a variety of chemically different carbons, the ^{13}C spectrum is a sum of different chemical shift anisotropy patterns, having different shapes and different isotropic centres. The resulting broadening arises from restrictions placed on molecular motion in the solid. Experimentally, it is possible to restore some of this motion by spinning the sample. The chemical shift anisotropy (σ_{izz}) can conveniently be expressed in terms of the angle of rotation of the sample with respect to the applied field:

M1 $$\sigma_{izz} = (3\cos^2\beta - 1)(\text{other terms}) + (\tfrac{3}{2}\sin^2\beta)\sigma_i$$

when β is chosen to be 54.7°, $3\cos^2\beta - 1 = 0$, and $\sigma_{izz} = \sigma_i$, the isotropic chemical shift, i.e. that which is observed in NMR of liquids. This results in high-resolution ^{13}C NMR spectra of solids, and the angle $\beta = 54.7°$ is referred to as the magic angle.

FURTHER READING

Andrew, E. R. (1971). *Prog. NMR Spectr.* **8,** 1.

Schaefer, J. and Stejskal, E. (1979). In *Topics in carbon-13 NMR spectroscopy* **3,** Chapter 4.

Magnetic moment The classical concept of an NMR active nucleus as a rotating charge gives rise to a nuclear magnetic moment. This is analogous to the magnetic moment possessed by a simple bar magnet or compass needle. An important principle in the classical theory of NMR (which gives rise to the **Bloch equations**) states that the rate of change of angular momentum (ρ) of the spinning nucleus, depends upon the torque ($\mu \times B$) exerted on the magnetic moment (μ) by the applied field (B):

M2 $$\frac{\mathrm{d}\rho}{\mathrm{d}t} = \mu B.$$

It is easily shown by classical mechanics that the torque exerted on a magnetic moment by a magnetic field inclined at an angle θ to the moment results in the precession of the nuclear magnetic moment about the direction of the field with a frequency given by the Larmor equation (see **Larmor precession**):

M3 $$\omega = \gamma B_0.$$

The quantum mechanical **expectation value** of μ has a time dependence which is exactly that shown by the classical magnetization (see **classical formalism**).

Magnetic resonance imaging See **imaging**.

Magnetization Magnetization is a term which is in general use in the description of pulsed NMR. Formally, magnetization is equivalent to the x, y, or z component **expectation values** of the angular momentum operators I_x, I_y, I_z (see **angular momentum**). The response from the ensemble of nuclei in an NMR sample is often referred to as a bulk magnetization vector, which at equilibrium lies along the $+z$ axis (Fig. M1). The rotations of this vector in cartesian space under the influence of r.f. pulses and delays comprises the **classical formalism**.

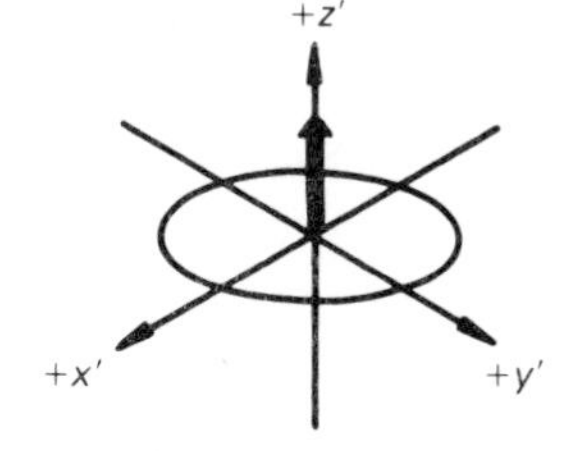

Fig. M1. The equilibrium bulk magnetization vector used in the classical description of NMR.

Magnetogyric ratio In NMR, we are concerned with magnetic systems that possess angular momentum. A system such as a nucleus may consist of many coupled particles. In any given state, the NMR properties of this nucleus may fundamentally be described by a total magnetic moment μ and a total angular momentum I. Both of these properties are vectors, and these may be taken as parallel, and as such may be described by

M4 $$\mu = \gamma I,$$

where γ is the magnetogyric ratio. For a given nucleus, γ is a constant.

Magnitude calculation See **absolute-value mode**.

Magnus expansion See **average Hamiltonian theory**.

Matrix algebra See Appendix 3.

Matrix representation In order to predict the results of NMR experiments, spectroscopists often employ the **density matrix** formalism. The **evolution** of the **spin system** under various **Hamiltonians** corresponding to delays or r.f. pulses is represented by the time evolution of the density matrix. The latter is given by the **Liouville–von Neumann equation**

M5 $$\dot{\sigma} = -i\hbar^{-1}[\mathcal{H}, \sigma].$$

Assuming that the Hamiltonian $\mathcal{H}$ in (M5) is time independent, then (M5) can be solved for $\sigma(t)$:

M6 $$\sigma(t) = \exp\{-i\mathcal{H}t\}\sigma(0)\exp\{i\mathcal{H}t\}$$

where the exponential operators (**propagators**) are formulated according to the relevant Hamiltonian which operates between $t=0$ and $t=t$. In the case where the Hamiltonian is time dependent then (M6) is not a solution of (M5) (see **average Hamiltonian theory**). In general, (M6) must be evaluated explicitly using the matrix representations of $\sigma(0)$, exp $\{-i\mathcal{H}t\}$, and $\exp\{i\mathcal{H}t\}$. In this section we illustrate how matrix representations for $\exp\{-i\mathcal{H}t\}$ and $\exp\{i\mathcal{H}t\}$ can be evaluated.

The form of $\mathcal{H}$ will depend upon whether an r.f. pulse or a free precession period (delay) is applied to the spin system. Let us first consider the case of an r.f. pulse of arbitrary flip-angle β applied along the x axis. The relevant Hamiltonian for this perturbation on a single spin is given by

M7 $$\mathcal{H} = (\beta/t)I_x$$

with an analogous expression for a r.f. pulse applied along the y axis. The corresponding exponential operator of this Hamiltonian is

M8 $$R = \exp\{-iI_x\beta\}$$

which is often abbreviated to R since the exponential operator can be thought of as a **rotation operator** which 'rotates' the density matrix. In order to express R in matrix form it is necessary to recast (M8) by expanding the exponent:

M9 $$\exp\{-\mathrm{i}I_x\beta\} = 1 - \mathrm{i}I_x\beta - \frac{I_x^2\beta^2}{2!} + \frac{\mathrm{i}I_x^3\beta^3}{3!} + \frac{I_x^4\beta^4}{4!} + \ldots.$$

Using the rules of operator powers (see Appendix 1), (M9) can be grouped into even and odd powers in I_x:

M10 $$\exp\{-\mathrm{i}I_x\beta\} = 1\left(1 - \frac{\beta^2}{2!\,2^2} + \frac{\beta^4}{4!\,2^4} - \frac{\beta^6}{6!\,2^6} + \ldots\right) - 2\mathrm{i}I_x\left(\beta - \frac{\beta^3}{3!\,2^3} + \frac{\beta^5}{5!\,2^5} - \ldots\right).$$

Each bracketed term on the right-hand side of (M10) can be equated with the Taylor series for cosine and sine, respectively. Thus

M11 $$\exp\{-\mathrm{i}I_x\beta\} = [\cos(\beta/2)\mathbf{1} - 2\mathrm{i}\sin(\beta/2)I_x],$$

where $\mathbf{1}$ is the **identity operator**. If the exponential operator in (M8) acts upon a group of spins i, then R becomes slightly more complicated:

M12 $$R = \exp\{-\mathrm{i}F_x\beta\} = \exp\left\{-\mathrm{i}\sum_{\mathrm{i}} I_{xi}\beta\right\}$$

i.e. for two spins I and S we would have

M13 $$R = \exp\{-\mathrm{i}(I_x + S_x)\beta\}$$

In expressions such as (M13) which contain more than one operator, it is permissible to express the exponent as a product of exponents according to the normal rules of algebra. However, this is possible only if the two operators commute (see **commutator**). In this case they clearly do, since I_x and S_x operate upon different spins. We can therefore write

M14 $$R = \exp\{-\mathrm{i}(I_x + S_x)\beta\} = \exp\{-\mathrm{i}I_x\beta\}\exp\{-\mathrm{i}S_x\beta\}$$

and using (M11) we can express $R = \exp\{-\mathrm{i}F_x\beta\}$ for two spins I and S as

M15 $$\begin{aligned}\exp\{-\mathrm{i}F_x\beta\} &= [\cos(\beta/2)\mathbf{1}_I - 2\mathrm{i}\sin(\beta/2)I_x)(\cos(\beta/2)\mathbf{1}_S - 2\mathrm{i}\sin(\beta/2)S_x]\\ &= [\cos^2(\beta/2)\mathbf{1}_I\mathbf{1}_S - 4\sin^2(\beta/2)I_xS_x\\ &\quad -2\mathrm{i}\sin(\beta/2)\cos(\beta/2)I_x\mathbf{1}_S\\ &\quad -2\mathrm{i}\sin(\beta/2)\cos(\beta/2)\mathbf{1}_IS_x].\end{aligned}$$

Analogous expressions exist for an arbitrary number of spins. Equation (M11) (for a single spin) or (M15) (for two spins) can now be used to obtain matrix representations for either $\exp\{-\mathrm{i}I_x\beta\}$ or $\exp\{-\mathrm{i}F_x\beta\}$ respectively. This is achieved by evaluating each element of the matrix according to

M16 $$R_{mn} = \langle m|\,A\,|n\rangle$$

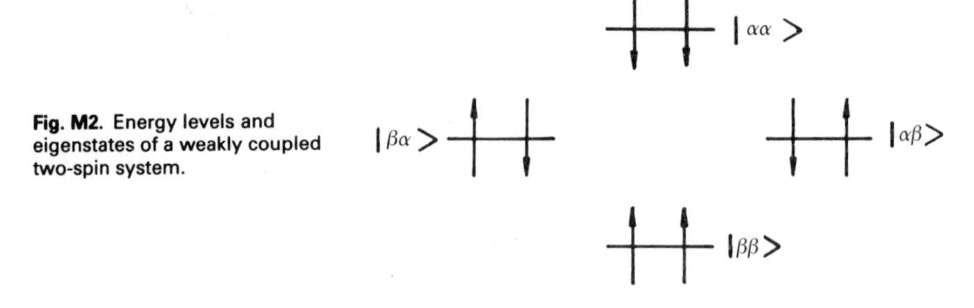

Fig. M2. Energy levels and eigenstates of a weakly coupled two-spin system.

where the **bra-ket notation** identifies the eigenstates ψ_m and ψ_n with the corresponding eigenvalues m and n. For example, a weakly coupled two-spin system can be described in terms of Fig. M2. We can construct a 4×4 matrix whose elements are labelled with these states:

$$R = \begin{array}{c} \\ |\alpha\alpha\rangle \\ |\alpha\beta\rangle \\ |\beta\alpha\rangle \\ |\beta\beta\rangle \end{array} \begin{array}{cccc} |\alpha\alpha\rangle & |\alpha\beta\rangle & |\beta\alpha\rangle & |\beta\beta\rangle \\ \left[\begin{array}{c} \\ \\ \\ \\ \end{array} \right. & & & \left. \begin{array}{c} \\ \\ \\ \\ \end{array} \right] \end{array} \tag{M17}$$

By inserting (M15) into (M16), we can evaluate each element of the matrix explicitly. For example, the upper left-hand element (R_{11}) of (M17) is evaluated according to

$$\begin{aligned} R_{11} = \langle \alpha\alpha |\, & \cos^2(\beta/2)\mathbf{1}_I\mathbf{1}_S - 4\sin^2(\beta/2)I_xS_x - 2\mathrm{i}\sin(\beta/2)\cos(\beta/2)I_x\mathbf{1}_S \\ & -2\mathrm{i}\sin(\beta/2)\cos(\beta/2)\mathbf{1}_IS_x\, |\alpha\alpha\rangle. \end{aligned} \tag{M18}$$

Although this expression appears complicated, it is actually very easy to evaluate. We can make things easier by expressing (M18) in a slightly different form:

$$\begin{aligned} R_{11} = {} & \langle \alpha\alpha |\ \cos^2(\beta/2)\mathbf{1}_I\mathbf{1}_S\, |\alpha\alpha\rangle = \mathrm{c}^2\langle \alpha\alpha |\, \mathbf{1}_I\mathbf{1}_S\, |\alpha\alpha\rangle \\ & + \langle \alpha\alpha |\, -4\sin^2(\beta/2)I_xS_x\, |\alpha\alpha\rangle = -4\mathrm{s}^2\langle \alpha\alpha |\, I_xS_x\, |\alpha\alpha\rangle \\ & + \langle \alpha\alpha |\, -2\mathrm{i}\sin(\beta/2)\cos(\beta/2)I_x\mathbf{1}_S\, |\alpha\alpha\rangle = -2\mathrm{isc}\langle \alpha\alpha |\, I_x\mathbf{1}_S\, |\alpha\alpha\rangle \\ & + \langle \alpha\alpha |\, -2\mathrm{i}\sin(\beta/2)\cos(\beta/2)\mathbf{1}_IS_x\, |\alpha\alpha\rangle = -2\mathrm{isc}\langle \alpha\alpha |\, \mathbf{1}_IS_x\, |\alpha\alpha\rangle \end{aligned} \tag{M19}$$

where $\mathrm{c} = \cos(\beta/2)$ and $\mathrm{s} = \sin(\beta/2)$. Each of the four terms on the right in (M19) can be readily evaluated using the rules for **angular momentum** operators. Remembering that I_x operates only on the state of spin I, and

S_x operates only on the state of spin S, we find:

M20
$$\begin{aligned}
c^2\langle\alpha\alpha|\,\mathbf{1}_I\mathbf{1}_S\,|\alpha\alpha\rangle &= c^2\langle\alpha\alpha\mid\alpha\alpha\rangle = c^2\\
-4s^2\langle\alpha\alpha|\,I_xS_x\,|\alpha\alpha\rangle &= -s^2\langle\alpha\alpha\mid\beta\beta\rangle = 0\\
-2isc\langle\alpha\alpha|\,I_x\mathbf{1}_S\,|\alpha\alpha\rangle &= -isc\langle\alpha\alpha\mid\beta\alpha\rangle = 0\\
-2isc\langle\alpha\alpha|\,\mathbf{1}_IS_x\,|\alpha\alpha\rangle &= -isc\langle\alpha\alpha\mid\alpha\beta\rangle = 0
\end{aligned}$$

and thus $R_{11} = c^2$. With practice each matrix element can be evaluated from (M18) by inspection. The full matrix representation of R is thus

M21
$$R = \begin{bmatrix} c^2 & -isc & -isc & -s^2\\ -isc & c^2 & -s^2 & -isc\\ -isc & -s^2 & c^2 & -isc\\ -s^2 & -isc & -isc & c^2 \end{bmatrix}$$

where we drop the matrix element labels since they are implied. R^{-1} can be calculated in an analogous manner, and will be seen to be equal to R with the imaginary elements changing sign.

In the case of free precession, assuming weak scalar coupling, the Hamiltonian for two spins I and S is

M22
$$\mathcal{H} = \mathcal{H}_Z + \mathcal{H}_J = \omega_I I_z + \omega_S S_z + 2\pi J I_z S_z$$

and the corresponding exponential operator corresponding to free precession is

M23
$$\exp\{-i\mathcal{H}t\} = \exp\{-i(\omega_I I_z + \omega_S S_z + 2\pi J I_z S_z)t\}.$$

Since I_z, S_z, and I_zS_z commute (see **commutator**), (M23) can again be expressed as a product of three exponentials:

M24
$$\exp\{-i\mathcal{H}t\} = \exp\{-i\omega_I I_z t\}\,.\,\exp\{-i\omega_S S_z t\}\,.\,\exp\{-i2\pi J I_z S_z t\}.$$

It is possible to calculate the matrix representation of (M24) by entirely analogous methods to those described above. However this is an unnecessary complication. Provided the **basis states** are eigenstates of the **Hamiltonian**, the exponential operators will always be diagonal. Since for the weak coupling case the basis functions in Fig. M2 are eigenstates of the weak coupling Hamiltonian (M22), we can immediately write

M25
$$\exp\{-i\mathcal{H}t\} = \begin{bmatrix} \exp\{-\mathcal{H}_{11}t\} & 0 & 0 & 0\\ 0 & \exp\{-i\mathcal{H}_{22}t\} & 0 & 0\\ 0 & 0 & \exp\{-i\mathcal{H}_{33}t\} & 0\\ 0 & 0 & 0 & \exp\{-i\mathcal{H}_{44}t\} \end{bmatrix}$$

where $\mathscr{H}_{mn}$ are the diagonal elements (**eigenvalues**) of the Hamiltonian (M22) (not the exponential form!) in its matrix representation which can be derived by inserting (M22) into (M16);

M26
$$\mathscr{H} = \begin{bmatrix} \frac{1}{2}(\omega_I + \omega_S) + \frac{1}{4}J & 0 & 0 & 0 \\ 0 & \frac{1}{2}(\omega_I - \omega_S) - \frac{1}{4}J & 0 & 0 \\ 0 & 0 & -\frac{1}{2}(\omega_I - \omega_S) - \frac{1}{4}J & 0 \\ 0 & 0 & 0 & -\frac{1}{2}(\omega_I + \omega_S) + \frac{1}{4}J \end{bmatrix}.$$

Clearly $\exp\{i\mathscr{H}t\}$ is defined in an analogous manner to (M25):

M27
$$\exp\{i\mathscr{H}t\} = \begin{bmatrix} \exp\{i\mathscr{H}_{11}t\} & 0 & 0 & 0 \\ 0 & \exp\{i\mathscr{H}_{22}t\} & 0 & 0 \\ 0 & 0 & \exp\{i\mathscr{H}_{33}t\} & 0 \\ 0 & 0 & 0 & \exp\{i\mathscr{H}_{44}t\} \end{bmatrix}.$$

One further matrix evaluation is required in order to extract the observable magnetization; that of F_x (see **density matrix**). This is simply derived by the operation of $F_x = I_x + S_x$ upon the basis functions, e.g.

M28
$$\begin{aligned} F_{x_{11}} &= \langle \alpha\alpha | \, I_x + S_x \, | \alpha\alpha \rangle \\ &= \langle \alpha\alpha | \, I_x \, | \alpha\alpha \rangle \\ &\quad + \langle \alpha\alpha | \, S_x \, | \alpha\alpha \rangle = 0, \end{aligned}$$

M29
$$\begin{aligned} F_{x_{12}} &= \langle \alpha\alpha | \, I_x + S_x \, | \alpha\beta \rangle \\ &= \langle \alpha\alpha | \, I_x \, | \alpha\beta \rangle \\ &\quad + \langle \alpha\alpha | \, S_x \, | \alpha\beta \rangle = \tfrac{1}{2}. \end{aligned}$$

The full matrix representation of F_x in the case of the two-spin system IS is thus

M30
$$F_x = \frac{1}{2} \begin{bmatrix} 0 & 1 & 1 & 0 \\ 1 & 0 & 0 & 1 \\ 1 & 0 & 0 & 1 \\ 0 & 1 & 1 & 0 \end{bmatrix}.$$

The above calculations demonstrate how to calculate the matrix forms of exponential operators in the **weak coupling** limit. However, in certain circumstances we sometimes need to calculate the results of experiments upon strongly coupled systems (see **strong coupling**) or upon systems which are effectively strongly coupled during some time period (see

homonuclear Hartmann–Hahn spectroscopy, total correlation spectroscopy (TOCSY)). Under these circumstances, the **weak coupling Hamiltonian** $2\pi J I_z S_z$ must be replaced by the full isotropic coupling Hamiltonian $\mathcal{H}_J = 2\pi J \mathbf{I} \cdot \mathbf{S} = 2\pi J(I_x S_x + I_y S_y + I_z S_z)$. The matrix representation of this Hamiltonian is difficult to obtain since the three terms in the Hamiltonian do not commute. If, however, we work in the **eigenbasis** of the strongly coupled system, rather than the **product basis** of Fig. M2, the calculation is simplified. This is because the matrix representation of the strong coupling Hamiltonian including the Zeeman term

M31 $$\mathcal{H} = \omega_I I_z + \omega_S S_z + 2\pi \mathbf{I} \cdot \mathbf{S}$$

is diagonal if the basis set is the eigenbasis. In the case of a strongly coupled two-spin system *IS*, the eigenbasis wave functions (those which diagonalize the Hamiltonian) can be calculated using the **variational method** (Fig. M3). We can use these basis functions directly as we did for the product functions in (M18), (M19), and (M20) to generate, for example, a rotation operator for an r.f. pulse applied along the x axis of the rotating frame:

M32 $$R = \begin{bmatrix} c^2 & -iusc & -ivsc & -s^2 \\ -iusc & c^2 & -s^2 & -iusc \\ -ivsc & -s^2 & c^2 & -ivsc \\ -s^2 & -iusc & -ivsc & c^2 \end{bmatrix}$$

where $u = \cos\theta + \sin\theta$, $v = \cos\theta - \sin\theta$, and $\tan 2\theta = J/(|\omega_A - \omega_B|)$. In an analogous manner to the weak coupling case, the exponential operator corresponding to evolution is diagonal:

M33 $$\exp\{-i\mathcal{H}t\} = \begin{bmatrix} \exp\{-i\mathcal{H}_{11}t\} & 0 & 0 & 0 \\ 0 & \exp\{-i\mathcal{H}_{22}t\} & 0 & 0 \\ 0 & 0 & \exp\{-i\mathcal{H}_{33}t\} & 0 \\ 0 & 0 & 0 & \exp\{-i\mathcal{H}_{44}t\} \end{bmatrix}$$

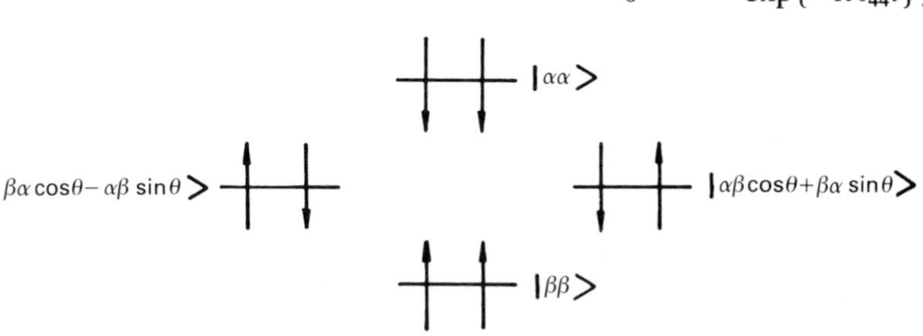

Fig. M3. Energy levels and eigenstates of a strongly coupled two-spin system.

where the $\mathcal{H}_{nn}$ are the diagonal elements (**eigenvalues**) of the matrix of the strong coupling Hamiltonian (M31) evaluated using the eigenbasis in Fig. M3:

M34
$$\mathcal{H} = \begin{bmatrix} \frac{1}{2}(\omega_I + \omega_S) + \frac{1}{4}J & 0 & 0 & 0 \\ 0 & -\frac{1}{4}J + C & 0 & 0 \\ 0 & 0 & -\frac{1}{4}J - C & 0 \\ 0 & 0 & 0 & -\frac{1}{2}(\omega_I + \omega_S) + \frac{1}{4}J \end{bmatrix}$$

where $C = \frac{1}{2}[(\omega_I - \omega_S)^2 + J^2]^{\frac{1}{2}}$. Similarly, matrices corresponding to F_x and F_y are calculated in an analogous manner to the weak coupling case by calculating the elements explicitly using the eigenbasis in Fig. M3:

M35
$$F_x = \begin{bmatrix} 0 & U & V & 0 \\ U & 0 & 0 & U \\ V & 0 & 0 & V \\ 0 & U & V & 0 \end{bmatrix}.$$

Actually, the matrix representations of exponential operators in the strong coupling case can be calculated in an alternative manner. If we define a matrix U and its inverse U^{-1} which diagonalizes the **strong coupling** Hamiltonian when it is evaluated in the product base (cf. M34):

M36
$$\mathcal{H} = \begin{bmatrix} \frac{1}{2}(\omega_I + \omega_S) + \frac{1}{4}J & 0 & 0 & 0 \\ 0 & \frac{1}{2}(\omega_I - \omega_S) - \frac{1}{4}J & \frac{1}{2}J & 0 \\ 0 & \frac{1}{2}J & -\frac{1}{2}(\omega_I - \omega_S) - \frac{1}{4}J & 0 \\ 0 & 0 & 0 & -\frac{1}{2}(\omega_I + \omega_S) + \frac{1}{4}J \end{bmatrix}$$

then U can be thought of as a matrix which converts from the product base to the eigenbase:

M37
$$\mathcal{H}_e = U \mathcal{H}_p U^{-1}$$

where $\mathcal{H}_e = $ (M34), $\mathcal{H}_p = $ (M36), and

M38
$$U = \begin{bmatrix} 1 & 0 & 0 & 0 \\ 0 & \cos\theta & \sin\theta & 0 \\ 0 & -\sin\theta & \cos\theta & 0 \\ 0 & 0 & 0 & 1 \end{bmatrix}.$$

Matrix representations evaluated in the product base may then be evaluated in the eigenbasis in a manner analogous to (M37) e.g.

M39
$$F_{x_e} = U F_{x_p} U^{-1}.$$

The reader may care to prove that evaluation of (M39) using (M30) and (M38) gives (M35). Either method may therefore be employed as convenient in calculations upon strongly coupled systems.

Maximum entropy processing In principle, the information content of a **Fourier transform** NMR spectrum can be increased by **convolution** (or deconvolution) of time series data (the **free induction decay**, FID) prior to Fourier transformation. Examples include increased signal-to-noise ratio by application of a matched filter, or resolution enhancement by a sine–bell function.

An entirely distinct procedure for the processing of NMR data, known as the maximum entropy method (MEM) is theoretically capable of achieving simultaneous resolution enhancement and increased signal-to-noise ratios. The basic principle of the method is quite straightforward. The FIDs derived from a series of trial spectra by inverse Fourier transformation are compared with the experimental FID. Most of the trial time-domain data can be rejected since they bear no resemblance to the experimental data. However, some of these trial data will match the experimental data quite closely, and in the absence of prior knowledge of the experimental spectrum, there is no reason to favour one of the corresponding trial spectra over all others. The most likely trial spectrum which matches the experimental spectrum is chosen on the grounds of minimum information content, i.e. maximum entropy. The maximum entropy solution gives an unbiased choice from amongst the possible candidates.

In practice, this procedure is performed iteratively by digital computers using a more efficient algorithm than that described above. The entropy, S, is defined as

M40 $$S = -\sum_{n=1}^{N} \left(\frac{\chi_n}{b}\right) \ln\left(\frac{\chi_n}{b}\right)$$

where χ_n is the intensity of the nth point in a trial spectrum digitized at N regular intervals and b is a parameter which incorporates information regarding knowledge about the spectrum baseline. Inverse Fourier transformation of (M40) gives

M41 $$y_m = \sum_{n=1}^{N} \exp(-2\pi i(n-1)(m-1)/N)\chi_n$$

where y_m is the mth complex intensity in the trial FID. The compatibility of the FID corresponding to the trial spectrum with the experimental signal is measured in terms of the χ^2 statistic:

M42 $$\chi^2 = \frac{1}{\sigma^2} \sum_{m=1}^{m=M/2} |y_m - d_m|^2 = M$$

where m is the number of data points. The quantity d_m is the mth complex intensity in the experimental FID and σ is the r.m.s. noise amplitude. The overall objective is to match y_m and d_m to within a tolerance specified by the noise level. The entropy S must be maximized with respect to χ_n. In practice the procedure requires a considerable amount of computing time. It is also important to realise that MEM is a non-linear method, and so in general information regarding intensity is not preserved.

FURTHER READING

For a description of MEM applied to NMR data, see

Sibisi, S., Skilling, J., Brereton, R., Laue, E., and Staunton, J. (1984). *Nature (London)* **311,** 446.

For a critical assessment of MEM, see

Davies, S. J., Bauer, C. J., Hore, P. J., and Freeman, R. (1988). *J. Magn. Reson.* **76,** 476.

Mixed state There exist quantum mechanical systems for which no experiment gives an unique result that can be predicted with certainty. Systems of this nature are described as being in a 'mixed' state, to distinguish them from 'pure' states. Mixed states can be represented by the incoherent superposition of pure states. In other words, to calculate the probability of a given result with a system in a mixed state, it is necessary to calculate the probability for each pure state and then take an average, in which each pure state is 'weighted' with a coefficient. NMR spectroscopists are interested in 'mixed' states, since in the NMR sample all the spins are not in an identical state. In order to predict the results of NMR experiments upon such mixed states, we therefore employ a statistical mechanical formalism (see **ensemble average**). The state of the spin system is then represented by the **density matrix**, and its equation of motion (see **Liouville–von Neumann equation**) allows us to determine the state of the spin system at any given time during an experiment. As an example, the spin orientation of a spin $\frac{1}{2}$ nucleus is represented by a density matrix with two rows and columns, corresponding to two **pure states** of opposite spin orientation.

Mixing time See **nuclear Overhauser effect spectroscopy**.

Modulation See **amplitude modulation**, **frequency modulation**, **phase modulation**.

Multiple-quantum coherence A system of n weakly coupled spins can be described by 2^n eigenstates formulated in terms of simple product functions (see **product basis**). For a two-spin $\frac{1}{2}$ system IS we therefore

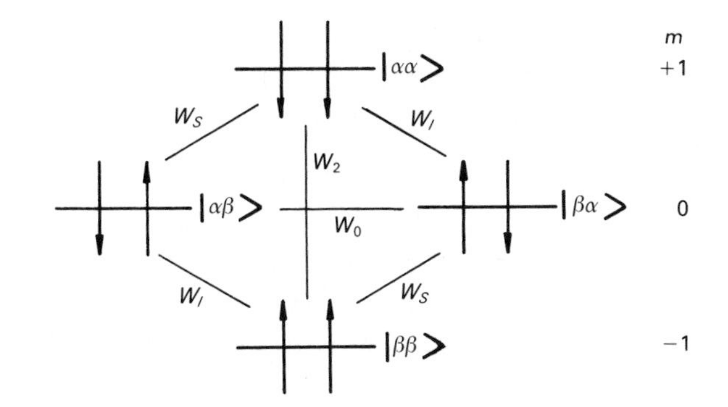

Fig. M4. The four energy levels and product functions of two coupled spins $\frac{1}{2}$.

find four energy levels (Fig. M4), where the eigenstates are labelled in the **bra-ket notation**. Each state is characterized by a value for the magnetic quantum number *m*, and a selection rule of **angular momentum** requires that only transitions between states with $\Delta m = \pm 1$ can lead to observable **magnetization**. These are the so-called 'allowed'' transitions, which correspond to W_I and W_S in Fig. M4. They are also often referred to as single-quantum transitions. In contrast, two further transitions can be identified in Fig. M4, corresponding to $\Delta m = 2$ (W_2) and $\Delta m = 0$ (W_0). These do not lead to observable magnetization in a simple pulse-and-collect NMR experiment, and are members of a class known as **forbidden transitions**. In this particular example W_2 is known as a double-quantum transition, W_0 is known as a zero-quantum transition, and collectively they are called multiple-quantum transitions. While **phase coherence** of single-quantum transitions can be adequately represented using the simple vector representation of the **classical formalism**, the phase coherence of multiple-quantum transitions (multiple-quantum coherence) cannot be pictured in this manner. It is necessary to employ the **density matrix** formalism for the description of such coherences. At thermal equilibrium, the density matrix of states is a 4×4 matrix with diagonal elements which represent the populations of the states:

$$\begin{array}{c} \\ |\alpha\alpha\rangle \\ |\alpha\beta\rangle \\ |\beta\alpha\rangle \\ |\beta\beta\rangle \end{array} \begin{array}{c} \begin{array}{cccc} |\alpha\alpha\rangle & |\alpha\beta\rangle & |\beta\alpha\rangle & |\beta\beta\rangle \end{array} \\ \begin{bmatrix} P_1 & 0 & 0 & 0 \\ 0 & P_2 & 0 & 0 \\ 0 & 0 & P_3 & 0 \\ 0 & 0 & 0 & P_4 \end{bmatrix} \end{array} . \tag{M43}$$

The off-diagonal elements indicate phase coherence 'in progress' between states. These are created as the density matrix evolves under the various **Hamiltonians** which operate during the course of an experiment. We can show matrix (M43) diagrammatically to show the characteristics of the off-diagonal elements;

$$\begin{bmatrix} \text{POP} & \text{SQC} & \text{SQC} & \text{DQC} \\ \text{SQC} & \text{POP} & \text{ZQC} & \text{SQC} \\ \text{SQC} & \text{ZQC} & \text{POP} & \text{SQC} \\ \text{DQC} & \text{SQC} & \text{SQC} & \text{POP} \end{bmatrix}. \quad \text{M44}$$

The elements SQC represent single-quantum coherence, and are equivalent to precessing transverse magnetization vectors in the classical formalism. In contrast, the labels ZQC and DQC represent zero- and double-quantum coherence, which do not have a classical equivalent, and they do not induce a signal in the receiver coils of the spectrometer. The presence of non-zero off-diagonal elements describes an ongoing coherence of the specified type. After a single pulse, for example (see **density matrix**) only SQC elements are occupied (together with the diagonal elements). Both ZQC and DQC elements are zero. In order to create the latter, it is necessary to apply a second perturbation to a non-equilibrium matrix, i.e. one which already possesses non-zero SQC elements which have not decayed due to relaxation. The simplest method by which this can be achieved is by the application of two 90° pulses separated by a delay (Fig. M5). A sequence of this type is found in for example **double-quantum filtered correlated spectroscopy**. This sequence creates all orders of multiple-quantum coherence in an n-spin system. If we can separate these orders, a whole variety of multiple-quantum experiments becomes available to us, allowing the unique properties of multiple-quantum coherences to be exploited in unravelling the complex spin system found in macromolecules. There are two ways in which we can separate the various orders of multiple-quantum coherence. The first uses a much more complex sequence than that shown in Fig. M5 to excite multiple-quantum coherence. The overall purpose of this sequence is to achieve **order-selective excitation**. The second relies upon a sequence such as that shown in Fig. M5 to create all orders of coherence, followed by order-selective detection of the required coherence. In principle, the first method is much more efficient, particularly for the large-order coherences. However, in systems with spin couplings measurable in Hz, the excitation sequence becomes extremely long, and the efficiency is lost due to relaxation between the pulses. This method is therefore restricted to systems where large dipolar couplings (measurable in kHz) are present, i.e. solids and liquid crystalline systems. In liquids the dipolar

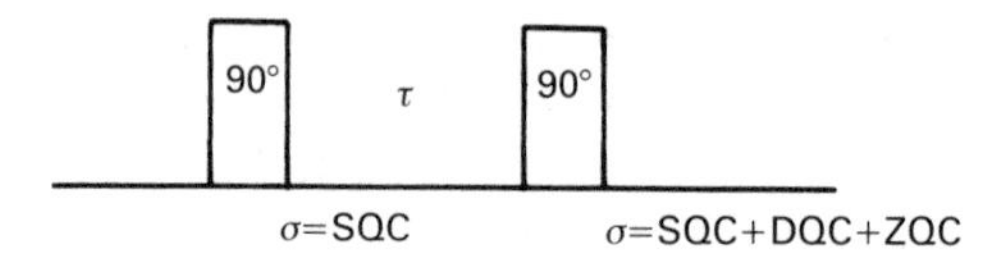

Fig. M5. Simplest pulse sequence for the creation of multiple-quantum coherence. SQC, DQC, and ZQC are single-quantum, double-quantum, and zero-quantum coherences respectively.

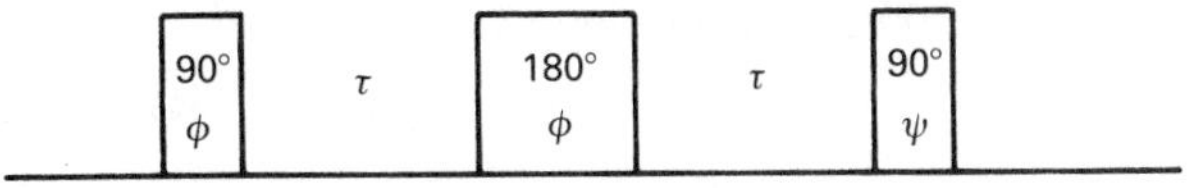

90° ϕ	τ	180° ϕ	τ	90° ψ

Fig. M6. A practical pulse sequence for the selective detection of arbitrary orders of multiple-quantum coherence.

couplings average to zero (see **averaging**) and the less efficient order-selective detection sequence is employed. In its simplest form, the order-selective detection sequence consists of Fig. M5, together with the relevant **phase cycling**. In experiments such as **double-quantum correlated spectroscopy**, a three-pulse sequence is used (Fig. M6) where $\psi = \phi$. This is the even-order-selective detection sequence, exciting coherences of order 0, 2, 4, 6, . . . etc. In order to detect selectively for example double-quantum coherence, we exploit the characteristic properties of each coherence order under the influence of phase cycling. Similarly, the pulse sequence of (M6) with $\psi = \phi + 90°$ is the odd-order-selective detection sequence, exciting coherences of order 1, 3, 5, 7, . . . etc., and we can selectively detect triple-quantum coherence with the relevant phase cycling. The basis of the phase cycling procedures is the behaviour of multiple-quantum coherence of order n under the influence of a phase shift of order ϕ:

M45 $$(n\text{QT})_x \xrightarrow{\phi I_z} (n\text{QT})_x \cos n\phi + (n\text{QT})_y \sin n\phi.$$

Thus a 90° phase shift rotates single-quantum coherence through 90°, double-quantum coherence through 180°, triple-quantum coherence through 270°, and so on. Zero-quantum coherence is invariant to a phase shift. Thus if we repeat sequence (M6) with ϕ and ψ initially 0°, and increment each by 90° we obtain the following for each even coherence order:

	0°	90°	180°	270°
0	$+x$	$+x$	$+x$	$+x$
2	$+x$	$-x$	$+x$	$-x$
4	$+x$	$+x$	$+x$	$+x$
6	$+x$	$-x$	$+x$	$-x$

Subtraction of each alternate experiment achieves selection of order 2 and 6. At the sample concentrations commonly used in biological NMR, sixth-order coherence is not observed due to the low excitation efficiency, and hence the sequence can be considered double-quantum coherence selective.

A similar set of experiments can be performed using the odd-order-selective sequence. In this case we can for example begin with $\phi = 0°$ and

$\psi = 90°$, and increment each by 60°:

	0	60	120	180	240	300
1	$+x$	$x+60°$	$x+120°$	$-x$	$-x+60°$	$-x+120°$
3	$+x$	$-x$	$+x$	$-x$	$+x$	$-x$
5	$+x$	$-x+120°$	$-x+60°$	$-x$	$x+120°$	$x+60°$
7	$+x$	$x+60°$	$x+120°$	$-x$	$-x+60°$	$-x+120°$
9	$+x$	$-x$	$+x$	$-x$	$+x$	$-x$

For similar reasons the sequence can be considered triple-quantum coherence selectively on subtraction of the data. However, neither sequence is complete since multiple-quantum coherence cannot be directly detected. A third pulse is required either immediately after the second 90° pulse (leading to **multiple-quantum filters**) or after a delay t_1 (see e.g. **double-quantum correlated spectroscopy**). This converts the selectively detected multiple-quantum coherence to observable single-quantum coherence. This basic set of principles is inherent in all multiple-quantum NMR experiments in liquids. The applications of the various methods together with detailed analyses are described under each experiment.

FURTHER READING

A good review of multiple quantum NMR is
Bodenhausen, G. (1981). *Progr. NMR Spectr.* **14,** 137.

See also

Braunschweiler, L., Bodenhausen, G., and Ernst, R. R. (1983). *Mol. Phys.* **48,** 535.

Ernst, R. R., Bodenhausen, G., and Wokaun, A. (1987). *Principles of NMR in one and two dimensions.* p. 449ff. Clarendon Press, Oxford.

Multiple-quantum filters An important aspect of NMR experiments upon spin systems which are not at thermal equilibrium is the creation of **multiple-quantum coherence**. These are of fundamental importance in a very useful class of experiments which contain multiple-quantum filters. The rationale in all of these experiments is to achieve editing of NMR spectra by using the characteristic properties of the multiple-quantum spectra of various spin systems. Some of the more useful experiments are recorded in two dimensions (see **double-quantum correlated spectroscopy**, **double-quantum filtered correlated spectroscopy**, **triple-quantum filtered correlated spectroscopy**). However, multiple-quantum filters can be employed in conventional one-dimensional NMR with equal success. Simply stated, a multiple-quantum filter can be thought of as a black box, into which the response from the spin system is fed. The output consists of a simplified response, which depends upon the coherence order selected, and upon the characteristics of the spin system under investigation. Before considering this in more detail, it is useful to illustrate the basic principle with an example. Let us postulate that the black box is set to filter **double-quantum coherence**. In other words, only responses from spin systems within which a state of double-quantum coherence can be created will pass the filter. If, for example, we were to examine the NMR response from a mixture of **spin systems** such as A and AX, then we would selectively detect the response from the AX spin system, since two coupled spins are required in order to create a state of double-quantum coherence. The response from the one-spin system is thus filtered out. Unfortunately the double-quantum filter would fail to remove responses from an AMX system, since double-quantum coherence is efficiently created in such a system. However, if we examine the principles in more detail, we can begin to see how this difficulty can be overcome.

In biological NMR we are mainly concerned with NMR of liquids, and thus the order-selective detection scheme of multiple quantum coherence is universally employed, despite its less than optimum sensitivity. The front-end of the pulse sequence designed for multiple-quantum filtration thus consists of three r.f. pulses and two delays (Fig. M7). The order of coherence filtration depends upon the choice of phases ϕ, and ψ (see **multiple-quantum coherence**). For example, if we wish to construct a double-quantum filter, the ϕ and ψ are both set to 0°, and are incremented sequentially by 90° at each transient. However, since multiple-quantum coherences cannot be detected directly (see **observable**, **forbidden transitions**), we require a further 90° r.f. pulse immediately after the third, to 'read' the phase properties of multiple-quantum coherence into observable single-quantum coherence. For a double-quantum filter, the resulting data are alternatively added and subtracted in sympathy with the phase cycle described above. The complete pulse sequence is shown in Fig. M8 where Δ is a small delay (several μs) to allow a clean shift of r.f. phase between the third and fourth pulses. The relevant phase cycle is as follows:

ϕ	ψ	receiver
0	0	+
90°	90°	−
180°	180°	+
270°	270°	−

As usual, this cycle is repeated four times with incrementation of

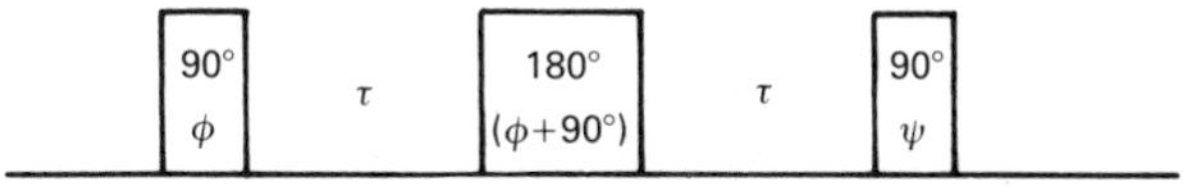

90° ϕ — τ — 180° $(\phi+90°)$ — τ — 90° ψ

Fig. M7. Three-pulse sequence for the creation of multiple-quantum coherence.

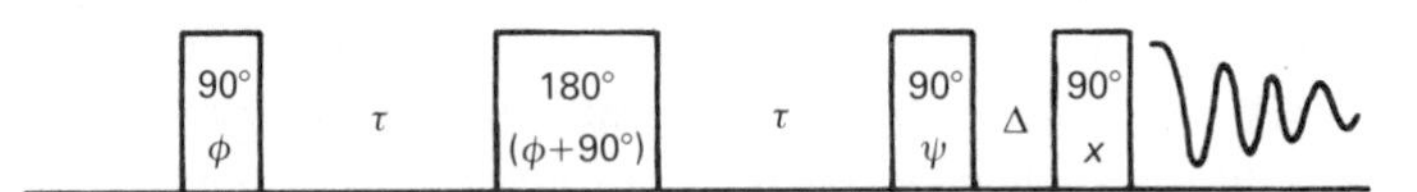

Fig. M8. Pulse sequence for the acquisition of NMR spectra filtered through double-quantum coherence.

CYCLOPS phase cycling at every fourth transient, giving a minimum of $16n$ scans.

The difficulty with a multiple-quantum filter scheme of this type is the dependence of the magnitude of the created multiple-quantum coherence upon the delay τ. It can be shown theoretically (see e.g. **double-quantum correlated spectroscopy**) that the efficiency of creation of double-quantum coherence using the pulse sequence in Fig. M8 is, for a loosely coupled two-spin system IS,

M46 $$M_{\mathrm{DQ}} \propto \sin(2\pi J_{IS}\tau).$$

This is of no concern if we are simply interested in a magnetically isolated two-spin system (see **DOUBTFUL**), but this is rarely the case in biological NMR. More probably we would employ a double-quantum filter to remove singlet resonances from the spectrum (derived for example from weak solvent lines or uncoupled methyl groups), at the same time hoping to leave the rest of the spectrum unperturbed. This is obviously impossible unless all spin couplings are of the same magnitude. One means by which the constraint defined by (M46) can be circumvented is to employ so-called 'accordion-like' preparation, whereby a group of experiments (of $16n$ scans each) is recorded, each with a different value of τ. This method is reasonably effective. However, there is an alternative method, which would appear to be more efficient in this regard. At the same time it points us in the direction of a scheme which might allow us to achieve true order selection of a given coherence for a specific type of spin system. Naturally, the increased performance is gained at the expense of additional complexity.

The basic principle of the alternative method, due to Sorensen *et al.*, is to modify the pulse sequence such that the efficiency of creation of multiple-quantum coherence exhibits a $\sin^2$ dependence with respect to τ. Thus, in the case of a double-quantum filter, (M46) becomes

M47 $$M_{\mathrm{DQ}} \propto \sin^2(2\pi J_{IS}\tau).$$

The pulse sequence with which this function can be generated consists essentially of an additional pulse train after the t_1 evolution period (Fig. M9). Antiphase magnetization created by the 90° pulse immediately before the t_1 period is partially refocused during the second evolution period 2τ. It can readily be demonstrated, using for example the **product operator formalism**, that this generates the desired $\sin^2$ dependence. If,

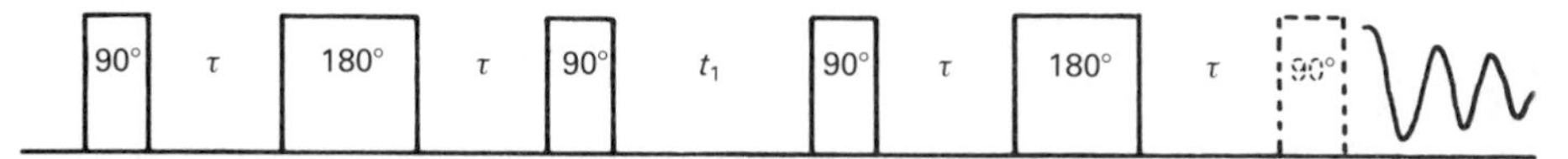

Fig. M9. Pulse sequence for uniform excitation of multiple-quantum coherence. The final optional 'purging pulse' removes multiplet distortions.

now, signal averaging is employed for variable τ, i.e. the value of τ is stochastically or sequentially varied for each experiment with a given t_1 increment, the average magnetization is proportional to $\overline{\sin^2(2\pi J_{IS}\tau)} = \frac{1}{2}$. Double-quantum coherence is thus created independent of the magnitude of J. The optional 'purging pulse' in Fig. M9 can be employed to remove undesirable multiplet distortions. A feature in common with all multiple-quantum filters such as those shown in Fig. M8 and M9 is their high-pass characteristic; that is, a multiple-quantum filter of order p is transparent to higher orders. A simple modification of the symmetrical sequence to Fig. M9 can impart a bandpass characteristic to the filter. This modification consists simply in the addition of a 180° pulse in the centre of the t_1 period (Fig. M10). This sequence exploits the fact that the p-spin coherences from N-spin systems with $N > p$ are split by couplings to the additional $N - p$ 'passive' spins, while the p-quantum coherence of a p-spin system is not. Thus, during the evolution period t_1 with a central π pulse to refocus chemical shifts, the p-quantum coherences of p-spin systems do not evolve, whereas the p-quantum p-spin coherences of spin systems $N > p$ evolve under the additional J couplings. Averaging of responses with variable t_1 may therefore eliminate the responses of larger spin systems. Although imperfect, a 'p-spin filter' such as this may be useful in unravelling the complex multiplet patterns found in the NMR spectra of biomolecules.

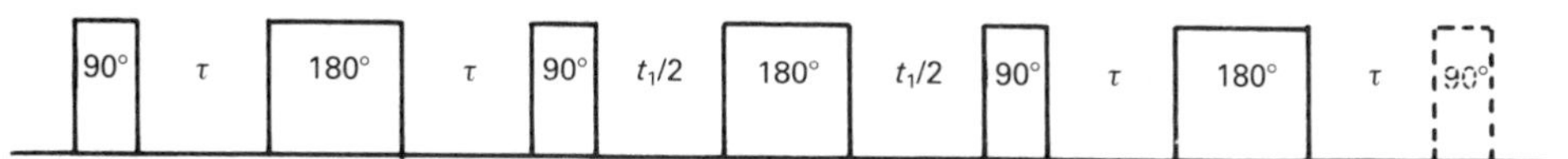

Fig. M10. Pulse sequence for 'bandpass' multiple-quantum filtration which is selective to order p. The final 'purging pulse' removes multiplet distortions.

FURTHER READING

Sorensen, O. W., Levitt, M. H., and Ernst, R. R. (1983). *J. Magn. Reson.* **55**, 104.

Multiple-quantum transition See **multiple-quantum coherence**.

N

NOE See **nuclear Overhauser effect.**

NOESY see **nuclear Overhauser effect spectroscopy**.

Noise The signal induced in the receiving coils of an NMR probe is typically in the range 10^{-9}–10^{-5} V. The Brownian motion of electrons in a conductor at room temperature generate e.m.f.s. in this range also. Only in the case of zero resistance and/or zero temperature are the latter thermal e.m.f.s equal to zero. Obviously they are undesirable, and short of performing experiments at 0 K, steps must be taken to ensure that the level of noise which is eventually detected (in the electronic sense of the word, see **detector**) is minimal. The r.m.s. noise e.m.f. over a bandwidth $\Delta\nu$ about the Larmor frequency of interest is given by

N1 $$(\bar{N}^2)^{\frac{1}{2}} = \sqrt{4kTr\,\Delta\nu}$$

where k is the Bolzmann constant, T is the absolute temperature, and r is the resistance of the source. In physical terms noise can be thought of as a function whose phase is a totally random function of frequency, but the amplitude is not, and has the RMS value defined by equation (N1). In contrast, the desired signal is phase coherent. We can therefore improve the quality of the signal (i.e. the signal-to-noise ratio) by using **signal averaging** procedures.

Noise figure In general, the signal obtained from the probe of an NMR spectrometer is of very small amplitude, and contains apart from the desired signal a certain amount of **noise**. The purpose of the spectrometer preamplifier (see **amplifier**) is to amplify the desired signal without distortion and without the addition of extra noise. A measure of the ability of the preamplifier to achieve this objective is given by the noise figure. If the RMS value of the noise derived from the signal source is given as N_S, and the extra noise introduced by the preamplifier has an r.m.s. value given by N_A, then the noise figure, F, is given by

N2 $$F = 10\log_{10}\left[\frac{N_A^2 + N_S^2}{N_S^2}\right],$$

where F is expressed in dB. A poor preamplifier has a noise figure greater than 3 dB, in which case the signal-to-noise ratio is degraded by a factor greater than 2. The number of acquisitions required to overcome the signal-to-noise degradation is thus quadrupled. A good preamplifier has a noise figure of less than 1 dB, corresponding to a degradation of less than 12%.

FURTHER READING

Hoult, D. I. (1978). *Prog. NMR Spectr.* **12,** 41.

Nonexponential relaxation See **relaxation**.

N-type peak See **antiecho**.

Nuclear Overhauser effect Originally, the nuclear Overhauser effect (NOE) was defined as a change in the integrated NMR absorption intensity of a nuclear spin when the NMR absorption of another spin is saturated (see **saturation**). It is worthwhile considering in simple physical terms how this effect might occur. Consider a two-spin system IS which is not J-coupled (although the analysis holds for **weak coupling**) (Fig. N1). We can define transition probabilities (W) per unit time between states as illustrated. The equilibrium populations of each level are governed by the **Boltzmann distribution**, and can be defined as follows:

$$P_4^0 = p + \delta, \qquad P_2^0 = P_3^0 = P, \qquad P_1^0 = P - \delta. \tag{N3}$$

Now, the NMR resonance of spin I is composed of transitions 4–2 and 3–1, and likewise for spin S, 4–3 and 2–1. The absorption intensity of the I spins must be proportional to the net population difference across the relevant transitions:

$$M_I = (P_4^0 - P_2^0) + (P_3^0 - P_1^0) = +2\delta. \tag{N4}$$

If the absorption intensity of spin S is now saturated by the application of a strong r.f. field at the Larmor frequency (see **Larmor precession**) of spin S, the populations are equalized across the S spin transitions, and since

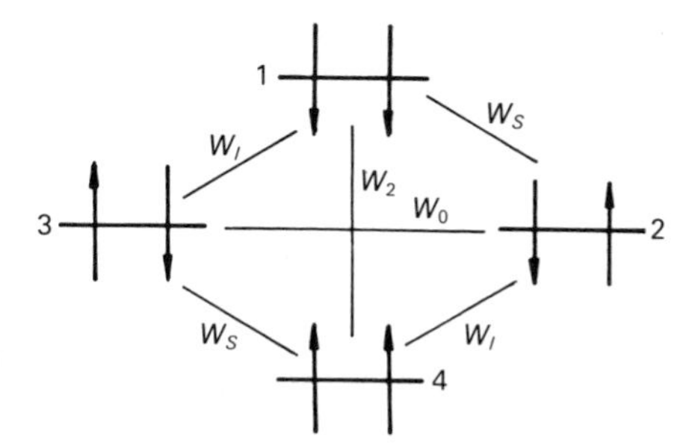

Fig. N1. Spin states and transition probabilities for a two-spin system IS.

the total number of spins must remain unchanged,

N5 $$P_4 = P_3 = P + \tfrac{1}{2}\delta \quad \text{and} \quad P_2 = P_1 = P - \tfrac{1}{2}\delta \quad \text{and} \quad M_I = +2\delta$$

In other words the absorption intensity of spin I is unchanged on saturation of spin S. However, we have not yet considered the transition probabilities between states. In the presence of the strong r.f. field upon spin S, W_S will not alter the spin state populations, since these are being made equal by the field. Also, the saturation of spin S equilibrates the transitions of spin I, that is,

$$P_4 - P_2 = P_4^0 - P_2^0$$

N6 and

$$P_3 - P_1 = P_3^0 - P_1^0$$

where the P's and P^0's represent the populations in the absence and presence of S spin saturation respectively. There will therefore be no net change in populations due to W_I alone. Conversely, the population difference $P_4 - P_1 = \delta$, whereas $P_4^0 - P_1^0 = 2\delta$. Thus, W_2 will effectively reestablish equilibrium during S spin saturation by equalizing P_4 and P_1; i.e., P_4 will be increased by an amount (say) Δ, whereas P_1 will decrease by a similar amount. Thus the I spin absorption intensity, in the presence of S spin saturation, becomes

N7 $$\begin{aligned} M_I &= (P_4 - P_2) + (P_3 - P_1) \\ &= (P + \tfrac{1}{2}\delta + \Delta - (P - \tfrac{1}{2}\delta)) + (P + \tfrac{1}{2}\delta - (P - \tfrac{1}{2}\delta - \Delta) \\ &= +2(\delta + \Delta) \end{aligned}$$

which is 2Δ greater than the equilibrium value. In a realistic case, all transition probabilities are effective. This can be seen clearly by using a more rigorous treatment. In using transition probabilities in the simple physical picture described above, we have actually been considering the effects of **spin–lattice relaxation** on the spin-state populations. Thus, a clearer insight into the mechanism of the NOE can be had by examining the theory of spin–lattice relaxation. Of particular importance is the relaxation between two dipolar coupled spins. As described under spin–lattice relaxation, the time evolution of the longitudinal magnetizations of two dipolar coupled spins I and S is given by the coupled differential equations

N8 $$\frac{\mathrm{d}\langle I_Z \rangle}{\mathrm{d}t} = -\rho_I(\langle I_Z \rangle - I_0) - \sigma_{IS}(\langle S_Z \rangle - S_0)$$

N9 $$\frac{\mathrm{d}\langle S_Z \rangle}{\mathrm{d}t} = -\rho_S(\langle S_Z \rangle - S_0) - \sigma_{SI}(\langle I_Z \rangle - I_0)$$

where

$$\rho_I = (2W_I + W_2 + W_0)$$

$$\rho_S = (2W_S + W_2 + W_0)$$

$$\sigma_{SI} = \sigma_{IS} = (W_2 - W_0)$$

and I_0, S_0, and $\langle I_Z \rangle$, $\langle S_Z \rangle$ are the equilibrium and transient magnetization components of spins I and S. In analogy to the physical picture given above, we can examine the effect of saturating the I spins. Under these conditions, $\langle I_Z \rangle = 0$. If we define 'steady-state' conditions, such that $\mathrm{d}\langle S_Z \rangle / \mathrm{d}t = 0$, then (N9) gives

N10 $$\langle S_Z \rangle = S_0 + \frac{\sigma_{IS}}{\rho_S} I_0.$$

Assuming I and S are like spins $\frac{1}{2}$, (almost invariably protons) then saturation of spin I increases the absorption intensity of spin S by (σ_{IS}/ρ_S) over the equilibrium value. This is the 'steady-state' NOE. Equation (N10) clearly shows the interplay between the transition probabilities in the generation of the NOE. Since σ and ρ depend upon the Larmor frequencies of the spins (ω), the correlation time of the internuclear vector (τ_C), and the internuclear distance (r), it follows that the magnitude of the NOE is dependent upon all of these factors. In particular assuming isotropic relaxation, we can define the situation where $\omega\tau_C \approx 1.118$, when $\sigma_{IS} = 0$, and no NOE is detectable. This is rationalized by noting that $W_2 = W_0$ under these conditions. In the **extreme narrowing** limit, i.e. $\omega^2\tau_C \ll 1$, W_2 is greater than W_0, and a positive NOE results, with a maximum intensity of 0.5. Conversely, in the **spin diffusion** limit, $\omega^2\tau_C^2 \gg 1$, W_0 becomes much larger than W_2, and a negative NOE results, with a maximum intensity of -1, i.e. the resonance line may disappear completely. In macromolecular NMR, the motion is generally within the spin diffusion limit, and negative NOEs are usually observed.

Apart from the 'steady-state' NOE, equations (N8) and (N9) are a general starting point in the calculation of a variety of phenomena known collectively as 'transient' NOEs. That is, the development of the NOE is monitored with respect to a variable time period. Experimentally, both steady-state and transient methods are capable of yielding information regarding molecular conformation by way of the internuclear distance dependence of the NOE. However, in biological spectroscopy of macromolecules these methods have given way to the more efficient two-dimensional nuclear Overhauser effect (NOESY) technique (see **nuclear Overhauser effect spectroscopy**). Like its one dimensional counterpart, the theory of NOESY has its roots in the transient solutions of (N8) and (N9).

In order to see how distance information can be obtained from one-dimensional NOE measurements, we will examine a typical example. Consider an experiment upon a two-spin $\frac{1}{2}$ system IS, where the magnetization of spin S is selectively inverted, after which the time development of the NOE to spin I is measured. This represents one of several means by which transient NOE can be measured. The initial conditions are $\langle I_z \rangle = I_0$ and $\langle S_z \rangle = -S_0$ at $t = 0$. Using these boundary conditions, (N8) and (N9) represent an initial value problem which has the analytical solutions

N11
$$\langle I_z \rangle = I_0 + C_1 \exp\{-\lambda_1 t\} + C_2 \exp\{-\lambda_2 t\}$$
$$\langle S_z \rangle = S_0 + \frac{\lambda_1 - \rho_I}{\sigma_{IS}} C_1 \exp\{-\lambda_1 t\} + \frac{\lambda_2 - \rho_I}{\sigma_{IS}} C_2 \exp\{-\lambda_2 t\}$$

where

$$\lambda_{1,2} = \tfrac{1}{2}\{(\rho_A + \rho_B) \pm [(\rho_A - \rho_B)^2 + 4\sigma_{IS}^2]^{\frac{1}{2}}\}$$

and

$$C_1 = -C_2 = -2S_0\sigma_{IS}/(\lambda_1 - \lambda_2).$$

Now consider the 'initial rate approximation', where t is very small. Under these conditions, we can write

N12
$$\langle I_z \rangle \approx I_0 + C_1(1 - \lambda_1 t) + C_2(1 - \lambda_2 t)$$

which reduces to

N13
$$\langle I_z \rangle = I_0 + 2S_0\sigma_{IS}t.$$

Thus, the initial slope of a plot of $\langle I_z \rangle$ against t (i.e. the NOE buildup rate) is proportional to σ_{IS}. Now under isotropic motion of the internuclear vector with a correlation time τ_c, and at a given Larmor frequency (see **spin–lattice relaxation**), σ is proportional to the inverse sixth power of the internuclear distance:

N14
$$\sigma_{IS} \alpha \frac{1}{r_{IS}^6}.$$

To extract structural information, therefore, the buildup rate of the NOE corresponding to an unknown distance is compared with that corresponding to a known distance, and the unknown distance is thus readily computed. This procedure can also be used in larger networks of dipolar coupled nuclei. However, it is essential in any application to ensure that the initial rate approximation is not violated.

See also **spin–lattice relaxation**, **spin diffusion**.

FURTHER READING

Noggle, J. H. and Schirmer, R. E. (1971). *The Nuclear Overhauser effect, chemical applications*. Academic Press, New York.

Nuclear Overhauser effect spectroscopy NOESY (See also **nuclear Overhauser effect**.) The NOESY experiment applied to protons is one of the most important techniques available in biological spectroscopy, since under the correct conditions a complete set of short-range (<5 Å) through space connectivities can be obtained for a macromolecule. This is therefore the primary NMR method for solving the complete solution structure of the molecule.

The NOESY experiment consists of three r.f. pulses, together with the ubiquitous phase cycle. Unlike the majority of two-dimensional experiments, NOESY can be understood classically (see **classical formalism**). The pulse scheme is shown in Fig. N2. We can follow each stage of the experiment diagrammatically. Starting with equilibrium magnetization of the spin system (which we will assume to be not J-coupled), the first 90° pulse creates XY magnetization (Fig. N3). The spins will now begin to precess in the rotating frame during t_1 with their characteristic Larmor frequencies, in complete analogy to classical one-dimensional NMR. If we consider just two spins IS with Larmor frequencies $+\delta\omega$ and $+2\delta\omega$ respectively from the transmitter **carrier**, then the situation for a finite value of t_1 will be Fig. N4. If, now, a second 90° pulse is applied along the $+x$ axis, the magnetization vectors will be rotated such that a component exists along the $-z$ axis (Fig. N5). During the subsequent mixing period τ_m, z-magnetization components exchange under the influence of cross-relaxation. The transverse components are not required and are removed by **phase cycling** or homospoil techniques. The magnetization vectors therefore have a component in the z direction only after either of these procedures. Finally, a third 90°x pulse regenerates observable magnetization (Fig. N6). If this sequence is repeated for a larger value of t_1, the the magnetization vectors would dephase further in Fig. N4. A smaller $-z$ component is thus created in Fig. N5, which would pass through zero and become positive for increasing values of t_1 (Fig. N7). These changes are 'read' by the final 90° pulse. In other words, an **amplitude modulation** of the magnetization is generated as a function of t_1. The frequency of this modulation is proportional to the Larmor precession frequency of the spin concerned; the magnetization of spin I would modulate at $\delta\omega$ Hz and of spin S at $2\delta\omega$ Hz. The purpose of the 90°–t_1–90° sequence is

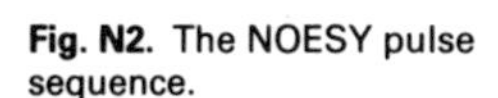

Fig. N2. The NOESY pulse sequence.

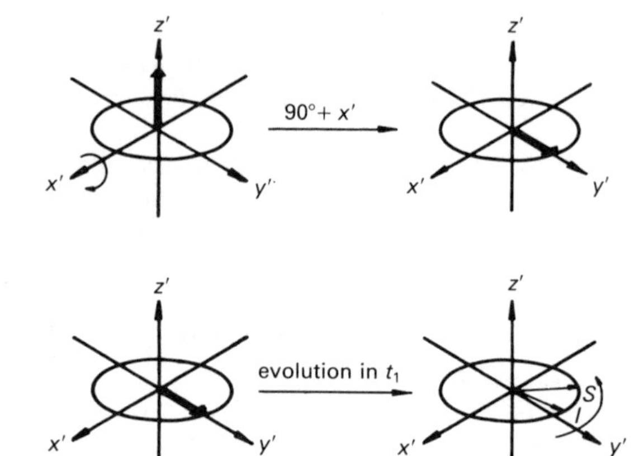

Fig. N3. The first r.f. pulse in the NOESY sequence creates transverse ($x'-y'$) magnetization in the rotating frame.

Fig. N4. Precession of magnetization vectors during t_1.

therefore to frequency-label the magnetization vectors, and then to rotate them along the $-z$ axis. After exchange of magnetization during τ_m, each vector then precesses with its characteristic Larmor precession frequency in the XY plane during t_2 after the third pulse. In analogy to **correlated spectroscopy** (COSY) we can therefore imagine four distinct events during the course of the NOESY pulse sequence. Firstly, the magnetization vector of spin I will precess wth its characteristic Larmor frequency $\delta\omega$ Hz during t_1. During the mixing time, a proportion of this magnetization is transferred to spin S, at a rate determined by **cross-relaxation** between the two spins. The transferred magnetization will thus precess at the Larmor frequency of spin S ($2\delta\omega$ Hz) during t_2. Magnetization which failed to 'migrate' during the t_1 period will continue to precess at $\delta\omega$ Hz during t_2. Applying an exactly analogous (and

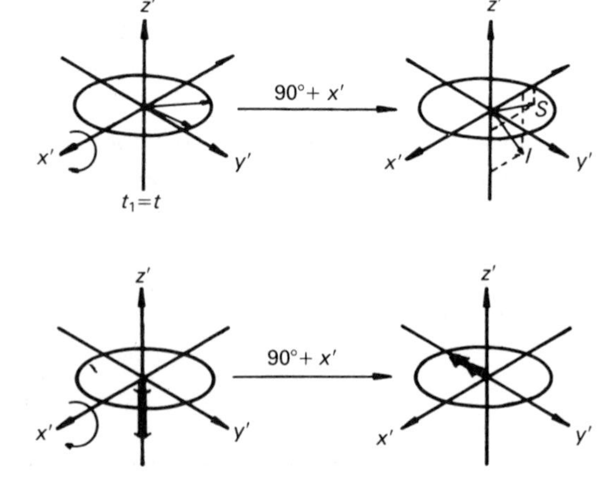

Fig. N5. The second pulse in the NOESY sequence creates longitudinal magnetization.

Fig. N6. After phase cycling or homospoil techniques, the third pulse in the NOESY sequence creates x–y magnetization.

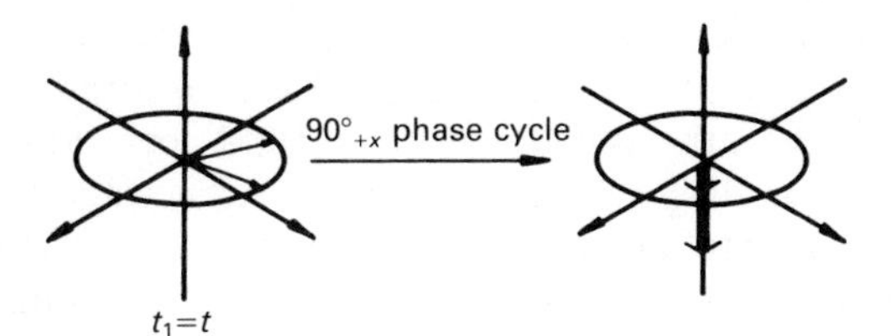

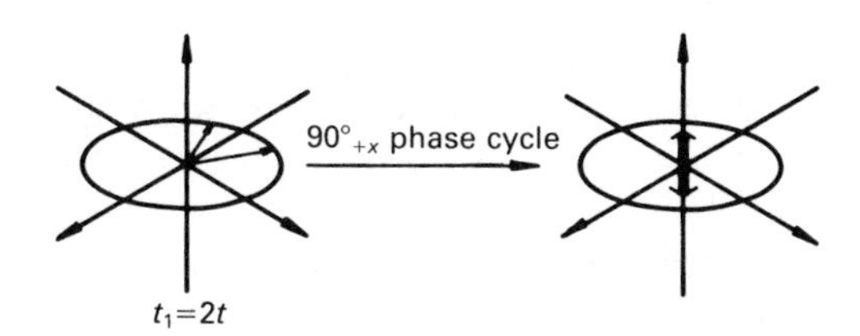

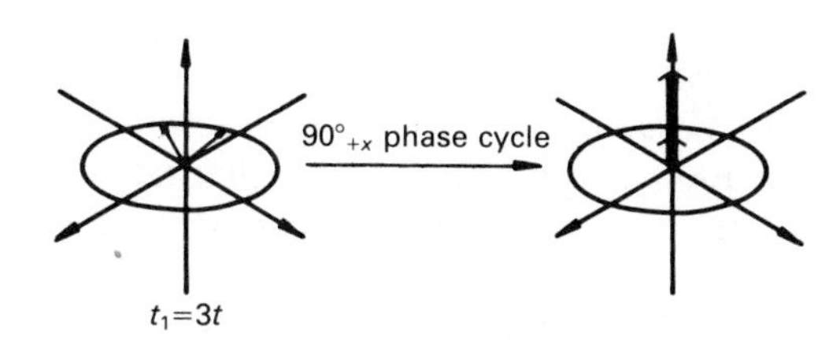

Fig. N7. The situation at the beginning of the mixing period (τ_m) of the NOESY sequence for three consecutive t_1 values.

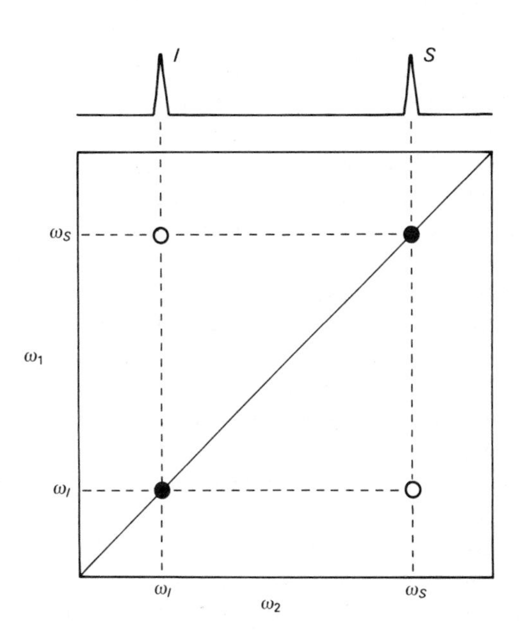

Fig. N8. The essential features of a NOESY experiment on two through-space coupled spins. The filled circles represent diagonal peaks and the open circles are crosspeaks.

symmetrical) argument to spin S we can predict the result of the experiment. After **two-dimensional Fourier transformation** with respect to t_1 and t_2, the **two-dimensional NMR** spectrum will resemble Fig. N8. We observe diagonal peaks which are generated by magnetization which fails to migrate during τ_m, and crosspeaks which are generated from the magnetisation transfer between the two spins. This transfer is a cross-relaxation process, commonly referred to as the **nuclear Overhauser effect**. Since this process depends in part upon the distance between the nuclei, the crosspeaks correlate resonances which are through-space coupled. We can therefore begin to see why NOESY is particularly useful in the determination of macromolecular structure.

The above shows in a qualitative manner how crosspeaks can be generated in the NOESY experiment. However, in any practical application, a variety of crosspeaks can be generated by mechanisms other than cross-relaxation, and these can cause unacceptable confusion in the qualitative interpretation of through-space coupling networks. In addition, as will become clear when we examine the mixing process in more detail, the analysis of NOESY spectra to provide quantitative distance information is also affected by such artefacts. In order to see where these artefacts come from, we must consider the NOESY experiment in rather more detail.

As in all two-dimensional spectra, **axial peaks** occur in NOESY, but these can be cancelled by **phase cycling**. However, additional crosspeaks may also occur in NOESY spectra of uncoupled spins which are not generated by cross-relaxation. These derive from chemical exchange within the sample. Such effects may arise for example from the flipping of the aromatic rings of tyrosine residues in proteins, whereby the ring protons experience two distinct environments. Crosspeaks may occur between resonances with chemical shifts corresponding to each environment. While in some circumstances exchange crosspeaks can give valuable information on the exchange process (see **exchange spectroscopy**), in NOESY they can cause undesirable complications. In the standard NOESY experiment, it is not possible to easily distinguish between exchange and cross-relaxation peaks, and the former certainly cannot be removed by phase cycling without also cancelling cross-relation peaks. Fortunately, however, in the systems of interest in biology, the problem is not significant since the experimenter is usually aware of the existence of chemical exchange in the sample. In cases where it is necessary to distinguish between peak types, an alternative experiment, **rotating frame Overhauser effect spectroscopy** (*ROESY*) can be employed.

Thus far we have considered artefacts which are generated in spin systems which are not J-coupled (see **spin coupling**). In any practical situation, we will inevitably attempt to observe cross-relaxation pathways via NOESY in systems of J-coupled spins. This generates an additional type of artefact known as J crosspeaks which are generated by **coherence transfer**. More specifically, the first two pulses in NOESY can generate single- and **multiple-quantum coherences** between coupled spins which are converted to observable magnetization by the third pulse. Since the creation of multiple-quantum coherence is a non-classical phenomenon, we must resort to a quantum mechanical description of the processes which lead to J crosspeaks. This is made more tractable with the use of the **product operator formalism**, since this allows us to follow the fate of the magnetization components during the course of the experiment.

If we consider a J-coupled two-spin $\frac{1}{2}$ system IS, the state of the density operator (see **density matrix**) at equilibrium is given by

$$\sigma_0 = I_z + S_z. \tag{N15}$$

After the first 90° pulse along the x axis, followed by evolution during t_1 under chemical shift and spin coupling terms, we can calculate an expression for the density operator using the simple rules of the product operator formalism:

$$\begin{aligned}\sigma_2 = {} & [-I_y \cos \omega_I t_1 + I_x \sin \omega_I t_1 - S_y \cos \omega_S t_1 + S_x \sin \omega_S t_1] \cos \pi J_{IS} t_1 \\ & +[+2I_xS_z \cos \omega_I t_1 + 2I_yS_z \sin \omega_I t_1 + 2I_zS_x \cos \omega_S t_1 \\ & +2I_zS_y \sin \omega_S t_1] \sin \pi J_{IS} t_1.\end{aligned} \tag{N16}$$

If a second 90° r.f. pulse is now applied along the x axis, the density operator takes the form

$$\begin{aligned}\sigma_3 = {} & [-I_z \cos \omega_I t_1 + I_x \sin \omega_I t_1 - S_z \cos \omega_S t_1 + S_x \sin \omega_S t_1] \cos \pi J_{IS} t_1 \\ & -[2I_xS_y \cos \omega_I t_1 + 2I_yS_x \cos \omega_S t_1 + 2I_zS_y \sin \omega_I t_1 \\ & +2I_yS_z \sin \omega_S t_1] \sin \pi J_{IS} t_1.\end{aligned} \tag{N17}$$

The terms $2I_xS_y$ and $2I_yS_x$ consist of a superposition of double- and zero-quantum coherence, which can be demonstrated by expanding (N17):

$$\begin{aligned}\sigma_3 = {} & [-I_z \cos \omega_I t_1 + I_x \sin \omega_I t_1 - S_z \cos \omega_S t_1 + S_x \sin \omega_S t_1] \cos \pi J_{IS} t_1 \\ & +\{\tfrac{1}{2}[(2I_xS_y \overset{(1)}{+} 2I_yS_x) - (2I_yS_x \overset{(2)}{-} 2I_xS_y)] \cos \omega_I t_1 \\ & +\tfrac{1}{2}[(2I_xS_y \overset{(3)}{+} 2I_yS_x) + (2I_yS_x \overset{(4)}{-} 2I_xS_y)] \cos \omega_S t_1 \\ & +2I_zS_y \sin \omega_I t_1 + 2I_yS_z \sin \omega_S t_1\} \sin \pi J_{IS} t_1\end{aligned} \tag{N18}$$

where terms (1) and (3) represent double-quantum coherence, and (2) and (4) represent zero-quantum coherence. Now, since we are only interested in longitudinal magnetization components during the mixing period τ_m, it is necessary to remove all components except $-I_z \cos \omega_I t_1$

and $-S_z \cos \omega_S t_1$. Note that these terms do indeed possess **amplitude modulation** during t_1, with their respective chemical shifts, as predicted from our simple classical treatment. In order to remove unwanted components we can phase cycle (see **phase cycling**) the first two pulses. If we phase cycle these by 90° each, i.e. XX, YY, $-X-X$, $-Y-Y$ and add each separate response then this will cancel coherences of order $1, 2, 3, 5, \ldots$ due to the characteristic phase properties of the various orders (see **phase cycling, multiple-quantum coherence**). It will also be necessary to repeat this procedure with the phase of the first and third pulses shifted by 180°, to cancel axial peaks. However, we will fail to separate zero-quantum coherence due to these procedures, since, like the longitudinal magnetization, it is insensitive to the phase shifts of the first two pulses. Therefore we find at the beginning of the mixing period

N19
$$\sigma_3 = (-I_z \cos \omega_I t_1 - S_z \cos \omega_S t_1) \cos \pi J_{IS} t_1 + (I_y S_x - I_x S_y) \times [\cos \omega_S t_1 - \cos \omega_I t_1] \sin \pi J_{IS} t_1.$$

The zero-quantum term $(I_y S_x - I_x S_y)$ evolves according to the normal rule for the evolution of zero-quantum coherence (see **product operator formalism**), and the longitudinal $(-I_z)$ terms mix under the effects of cross-relaxation. After the final 90° X pulse, the **observable** magnetization is

N20
$$\sigma_4 = [I_y a_{II} \cos \omega_I t_1 + S_y a_{SS} \cos \omega_S t_1 + I_y a_{SI} \cos \omega_S t_1 + S_y a_{IS} \cos \omega_I t_1] \times \cos \pi J_{IS} t_1 + (I_z S_x - I_x S_z) \cos (\omega_I - \omega_S) \times \tau_m (\cos \omega_S t_1 - \cos \omega_I t_1) \sin \pi J_{IS} t_1.$$

The terms in σ_4 represent diagonal peaks proportional to the mixing coefficients a_{II} and a_{SS}, and NOE crosspeaks proportional to a_{SI} and a_{IS}. These are all in phase with respect to J_{IS}. Also, we find diagonal and crosspeaks which are antiphase with respect to J_{IS}. These are the J crosspeaks derived from zero-quantum coherence which could not be removed by phase cycling. These must therefore be eliminated using alternative methods, and there are several techniques available. The simplest method exploits the fact that the J crosspeaks are in antiphase with respect to J_{IS}, whereas the NOESY peaks are in phase. We can therefore broaden the resonance lines using an exponential weighting function (see **convolution**), whereby mutual cancellation of antiphase components occurs. This method, known as digital filtering, is not particularly useful since it causes unacceptable loss in resolution. A second method of removing J crosspeaks relies upon the fact that J crosspeaks are derived from the evolution of coherent components during the mixing time. The characteristic dependence of such coherent transfer processes during the mixing period is different from the incoherent transfer processes due to the **nuclear Overhauser effect**. The former shows an oscillatory dependence on the mixing time, whereas the latter is a slowly varying process. These can therefore be separated by incrementing τ_m from experiment to experiment within the scheme of NOESY, in parallel within the evolution time, i.e.

N21 $$\tau_m = \tau_m^0 + kt_1$$

where $\tau_m^0 = \tau_m$ at $t_1 = 0$, and k is a constant which is selected such that the variation in τ_m is small compared with t_1, thus preventing severe perturbation of the incoherent transfer process. This 'incremented mixing technique' leads to a displacement of all J crosspeaks from their original positions along the ω_1 direction. This destroys the inherent symmetry of the J crosspeak pattern with respect to the diagonal, and they can therefore be eliminated by symmetrization. (Alternative methods for J-crosspeak suppression exist, and these may be found under Further reading.)

If the NOESY experiment is performed using phase-sensitive manipulation of the data, the presence of J crosspeaks is less likely to confuse the interpretation of incoherent transfer pathways, since the antiphase nature of the former are readily apparent in cross-sections through either ω_1 or ω_2. In addition, these have zero integrated intensity, and should not in theory contribute to the integrated intensity of NOE crosspeaks. Their removal is therefore of less importance in phase-sensitive NOESY spectra.

The complete phase cycle for phase-sensitive NOESY is therefore as follows:

P1	P2	P3	Receiver	
X	X	X	X	
Y	Y	X	X	
$-X$	$-X$	X	X	
$-Y$	$-Y$	X	X	location 1
$-X$	X	$-X$	X	
$-Y$	Y	$-X$	X	
X	$-X$	$-X$	X	
Y	$-Y$	$-X$	X	
Y	X	X	X	
$-X$	X	X	X	
$-Y$	$-X$	X	X	
X	$-Y$	X	X	location 2
$-Y$	X	$-X$	X	
X	Y	$-X$	X	
Y	$-X$	$-X$	X	
$-X$	$-Y$	$-X$	X	

The phase cycle X, Y, $-X$, $-Y$ on P1 and P2 cancels multiple-quantum coherence. The cycle X, $-X$ on P1 and P3 cancels axial peaks. The cycle is repeated with the phase of all pulses preceding t_1 incremented by 90° in common with most **phase-sensitive experiments**. The 16-step sequence is then repeated fourfold with **CYCLOPS** phase incrementation, giving a minimum of $64n$ scans.

Finally, we analyse the incoherent transfer mechanism to see how quantitative distance information is obtained from NOESY. In order to illustrate the mixing process of the NOESY experiment in more detail, we must first examine the longitudinal (T_1) relaxation behaviour of dipolar-coupled spins. This is treated in detail under the heading **spin-lattice relaxation**, and a brief summary of T_1 relaxation for two coupled spins is sufficient here. The rate of change of the z magnetization of two dipolar coupled spins I and S is given by

N22
$$\langle \dot{I}_z \rangle = -\rho_I(\langle I_z \rangle - I_0) - \sigma_{IS}(\langle S_z \rangle - S_0)$$
$$\langle \dot{S}_z \rangle = -\rho_S(\langle S_z \rangle - S_0) - \sigma_{SI}(\langle I_z \rangle - I_0).$$

These equations are sometimes expressed in the equivalent matrix form (see Appendix 3):

N23
$$\begin{matrix} \langle \dot{I}_z \rangle \\ \langle \dot{S}_z \rangle \end{matrix} = \begin{bmatrix} -\rho_I & -\sigma_{IS} \\ -\sigma_{SI} & -\rho_S \end{bmatrix} \begin{bmatrix} \langle I_z \rangle - I_0 \\ \langle S_z \rangle - S_0 \end{bmatrix}$$

$\langle I_z \rangle$ and $\langle S_z \rangle$ represents the **expectation values** of the longitudinal magnetization of spins I and S respectively, and I_0 and S_0 are the corresponding equilibrium magnetization. The ρ's represent the direct relaxation rates of the spins, whereas the σ's represent the cross-relaxation rates. The latter terms are responsible for the **nuclear Overhauser effect**—each spin 'senses' the relaxation of the other. In order to extract any useful information from (N22) we must solve the equations. They are known in mathematics as coupled differential equations, and their solution is dependent upon the boundary conditions imposed at $t = 0$. In the case of the NOESY experiment, we can derive these by considering for example a cross-section through the spectrum at $\tau_m = 0$ where the I spin resonance is on the diagonal. Since the I spin diagonal peak will be of maximum intensity, we can define $(I_z - I_0) = 1$. Since no cross-relaxation has taken place at $\tau_m = 0$, there is zero cross peak intensity and $(S_z - S_0) = 0$. The analytical solution of (N22) under these conditions is rather bulky, and the analogous equations for multispin systems have very complex analytical solutions. It is therefore convenient to solve them numerically. A system frequently encountered in biological NMR is the three-spin system such that the shown in Fig. N9, with typical internuclear distances. A numerical solution of the equations corresponding to this system with $(I_z - I_0) = 1$, $(S_z - S_0) =$

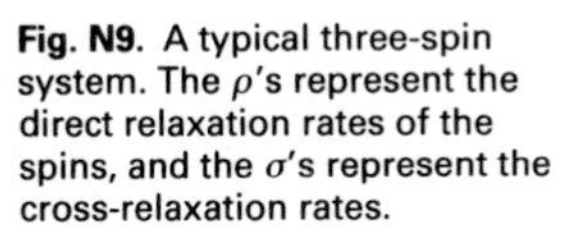

Fig. N9. A typical three-spin system. The ρ's represent the direct relaxation rates of the spins, and the σ's represent the cross-relaxation rates.

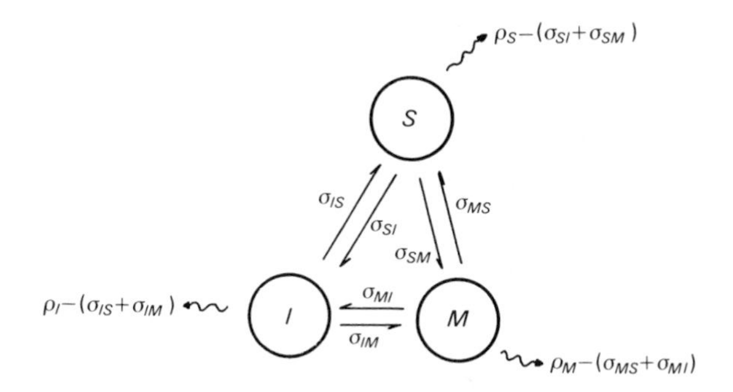

$(M_z - M_0) = 0$, and equal ρ's for the three nuclei gives the time development of the crosspeak intensities shown in Fig. N10.

The I spin diagonal peak intensity governed by a_{II} decays with increasing τ_m, whereas the S and M spin crosspeak intensities generated by a_{IS} and a_{IM} increase before decaying with increasing τ_{m}. The importance of the time development of crosspeaks intensities is that the initial buildup rates of the S and M spin crosspeak intensities (i.e. at $\tau_m = 0$) are proportional to σ_{IS} and σ_{IM}. If, therefore, a_{IM} corresponds to a known fixed internuclear distance r_{IM}, r_{IS} can be calculated from the

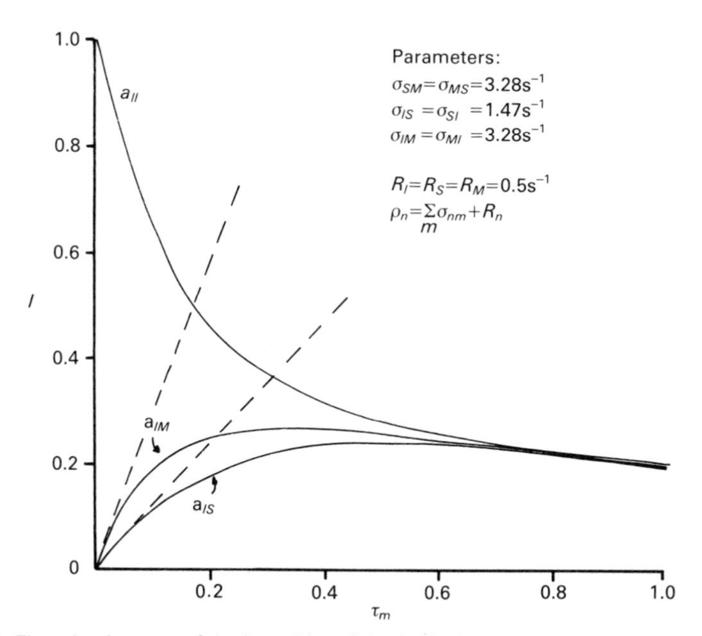

Fig. N10. Time development of the intensities of the I spin diagonal peak (a_{II}) and the S and M spin crosspeaks (a_{IS} and a_{IM}) as a function of the mixing time (τ_{m}) of the NOESY sequence. The Rs are the total direct relaxation rates of the spins in obvious notation.

r^{-6} dependence of σ:

N24 $$\frac{r_{IM}}{r_{IS}} = \left[\frac{\sigma_{IS}}{\sigma_{IM}}\right]^{\frac{1}{6}}.$$

This can be demonstrated by inserting the relevant σ's in Fig. N10. This is the principle method by which quantitative distance information is obtained in biological NMR. A series of NOESY spectra is recorded as a function of mixing time in order to generate experimental plots similar to those obtained theoretically in Fig. N10. Alternatively, if the experimenter can be confident that the measured crosspeak intensities in a single NOESY experiment for a given mixing time were developed within the initial rate approximation, then quantitative distance information can be obtained with good accuracy by measurement of relative crosspeak intensities rather than initial rates:

N25 $$\frac{r_{IM}}{r_{IS}} = \left[\frac{a_{IS}}{a_{IM}}\right]^{\frac{1}{6}};$$

initial rate approximation only!!

FURTHER READING

For a detailed description of NOESY/exchange spectroscopy, see

Macura, S. and Ernst, R. R. (1980). *Mol. Phys.* **41,** 95.

Ernst, R. R., Bodenhausen, G. and Wokaun, A. (1987). *Principles of NMR in one and two dimensions,* Chapter 9 and references therein, Clarendon Press, Oxford.

Nyquist frequency See **aliasing**.

Observable Of the many transitions which can occur between the energy levels of a multispin system, only those which result in a change in the magnetic quantum number $\Delta m = \pm 1$ can generate a signal in the receiver coils of the spectrometer. These are the so-called allowed transitions. When we calculate the result of a pulse sequence upon this spin system using one of the available quantum mechanical formalisms for the description of pulsed NMR, it follows that we must determine which terms can give rise to detectable magnetization. These terms are known collectively as observables. In the case of the density matrix formalism, we compute the 'observable' elements of the density matrix by forming the trace of the product of the density matrix with the relevant observable operator F_x or F_y:

O1 $$\langle M_x \rangle = \mathrm{Tr}\{\sigma F_x\}, \qquad \langle M_y \rangle = \mathrm{Tr}\{\sigma F_y\}.$$

Equivalently, in the **product operator formalism**, we find that only terms in I_x and I_y can give rise to an observable signal. Terms such as $I_x S_z$ are excluded since this represents antiphase magnetization whose integrated intensity is zero. However, $I_x S_z$ will evolve during the acquisition period (if present at $t_2 = 0$) to generate an observable signal.

Off-resonance decoupling Off-resonance decoupling has been used to assign heteronuclear spin systems by scaling spin–spin interactions. A strong decoupling field is applied outside the spectrum of the nucleus of interest, e.g. protons. Partial decoupling due to the offset dependence of the field leads to a scaling of the multiplets of the heteronucleus which is dependent upon the decoupler offset. The scaling factor may conveniently be computed using **average Hamiltonian theory**, which leads to the zero-order Hamiltonian

O2 $$\bar{\mathcal{H}}_0 = \sum_{k,l} 2\pi J_{kl} \cos\theta_k I_{kz'} S_{lz} + \text{other terms}$$

where the prime indicates operators quantized along different effective fields. From (O2) it is clear that each heteronuclear spin coupling J_{kl} is scaled by a factor $\cos\theta_k$, where

O3 $$\theta_k = \tan^{-1}[\gamma B_2/(\omega_2 - \omega_{I_k})].$$

B_2 is the strength of the decoupling field, and $(\omega_2 - \omega_{I_k})$ is the offset of the decoupling field from the I_kth resonance line. Note that θ_k may be different for each spin I_k. For strong r.f. fields, $|\gamma B_2| \gg |(\omega_2 - \omega_{I_k})|$, the residual coupling constants can be approximated by

$$J^{\mathrm{r}}_{kl} \approx J_{kl} \left| \frac{(\omega_2 - \omega_{I_k})}{\gamma B_2} \right|. \tag{O4}$$

Before the advent of **heteronuclear correlation spectroscopy**, observation of changes in the scaling factors $\cos \theta_k$ were used to correlate I spin and S spin spectra by systematically varying the position of the decoupler resonance frequency ω_2 relative to the I spin spectrum.

Off-resonance effects In **Fourier transform** NMR, it is usually assumed that the amplitude of the applied r.f. pulse is sufficient to excite uniformly all resonances within the range of interest, i.e. across the spectral width. In some situations, the widths of the spectra under investigation are comparable to the maximum available field strength γB_1, and the criterion for uniform excitation:

$$|\gamma B_1| \gg |\omega_I - \omega_{\mathrm{r.f.}}| \tag{O5}$$

does not hold. Under these conditions off-resonance effects become important. The magnetization is rotated about a tilted effective field, which depends upon the resonance frequency $|\omega_0 - \omega_{\mathrm{r.f.}}|$ in the **rotating frame**. This results in intensity and phase anomalies. The tilted effective field is determined by the offset field:

$$\Delta B_0 = B_0 + (\omega_{\mathrm{r.f.}}/\gamma) = \frac{-(\omega_0 - \omega_{\mathrm{r.f.}})}{\gamma} \tag{O6}$$

along the z axis and by the r.f. field B_1 in the transverse plane. The amplitude of the effective field is thus

$$B_{\mathrm{eff}} = \{B_1^2 + (\Delta B_0)^2\}^{\frac{1}{2}} \tag{O7}$$

and has a tilt-angle θ with respect to the z axis which is given by

$$\tan \theta = B_1/\Delta B_0. \tag{O8}$$

The effective flip-angle during a pulse of duration τ_{p} is

$$\beta_{\mathrm{eff}} = -\gamma B_{\mathrm{eff}} \tau_{\mathrm{p}}. \tag{O9}$$

The magnetization components after the pulse can be computed in terms of θ and β_{eff} to give

$$\begin{aligned} M_x &= M_0 \sin \beta_{\mathrm{eff}} \sin \theta, \\ M_y &= M_0 (1 - \cos \beta_{\mathrm{eff}}) \sin \theta \cos \theta, \\ M_z &= M_0 [\cos^2 \theta + \cos \beta_{\mathrm{eff}} \sin^2 \theta]. \end{aligned} \tag{O10}$$

The transverse magentization of an r.f. pulse applied along the $-y$ axis is no longer along the x axis as for the on-resonance condition ($\theta = \pi/2$, $\Delta B_0 = 0$), but has a phase shift ϕ which depends upon resonance offset and the effective rotation angle:

O11
$$\tan\phi = \frac{M_y}{M_x} = \frac{(1-\cos\beta_{\text{eff}})\sin\theta}{\sin\beta_{\text{eff}}} \frac{|\omega_{\text{I}} - \omega_{\text{r.f.}}|}{-\gamma B_1}.$$

In addition, for $\theta \neq \pi/2$, it is not possible to orient the magnetization exactly into the $-z$ direction, and hence spin inversion is impossible with a single pulse. Off-resonance effects can be compensated by **composite pulses.**

Offset In an NMR spectrometer, various situations arise where it is desirable to apply a frequency offset in order to move the spectrum within the sweep-width of the receiver. This frequency offset is often achieved by moving the transmitter frequency with respect to the receiver. Thus, if the transmitter frequency is equal to that of the receiver, then on Fourier transformation of the free induction decay, the transmitter **carrier** will lie in the centre of the spectrum. If the transmitter frequency is now shifted by $\pm\Omega$ Hz with respect to the receiver, then the carrier will lie at an offset $\pm\Omega$ Hz. The application of an offset is desirable for several reasons. In many cases it is used to centre the spectrum within the receiver 'window'. Alternatively, it may be desirable to place the transmitter carrier at a given position in the spectrum in order to alleviate certain **off-resonance effects**. A similar procedure is employed where the spectrometer is equipped with a second irradiation frequency (decoupler). Here, it is essential to have the capability to irradiate a given resonance line selectively. This may be a solvent resonance, or a resonance of interest for **difference spectroscopy**. See also **d.c. offset**.

Operator In quantum mechanics, we are often confronted with the task of calculating the result of a given measurement upon a system. We achieve this by solving the **Schrödinger equation** for the system. In its simplest form, the Schrödinger equation may be written

O12
$$\mathcal{H}\psi = E\psi.$$

Here, ψ is known as the wavefunction for the system, and $\mathcal{H}$ is an operator. To each physical observable exists an operator. For example, in NMR we are particularly interested in the transition energies of the spin system, and so $\mathcal{H}$ is the energy operator, or **Hamiltonian** for the system. When $\mathcal{H}$ operates upon ψ, it generates a result E, which is known as the eigenvalue, of which there may be several, and leaves the system unchanged in the state ψ. As a simple example of an operator, consider the equation

$$\frac{\mathrm{d}e^{2x}}{\mathrm{d}x} = 2e^{2x}. \quad \text{(O13)}$$

Here, the operator is $\mathrm{d}/\mathrm{d}x$, the 'wavefunction' is $\exp(2x)$ and the eigenvalue is 2. Operators in NMR are rather more complex than this simple example would suggest (see **Hamiltonian**) but nevertheless the basic principle remains. In general, operators obey the usual rules of algebra, but they have the additional property of commutation (see **commutator**). If two operators do not commute, then certain manipulations become more complex. For example, consider the equation

$$\exp\{\mathrm{i}(A+B)\} = \exp\{\mathrm{i}A\}\exp\{\mathrm{i}B\}, \quad \text{(O14)}$$

which is perfectly correct according to the rules of algebra. If, however, A and B are two non-commuting operators, then (O14) is not valid. This has important consequences with regard to calculations involving for example strongly coupled systems (see **strong coupling**).

Order-selective detection See **multiple quantum coherence**.

Order-selective excitation NMR experiments involving the indirect detection of **multiple-quantum coherence** have been shown to be of great value in unravelling the complex spin-coupling networks found in macromolecules. Unfortunately, the advantages of multiple-quantum NMR must be offset against a decrease in sensitivity, which becomes increasingly severe as the multiple-quantum order increases. This loss in sensitivity is a direct consequence of the manner in which the experiment is performed. The indirect detection of multiple-quantum transitions in liquids essentially involves the creation of all orders of multiple-quantum coherence. There is essentially no selection in terms of the required coherence, save the even/odd order selectivity which may be achieved using the conventional excitation pulse sequence (see **multiple-quantum coherence**). Selectivity is achieved during detection where (essentially) all orders of coherence apart from the required coherence are cancelled by phase cycling. Consequently this approach is referred to as the order-selective detection scheme. It is highly inefficient since the vast majority of created coherences (which all derive from the same initial magnetization) are cancelled, and the effective signal contained with a given coherence order represents a fraction of the available magnetization after reconversion to single-quantum coherence. An obvious means by which the scheme could be improved would be to arrange for the distribution of the total spectral intensity between a few orders of coherence. This is achieved using order-selective excitation. Unfortunately, the procedure is theoretically and experimentally demanding, and thus far has enjoyed popularity only in solid state NMR, where the large dipolar couplings allow for the efficient creation of very high multiple-quantum orders. In liquids, we are restricted to scalar couplings which are usually measurable in tens of Hz, and the order-selective excitation scheme loses its appeal in view of the relatively lengthy pulse trains required by the excitation sequence.

Order-selective excitation sequences have been described by Pines and coworkers, using **average Hamiltonian theory** to derive the properties of the required **propagators** in the excitation sequence. Starting with a cyclic sequence of pulses and delays, it is possible to produce a sequence which is n-quantum selective to the zeroth order (average) term in the average Hamiltonian expansion (see **average Hamiltonian theory**). If the cyclic sequence has a duration $\Delta\tau_p$, associated with it will be an effective Hamiltonian $\mathscr{H} = \bar{\mathscr{H}}^0 + \bar{\mathscr{H}}^1 \ldots \bar{\mathscr{H}}^n$, and a propagator $U_0 = \exp\{-i\mathscr{H}_0\Delta\tau_p\}$. At the end of the $\Delta\tau_p$ interval, the sequence is repeated with the transmitter phase shifted by $\phi = 2\pi/n$ about the z axis, giving a new effective Hamiltonian during the subsequent τ_p interval. In practice, the excitation pulse sequence is designed so that all higher-order terms of the average Hamiltonian expansion are minimized. In particular, by designing a symmetric pulse sequence, all odd terms ($\bar{\mathscr{H}}^1$, $\bar{\mathscr{H}}^3 \ldots$) of the expansion vanish. In the absence of relaxation, unlimited phase cycling can be applied, and sequences selective to arbitrarily high order (n) may be designed. In real systems, however, limited phase cycling can be applied since relaxation effects invalidate the average Hamiltonian calculation.

FURTHER READING

For a detailed description of the theory of selective excitation, see

Warren, W. S., Weitekamp, D. P., and Pines, A. (1980). *J. Chem. Phys.* **73,** 2084.

Orthogonal See **orthonormal**.

Orthonormal When calculating the result of a given NMR experiment, it is always necessary to begin with the **basis states** representing the energy levels of the spin system. These are conventionally described in terms of the functions β and α to characterize the parallel and antiparallel orientations of the nuclear magnetic moment with respect to the static magnetic field. We define the properties of the **angular momentum** operators as postulates which describe the results of their application on the wavefunctions α and β. The wavefunctions themselves are further defined to be orthonormal. That is, they are orthogonal and normalized.

These properties are described by the integrals

O15 $$\int \alpha\alpha \, \mathrm{d}v = \int \beta\beta \, \mathrm{d}v = 1 \text{(normalization condition)}$$

O16 $$\int \alpha\beta \, \mathrm{d}v = \int \beta\alpha \, \mathrm{d}v = 0 \text{ (orthogonality)}$$

where the integral is over all space. These conditions can be represented in a more operational manner by the **bra-ket notation**:

O17 $$\langle \alpha \mid \alpha \rangle = \langle \beta \mid \beta \rangle = 1,$$

O18 $$\langle \alpha \mid \beta \rangle = \langle \beta \mid \alpha \rangle = 0.$$

In either case, the significance is the same: an individual nucleus can exist in either the α or the β state and the probability of its existence in one of the two states is exactly unity (when integrated over all space). The above integrals are of practical importance in the derivation of the **matrix representation** of certain operators. Here, we often find integrals of the form

O19 $$C_n \langle \alpha\alpha \mid \alpha\alpha \rangle = C_n$$

O20 $$C_m \langle \alpha\beta \mid \alpha\alpha \rangle = 0$$

where the C's are coefficients (often trigonometric functions). Due to the orthogonality condition, only the first coefficient survives.

Oscillator See **damped oscillator**.

P

Paramagnetic centre Resonances of nuclei in paramagnetic complexes often show large shifts from those in diamagnetic complexes. These shifts result from interaction with the unpaired electron. Two classes of shift may in general be distinguished: contact shift and pseudo-contact (dipolar) shift.

Contact shifts result from delocalization of unpaired electron spin density at the resonating nucleus, which is usually transmitted through chemical bonds. The contact shift is sometimes referred to as the Fermi or isotropic contact interaction, and for the first-row transition metals is given by

P1
$$\frac{(\omega_{\mathrm{P}} - \omega_{\mathrm{D}})}{\omega_{\mathrm{I}}} = -\left(\frac{A}{\hbar}\right) \frac{g\beta S(S+1)}{3kT\gamma_I}$$

where $A/\hbar$ is the hyperfine coupling constant (rad s^{-1}), g is the (assumed isotropic) Lande g factor, T is the absolute temperature, k is the Boltzmann constant, γ_I is the magnetogyric ratio of the hydrogen nuclei in rad s^{-1} G^{-1}, β is the Bohr magneton, S is the total electron spin, ω_{P} is the shift in the paramagnetic complex, ω_{D} is the shift in the diamagnetic complex, and ω_{I} is the irradiating frequency.

Pseudo-contact shifts derive from the failure of the dipolar interaction between the unpaired electron spin and a given nucleus to average to zero, i.e. the magnetic field produced by the unpaired electron is anisotropic. For transition metals the magnitude of the pseudo-contact shift is given by

P2
$$\frac{(\omega_{\mathrm{P}} - \omega_{\mathrm{D}})}{\omega_{\mathrm{I}}} = \frac{\beta^2 S(S+1)}{6kT} \cdot r^{-3} F'$$

where $F' = (g_z^2 - g^2)(3\cos^2\theta - 1) + (g_x^2 - g_y^2)\sin^2\theta\cos 2\phi$ and where $g^2 = \frac{1}{3}(g_x^2 + g_y^2 + g_z^2)$. θ and ϕ are defined in normal spherical coordinates; $\cos\theta = z/r$, $\sin\theta\cos\phi = x/r$, $\sin\theta\sin\phi = y/r$.

In addition to large chemical shifts, the relaxation times in a diamagnetic liquid are often reduced when small concentrations of paramagnetic ions are added. A simple qualitative explanation for this is that the **magnetic moments** of unpaired electrons are ~10^3-fold greater than nuclei magnetic moments, so the local fields generated are much greater.

These in turn generally lead to more efficient relaxation. In dilute solution, the relaxation is often dominated by pairwise electron–nuclear dipole–dipole interactions, or occasionally by scalar or hyperfine coupling through bonds. The relaxation times T_1 (see **spin–lattice relaxation**) and T_2 (see **spin–spin relaxation**) of nuclei bound near a paramagnetic site are usually well described by

P3
$$\frac{1}{T_1'} = \frac{2}{15}\frac{\gamma_I^2 g^2 S(S+1)\beta^2}{r^6}\left(\frac{3\tau_c}{1+\omega_I^2\tau_c^2} + \frac{7\tau_c}{1+\omega_S^2\tau_c^2}\right) + \tfrac{2}{3}S(S+1)\left(\frac{A}{\hbar}\right)^2\left(\frac{\tau_e}{1+\omega_S^2\tau_e^2}\right),$$

P4
$$\frac{1}{T_2'} = \frac{1}{15}\frac{\gamma_I^2 g^2 S(S+1)\beta^2}{r^6}\left(4\tau_c + \frac{3\tau_c}{1+\omega_I^2\tau_c^2} + \frac{13\tau_c}{1+\omega_S^2\tau_c^2}\right) + \tfrac{1}{3}S(S+1)\left(\frac{A}{\hbar}\right)^2\left(\frac{\tau_e}{1+\omega_S^2\tau_e^2} + \tau_e\right).$$

The first term in each equation arises from dipole–dipole electron (S) and nuclear (I) spin interactions, characterized by a **correlation time** τ_c. The second term in each equation arises from modulation of the scalar interaction, which is characterized by a correlation time τ_e. The electronic and nuclear **Larmor precession** frequencies are given by ω_S and ω_I respectively, γ_I, β and S are defined above, r is the distance between the nucleus and the paramagnetic ion, and $A/\hbar$ is the electron–nuclear hyperfine coupling constant in Hz. The correlation times are defined as

P5
$$\frac{1}{\tau_c} = \frac{1}{\tau_s} + \frac{1}{\tau_m} + \frac{1}{\tau_R}$$

P6
$$\frac{1}{\tau_e} = \frac{1}{\tau_s} + \frac{1}{\tau_m}$$

where τ_m is the lifetime of a nucleus in the bound site, τ_R is the rotational correlation time of the bound paramagnetic ion and τ_S is the electron-spin relaxation time.

The practical application of these equations is subject to several assumptions, which are discussed in detail by Dwek (1973). The possibility of obtaining structural and kinetic information in biochemical systems from studying effects caused by paramagnetic probes was first realized in 1962. In principle, structural information obtained by use of one paramagnetic probe can be combined with that of a second. If the distance between the probes is known, structural information can be obtained by a 'triangulation' procedure. However, paramagnetic probes have not enjoyed great favour in recent years, possibly due to the difficulty in the interpretation of their effects. In addition, the advent of

two-dimensional NMR has allowed structural information to be obtained in macromolecules in a much more straightforward manner. Nevertheless, one approach which may be of value in the future is a combination of these approaches, and this may allow detailed structural information to be obtained on larger macromolecules than is possible at present.

FURTHER READING

For a comprehensive discussion of the use of paramagnetic probes, see

Dwek, R. A. (1973). *NMR in biochemistry*. Clarendon Press, Oxford, and references therein

Partition function The partition function or 'sum of states' Z for a system with energy levels E_n and degeneracies M_i in thermal equilibrium with a bath of temperature T is given by

P7 $$Z = \sum_n M_n \exp(-E_n/kT)$$

where k is the Boltzmann constant. The value of this expression is that it allows us to calculate the populations of the energy levels at thermal equilibrium. For example, in the case of a two-spin $\frac{1}{2}$ system, there are four energy levels given by the product functions $|\alpha\alpha\rangle$, $|\alpha\beta\rangle$, $|\beta\alpha\rangle$, $|\beta\beta\rangle$ (Fig. P1). If the energies of states 2 and 3 are taken as zero, and the energies of states 1 and 4 are taken as $\omega\hbar$ and $-\omega\hbar$ respectively (where $\hbar = h/2\pi$), then Z will be the sum over the four states ($n = 4$),

P8 $$Z = \exp(\omega\hbar/kT) + \exp(0) + \exp(0) + \exp(-\omega\hbar/kT).$$

Since $\omega\hbar$ is small compared with kT in an NMR experiment at normal temperature, then $\exp(\pm\omega\hbar/kT) \sim 1$. Thus, $Z \sim 4$. The populations of the four states may therefore be calculated in terms of probabilities,

P9 $$\begin{aligned} P_1 &= \tfrac{1}{4}\exp(-\omega\hbar/kT) \sim \tfrac{1}{4}(1-(\omega\hbar/kT)) \\ P_2 &= \tfrac{1}{4}\exp(0) = \tfrac{1}{4} \\ P_3 &= \tfrac{1}{4}\exp(0) = \tfrac{1}{4} \\ P_4 &= \tfrac{1}{4}\exp(+\omega\hbar/kT) \sim \tfrac{1}{4}(1+(\omega\hbar/kT)). \end{aligned}$$

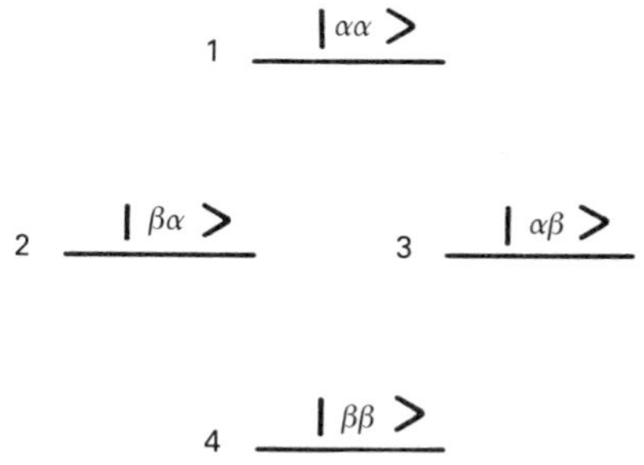

1 $|\alpha\alpha\rangle$

2 $|\beta\alpha\rangle$ 3 $|\alpha\beta\rangle$

4 $|\beta\beta\rangle$

Fig. P1. The four energy levels and product functions of a weakly coupled two-spin $\frac{1}{2}$ system.

From (P9), we can then derive an expression for the **density matrix** at thermal equilibrium, (σ_0) which is the usual starting point for most calculations in pulsed NMR:

P10
$$\sigma_0 = \tfrac{1}{4}\begin{bmatrix} 1-\delta & 0 & 0 & 0 \\ 0 & 1 & 0 & 0 \\ 0 & 0 & 1 & 0 \\ 0 & 0 & 0 & 1+\delta \end{bmatrix} = \tfrac{1}{4}\mathbf{1} + \tfrac{1}{4}\delta\begin{bmatrix} -1 & 0 & 0 & 0 \\ 0 & 0 & 0 & 0 \\ 0 & 0 & 0 & 0 \\ 0 & 0 & 0 & +1 \end{bmatrix}$$

where $\delta = \omega\hbar/kT$ and $\mathbf{1}$ is the **identity operator**. The identity operator is usually omitted from density matrix calculations proper, since it commutes with all operators and can never give rise to observable magnetization.

Pauli-spin matrices The Pauli-spin matrices are the matrix representations of the single-spin **angular momentum** operators I_x, I_y, and I_z:

P11
$$I_x = \tfrac{1}{2}\begin{bmatrix} 0 & 1 \\ 1 & 0 \end{bmatrix}, \quad I_y = \tfrac{1}{2}\begin{bmatrix} 0 & \mathrm{i} \\ -\mathrm{i} & 0 \end{bmatrix}, \quad I_z = \tfrac{1}{2}\begin{bmatrix} 1 & 0 \\ 0 & -1 \end{bmatrix}.$$

These are quite useful in NMR since the matrix representations of operator products can be generated from them by direct product (see Appendix 3). For this purpose it is useful to include the matrix representation of the **identity operator**:

P12
$$E = \begin{bmatrix} 1 & 0 \\ 0 & 1 \end{bmatrix}.$$

The matrix representation of $2I_xS_z$, for example, is calculated as follows:

P13
$$2I_xS_z = 2[I_x \otimes S_z] = 2\begin{bmatrix} 0 & \tfrac{1}{2} \\ \tfrac{1}{2} & 0 \end{bmatrix} \otimes \begin{bmatrix} \tfrac{1}{2} & 0 \\ 0 & -\tfrac{1}{2} \end{bmatrix} = \begin{bmatrix} 0 & 0 & \tfrac{1}{2} & 0 \\ 0 & 0 & 0 & -\tfrac{1}{2} \\ \tfrac{1}{2} & 0 & 0 & 0 \\ 0 & -\tfrac{1}{2} & 0 & 0 \end{bmatrix}$$

and the matrix representation of I_x in the **product operator formalism** is

$$I_x = I_x \otimes E$$

$$= \tfrac{1}{2}\begin{bmatrix} 0 & 1 \\ 1 & 0 \end{bmatrix} \otimes \begin{bmatrix} 1 & 0 \\ 0 & 1 \end{bmatrix}$$

P14
$$= \tfrac{1}{2}\begin{bmatrix} 0 & 0 & 1 & 0 \\ 0 & 0 & 0 & 1 \\ 1 & 0 & 0 & 0 \\ 0 & 1 & 0 & 0 \end{bmatrix}.$$

Each matrix for the other operator products is calculated in an analogous manner. This method is an entirely equivalent alternative to forming the **matrix representation** by explicit computation of the effects of the **angular momentum** operators on the eigenfunctions of the spin system of interest.

Phase In many forms of spectroscopy, the concept of phase has no relevance since the perturbing field is not coherent. In NMR, however, we apply a phase-coherent r.f. field to perturb the spins, and the phase of the detected **magnetization** can be expressed relative to this field. This leads directly to the observation of different **lineshapes** in phase and 90° out of phase with perturbing radiation. The introduction of the term 'phase' in the present context implies an inherent angular property. However, phase can also be represented with respect to time. Consider the function $A = \sin(\omega t)$. A plot of A against t gives the familiar sinusoidal oscillation or sine wave (Fig. P2) where ω is the frequency of the oscillation in rad s^{-1}. If we now add a constant factor ϕ, then the new function is given by $A = \sin(\omega t + \phi)$, where again ϕ is a constant angular function expressed in radians. For example, if ϕ is equal to $\pi/2$ radians (90°), then a plot of A against t would look like that shown in Fig. P3. The function has the same frequency as that in Fig. P2, but it starts at the maximal value of A rather than zero—it is a cosine wave. The factor ϕ is obviously responsible for this change, and it is termed the phase factor. In this example, a phase factor of $\pi/2$ radians 'converts' a sine wave to a cosine wave. The two waveforms are thus said to be $\pi/2$ radians (or 90°) out of phase. Another way of visualizing this is by considering the sinewave to 'lead' the cosine wave in time. We can see this more readily by combining both waveforms (Fig. P4). The dotted line shows that the sine wave

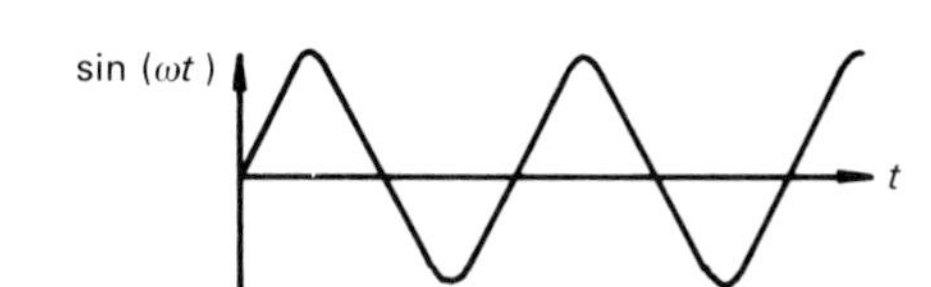

Fig. P2. Plot of the function $\sin(\omega t)$ vs. t.

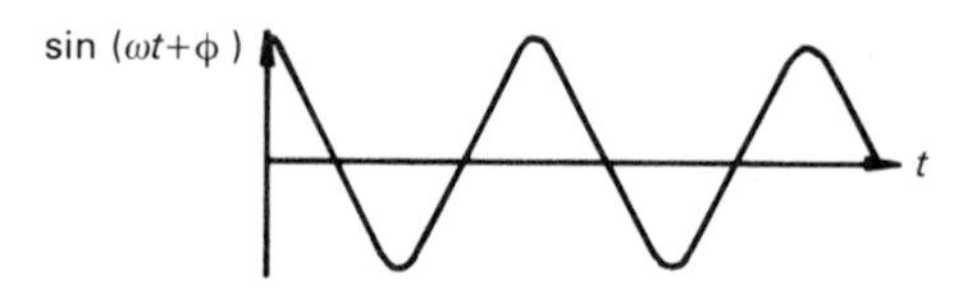

Fig. P3. Plot of $\sin(\omega t + \phi)$ vs. t, where $\phi = \pi/2$ radians.

completes a quarter of a cycle before the cosine wave begins. Since the x axis is time, this is equivalent to imposing a time delay on the cosine wave. This time delay is known as a phase shift. There are many occasions during the execution of an NMR experiment or during the detection period that phase shifts are introduced deliberately into either the exciting radiation or into the signal path of the NMR receiver. These phase shifts are all achieved instrumentally with a phase shifter. Their purpose is to selectively excite or detect oscillating off-diagonal elements of the **density matrix**. A simple example is the detection of magnetization which is either parallel or perpendicular to the axis along which the excitation is applied in the **rotating frame**. This is achieved instrumentally by applying a phase shift to the reference of the receiver phase-sensitive detectors. We can calculate the effects of the phase shifts using the **classical formalism** in simple cases, or an appropriate quantum mechanical formalism where the consequences of phase shifts are included in the relevant operators.

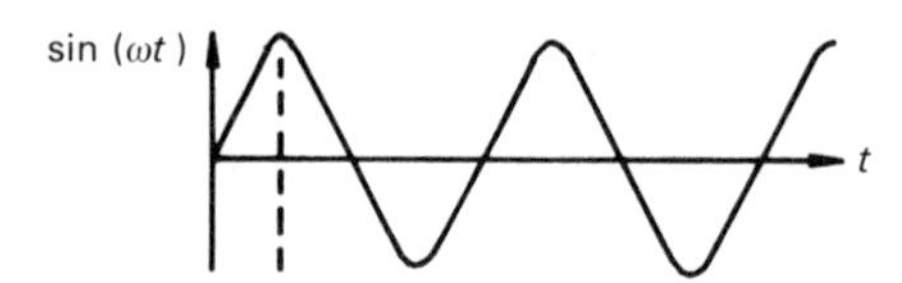

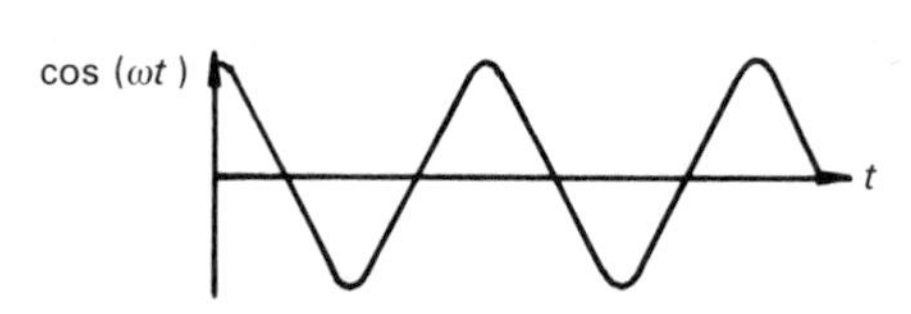

Fig. P4. A sine wave can be thought of as a function which leads a cosine wave in time by a quarter cycle.

Phase coherence Due to the large number of nuclear spins in an NMR sample, we can often use a simple classical treatment of the NMR phenomenon. In particular we can introduce the term **magnetization** and represent it by a vector. The components of this vector which are of interest are M_z, which lies along the direction of B_0, and M_x and M_y which are mutually orthogonal to each other and to M_z. At thermal equilibrium, there is a net excess of spins aligned along the field direction, giving rise to a finite value of M_z. However, we also find M_{xy} components since the spins do not align perfectly along B_0. These

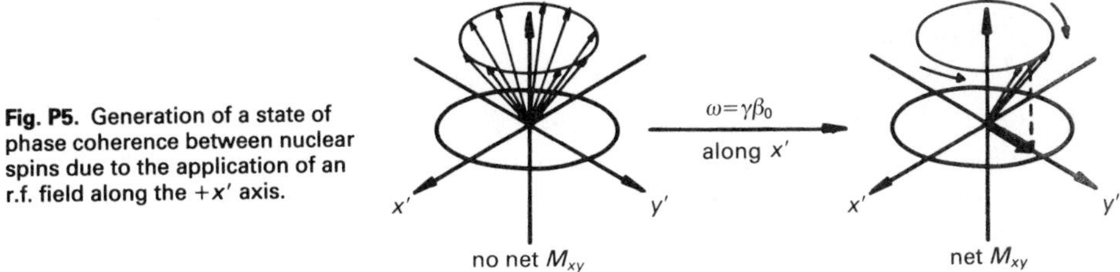

Fig. P5. Generation of a state of phase coherence between nuclear spins due to the application of an r.f. field along the $+x'$ axis.

components are randomly distributed about the x–y plane at equilibrium and $M_{xy}=0$. On application of an r.f. field at the **Larmor frequency** $\omega=\gamma B_0$, the spins resonate and a state of **phase coherence** is obtained with a net component of M in the x–y plane (Fig. P5). In the event that the phase coherence is generated by single-quantum transitions, we speak of single-quantum coherence, which is identical to the transverse magnetization M_{xy}. Equivalently, the presence of single-quantum off-diagonal elements σ_{nm} of the **density matrix** show phase coherence ongoing between states n and m. In addition, we can often create off-diagonal elements of the density matrix corresponding to double-quantum transitions or zero-quantum transitions. Such **multiple-quantum coherence** cannot be understood classically, and indeed multiple-quantum coherence does not generate an observable signal in the receiver coils of the spectrometer. It should be remembered that phase coherence is an ensemble property of the spin system, and it is not possible to refer to the 'coherence' of a single spin.

FURTHER READING

Bax, A. (1982). *Two dimensional NMR in liquids*. Delft University Press, Dordrecht.

Phase correction The NMR spectrum obtained by **Fourier transformation** of the **free-induction decay** does not in general consist of pure absorption-mode lineshapes. There are several reasons for this, but primary amongst these is the requirement for a small time delay between the application of the r.f. pulse and the acquisition of the free induction decay. This delay is required for instrumental reasons, i.e. to prevent blocking and desensitization of the receiver circuitry. During this delay, transverse magnetization which would normally lie along e.g. the y' axis after the pulse, begins to precess slowly in the x'–y' plane, and acquires a frequency-dependent phase shift. Each resonance therefore consists of an admixture of absorption-mode and dispersion-mode **lineshapes**. Fortunately, pure absorption-mode lineshapes can be restored using a simple software correction, which usually consists of a constant phase correction together with a frequency-dependent phase correction. The phase correction requires both real and imaginary parts (see **complex number**) of the spectrum. A phase correction ϕ corresponds with the following manipulations:

P15 $$\mathrm{Re}(k) = -\mathrm{Im}(j) \sin \phi + \mathrm{Re}(j) \cos \phi$$

P16 $$\mathrm{Im}(k) = \mathrm{Re}(j) \sin \phi + \mathrm{Im}(j) \cos \phi$$

where Re(k) and Im(k) represent the real and imaginary parts of each point in the spectrum following phase correction, and Re(j) and Im(j) represent those parts before correction.

Phase cycling (see also coherence transfer pathways) An important aspect of modern NMR experiments is the concept of phase cycling. This refers to the means by which unwanted signals in an NMR experiment are separated on the basis of their characteristic phase properties. These signals might perhaps be derived from imbalance in the spectrometer hardware (see **CYCLOPS**) or may be generated in a multipulse NMR experiment (see **axial peak**). Other signals which are often removed by phase cycling and which cannot strictly be described as artefacts are those involving for example **multiple-quantum coherence**, in which a particular coherence pathway is selected. The removal of these unwanted signals by phase cycling relies upon the fact that in NMR we are dealing with states of **phase coherence**. Thus it is possible to refer to a given class of signals with a given phase with respect to the applied irradiation, which itself is phase coherent. Thus in simple one-dimensional pulse and collect experiments we refer to an r.f. pulse applied along an arbitrary axis in the **rotating frame**, and to detection along a second axis, which is often orthogonal to the first. The selection of a particular r.f. phase may be accomplished using a phase shifter, which essentially imparts a time delay into either the transmitter reference signal, the receiver, or both. In practice, this time delay is incremented at each transient during **signal averaging**, and the transmitter or receiver can then be thought of as 'cycling' or rotating with respect to the rotating frame (Fig. P6). The behaviour of each type of signal during this procedure is different, resulting in the selective detection of the required signal. A detailed description of such behaviour is given under each separate subheading (see e.g. **axial peak**, **double-quantum correlated spectroscopy**).

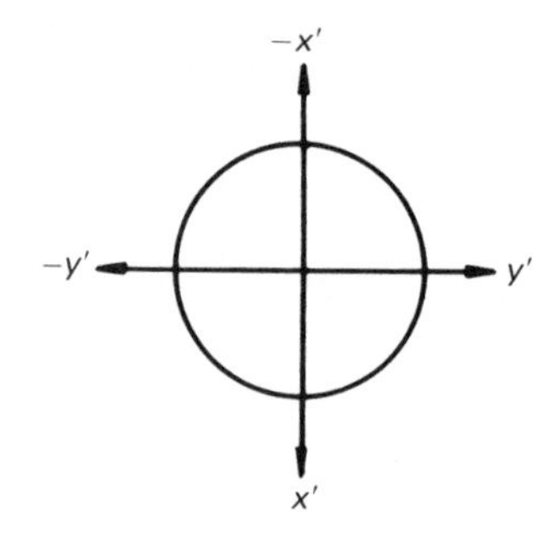

Fig. P6. The x', y', $-x'$, $-y'$ axes in the rotating frame are often used to identify the phase of either the transmitter or receiver reference.

Phase-locked loop The phase-locked loop (PLL) appears in various guises in an NMR spectrometer. A block diagram of a simple PLL is shown in Fig. P7. The output (A) of a voltage-controlled oscillator (VCO) is constantly compared with the frequency of the master reference oscillator (MRO). Any unwanted frequency change or drift in frequency of the VCO with respect to the MRO is detected by the **phase-sensitive detector** PSD.

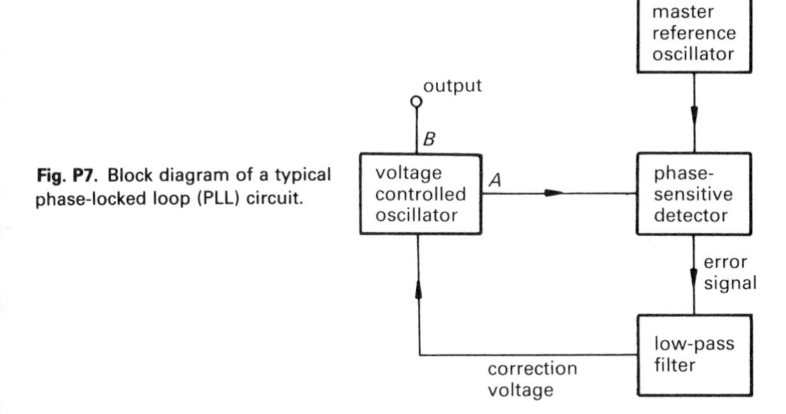

Fig. P7. Block diagram of a typical phase-locked loop (PLL) circuit.

When a phase difference exists, an error voltage is generated which is proportional to the cosine of the phase difference between the signals. This voltage is filtered by a low-pass filter (LPF), and the resulting d.c. voltage is fed to the VCO to return it to the correct frequency, i.e. that which results in no phase difference with respect to the MRO. The long-term stability of the PLL output is thus that of the MRO, which is generally a highly stable crystal oscillator. A more practical PLL contains a series of dividers by which a range of discrete frequencies is available, each with the stability of the MRO. A typical circuit is illustrated in Fig. P8. The value of the VCO is that it is possible to generate all the

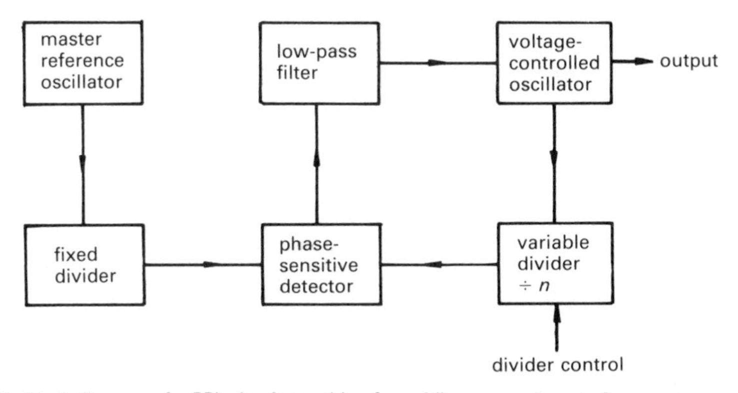

Fig. P8. Block diagram of a PPL circuit capable of providing many discrete frequencies.

frequencies in an NMR spectrometer from the same reference MRO. Thus, all frequency determining circuits in the spectrometer have the same long-term stability. More importantly, each separate signal is phase-locked. If this were not the case, it would be impossible to phase cycle the transmitter frequency for example, while holding constant the receiver phase, since no constant phase relationship would exist between the two.

A second important function of the PLL is in the field-frequency **lock** circuitry of the spectrometer.

Phase modulation An inherent property of most two-dimensional NMR experiments is the presence of amplitude-modulated time-domain signals during the t_1 interval. There is therefore no sign discrimination after Fourier transformation, and signals will be found at $\pm\omega_1$. This is simply demonstrated by considering (for instance) a cosine-modulated component:

P17 $$S_c(t_1, t_2) = \cos(\omega_1 t_1)\exp\{i\omega_2 t_2\}.$$

Using the identity $\cos(x) = \frac{1}{2}[\exp(ix) + \exp(-ix)]$ we find

P18 $$S_c(t_1, t_2) = \tfrac{1}{2}[\exp\{i\omega_1 t_1\} + \exp\{-i\omega_1 t_1\}]\exp\{i\omega_2 t_2\}.$$

Fourier transformation with respect to t_1 and t_2 gives

P19 $$S_c(\omega_1, \omega_2) = \tfrac{1}{2}[\mathrm{Abs}(\omega_1) + i\,\mathrm{Dis}(\omega_1) + \mathrm{Abs}(-\omega_1) + i\,\mathrm{Dis}(-\omega_1)][\mathrm{Abs}(\omega_2) + i\,\mathrm{Dis}(\omega_2)]$$

where Abs and Dis represent absorption and dispersion Lorentzian lines respectively (see **lineshape**) of which the real part is

P20 $$\mathrm{Re}\,S_c(\omega_1, \omega_2) = \tfrac{1}{2}[\mathrm{Abs}(\omega_1)\,\mathrm{Abs}(\omega_2) - \mathrm{Dis}(\omega_1)\,\mathrm{Dis}(\omega_2) + \tfrac{1}{2}[\mathrm{Abs}(-\omega_1)\,\mathrm{Abs}(\omega_2) - \mathrm{Dis}(-\omega_1)\,\mathrm{Dis}(\omega_2)].$$

Each of the pair of terms on the right-hand side of (P20) is a phase-twist lineshape, one at ω_1, ω_2, the other at $-\omega_1$, ω_2. The sign of the signals in ω_1 has not been determined. However, we can obtain frequency discrimination in ω_1 by recording a second component which has sinusoidal modulation:

P21 $$S_s(t_1, t_2) = \sin(\omega_1 t_1)\exp\{i\omega_2 t_2\}.$$

This is achieved by shifting the required coherence which evolves during t_1 by $\pi/2$ radians. Thus all pulses which precede t_1 are shifted by 90° in an experiment involving single-quantum evolution during t_1. Multiple-quantum evolution requires smaller phase shifts (see **multiple-quantum coherence**). The two signals are combined, with a $\pi/2$ radian receiver phase shift for the collection of the second component:

$$S(t_1, t_2) = S_c(t_1, t_2) + \exp\{i(\pi/2)\}S_s(t_1, t_2)$$

P22 $$= [\cos \omega_1 t_1 + i \sin \omega_1 t_1] \exp\{i\omega_2 t_2\}$$

$$= \exp\{i\omega_1 t_1\} \exp\{i\omega_2 t_2\}.$$

Upon double Fourier transformation, the real part of the spectrum is

P23 $$\mathrm{Re}[S(\omega_1, \omega_2)] = (\mathrm{Abs}\ \omega_1\ \mathrm{Abs}\ \omega_2 - \mathrm{Dis}\ \omega_1\ \mathrm{Dis}\ \omega_2)$$

which is a single phase-twist line at $+\omega_1$, ω_2. This results from the conversion of the amplitude-modulated signal $\cos \omega_1 t_1$ to a phase-modulated signal $\exp(i\omega_1 t_1)$. However, the undesirable phase-twist lineshape is retained. This can be overcome using so-called **phase-sensitive experiments**, which have all but replaced methods involving phase modulation.

FURTHER READING

Keeler, J. and Neuhaus, D. (1985). *J. Magn. Reson.* **63,** 454.

Phase-sensitive detector A phase-sensitive detector (PSD) can be thought of as a frequency-changing device which converts the input frequency to a lower (often very low) frequency. It achieves this by multiplying the input signal alternately by ±1. The name of the device arises from the fact that the output signal is a function of the phase difference between the input signal and the reference. For example, if the input signal ε is a sinusoidal oscillation of amplitude A and frequency ω_0 with a phase difference σ with respect to the reference ω_r,

P24 $$\varepsilon = A \sin(\omega_0 t + \sigma)$$

then the output signal for $\omega_0 = \omega_r$ is constant, and is given by

P25 $$\varepsilon F(\omega) = (2A/\pi) \cos \sigma,$$

i.e. it is proportional to the cosine of the phase difference. Phase-sensitive detectors find many applications in NMR spectrometers. An example of its use is in a single-sideband detector such as that shown in Fig. P9. The input signal is split and fed to two PSDs which are fed with reference signals 90° out of phase. The output of the first PSD is given by

P26 $$\psi_1 = A \cos(\{\omega_0 - \omega_r\}t + \sigma)$$

and of the second by

P27 $$\psi_2 = A \cos(\{\omega_0 - \omega_r\}t + (\sigma - 90°))$$

or

P28 $$\psi_2 = A \sin(\{\omega_0 - \omega_r\}t + \sigma).$$

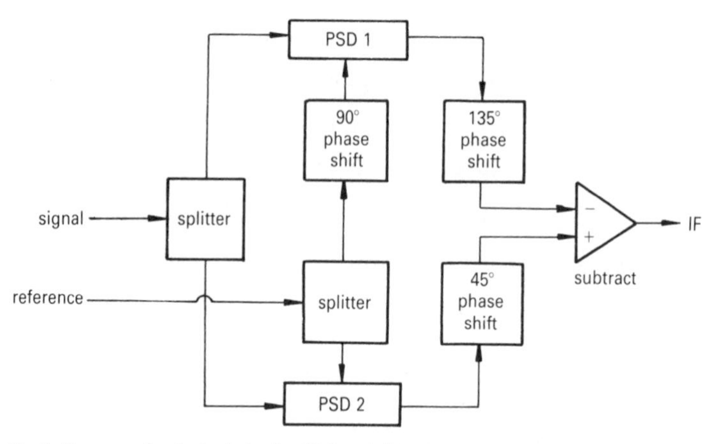

Fig. P9. Block diagram of a typical single-sideband detector.

In other words, we are detecting the signal with two detectors which are orthogonal to each other, which is equivalent to using two pairs of orthogonal coils in the probe. This is known as a **quadrature detection** system. It allows the signs of the precession frequencies in NMR to be discriminated. Since the reference which is fed to the PSDs is generally of the same frequency (plus or minus the **offset**) as that of the transmitter, then the PSDs detect the frequency differences of the Larmor precession frequencies of the spins with respect to the reference. This of course is the electronic equivalent of detection in the **rotating frame** of coordinates, which explains why the latter is not an artificial means of describing simple NMR experiments.

FURTHER READING

Hoult, D. I. (1978). *Progr. NMR Spectr.* **12,** 41.

Phase-sensitive experiments An amplitude-modulated (see **amplitude modulation**) time-domain signal from a two-dimensional NMR experiment can be described as

$$S_{\cos}(t_1, t_2) = \cos(\omega_1 t_1) \exp\{i\omega_2 t_2\} \tag{P29}$$

where we neglect relaxation terms and phase factors. This function is a common characteristic of many two-dimensional experiments. Unfortunately, it contains no information regarding the signs of the frequencies in ω_1. This can be shown explicitly by **Fourier transformation** of (P29), after first using the identity

$$\cos(\omega_1 t_1) = \tfrac{1}{2}[\exp\{i\omega_1 t_1\} + \exp\{-i\omega_1 t_1\}];$$

$$S(\omega_1, \omega_2) = \tfrac{1}{2}[\mathrm{Abs}(\omega_1) + i\,\mathrm{Dis}(\omega_1) + \mathrm{Abs}(-\omega_1) + i\,\mathrm{Dis}(-\omega_1)][\mathrm{Abs}(\omega_2) + i\,\mathrm{Dis}(\omega_2)]. \tag{P30}$$

The real part of the spectrum is

$$\text{Re}[S(\omega_1, \omega_2)] = \tfrac{1}{2}[(\text{Abs}(\omega_1)\,\text{Abs}(\omega_2) - \text{Dis}(\omega_1)\,\text{Dis}(\omega_2)) + (\text{Abs}(-\omega_1)\,\text{Abs}(\omega_2) - \text{Dis}(-\omega_1)\,\text{Dis}(\omega_2)], \tag{P31}$$

where in (P30) and (P31) the abbreviations Abs and Dis are used for the absorption and dispersion components respectively. Equation (P31) shows that two lines are produced at ω_1, ω_2 and $-\omega_1$, ω_2 and thus the signs of the frequencies in ω_1 have not been discriminated. In addition, it is seen that each lineshape is composed of an admixture of absorption and dispersion components. This is the so called phase-twist lineshape. It is highly undesirable in that it is impossible to phase resonance lines in the two-dimensional spectrum to pure absorption mode, and the dispersion-mode contributions result in broad wings along both axes. Fortunately, there is a simple method by which the phase-twist lineshape can be avoided. If the transmitter **carrier** is positioned at one end of the spectrum, then sign discrimination during ω_1 is unimportant. The spectrum can then be 'folded' about $\omega_1 = 0$ to give a double absorption lineshape. Such a spectrum can be generated experimentally by zeroing the imaginary part of the data matrix prior to a complex transform with respect to t_1. Equation (P30) then becomes

$$S(\omega_1, \omega_2) = \tfrac{1}{2}[\text{Abs}(\omega_1) + \text{i}\,\text{Dis}(\omega_1) + \text{Abs}(-\omega_1) + \text{i}\,\text{Dis}(-\omega_1)]\,\text{Abs}(\omega_2) \tag{P32}$$

of which the real part is

$$\text{Re}[S(\omega_1, \omega_2)] = \tfrac{1}{2}[\text{Abs}(\omega_1)\,\text{Abs}(\omega_2) + \text{Abs}(-\omega_1)\,\text{Abs}(\omega_2)]. \tag{P33}$$

Pure absorption lineshapes are obtained, although no sign discrimination in ω_1 is available. An unfortunate problem with this approach is that the data matrix is increased fourfold in size by placing the transmitter carrier to one end of the spectrum. Early attempts to avoid this problem involved the use of **phase modulation** during t_1 to achieve sign discrimination. However, this unfortunately reintroduces the phase-twist lineshape. The requirement is therefore for a mechanism which allows sign discrimination in t_1 together with the retention of pure absorption lineshapes. This is achieved by so-called phase-sensitive experiments. The key principle in such experiments is to record a second amplitude-modulated component (like P29) but which has sine rather than cosine modulation:

$$S_{\text{sin}}(t_1, t_2) = \sin(\omega_1 t_1)\exp\{\text{i}\omega_2 t_2\}. \tag{P34}$$

This is achieved experimentally by phase-shifting the required coherence by $\pi/2$ radians (90°). For example, in a standard COSY experiment, it is necessary to record two experiments for each t_1 value (Fig. P10). The 90°

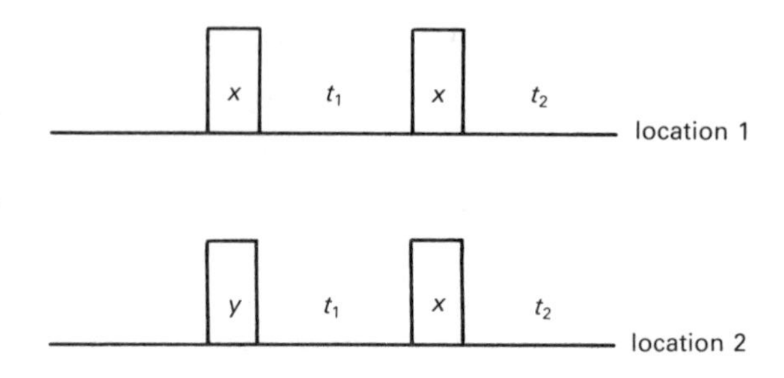

Fig. P10. Diagrammatic representation of pulse sequence for the acquisition of homonuclear phase-sensitive COSY spectra. The FIDs from two separate experiments (with the same t_1 value) are stored in separate memory locations.

phase shift on the first pulse ensures that two components are generated with sine and cosine amplitude modulation. These components are kept in separate locations in computer memory. Prior to the second Fourier transformation the real parts of the two data sets are combined and the imaginary parts are discarded, giving

$$\begin{aligned} S(t_1, \omega_2) &= \mathrm{Re}[S_{\cos}(t_1, \omega_2)] + \mathrm{i}\,\mathrm{Re}[S_{\sin}(t_1, \omega_2)] \\ &= \cos(\omega_1 t_1)\,\mathrm{Abs}(\omega_2) + \mathrm{i}\sin(\omega_1 t_1)\,\mathrm{Abs}(\omega_2) \end{aligned} \quad \text{P35}$$

which upon Fourier transformation gives for the real part of the spectrum

$$\mathrm{Re}[S(\omega_1, \omega_2)] = \mathrm{Abs}(\omega_1)\,\mathrm{Abs}(\omega_2). \quad \text{P36}$$

This final Fourier transform is often referred to as 'hypercomplex' Fourier transformation. The result is the same as (P33) except that sign discrimination is achieved in ω_1. The various permutations we have described are illustrated diagrammatically in Fig. P11.

A second method is available with which to obtain data in the phase-sensitive mode, which can be employed on spectrometers only equipped for real Fourier transforms. This method is based upon the **time-proportional phase incrementation** routine (TPPI) and is described thereunder. Although phase-sensitive experiments lead to a dramatic improvement in spectral quality, it must be realized that not all two-dimensional experiments will yield pure absorption-mode lineshapes when recorded in the 'phase-sensitive' manner. This is because in some cases the lineshapes are inherently not of pure absorption mode. Indeed, the COSY experiment which we used as our example has dispersion-mode lineshapes along the diagonal. Phase sensitive manipulation is still worthwhile, however, since the crosspeaks are always of (antiphase) pure absorption mode. Other types of experiment, notably NOESY, are of pure absorption mode throughout, and phase-sensitive manipulation is particularly valuable in this case. The remainder in general have diagonal and crosspeak lineshapes which are composed of various admixtures of absorption and dispersion mode, dependent upon the **coherence transfer pathways** within the molecule.

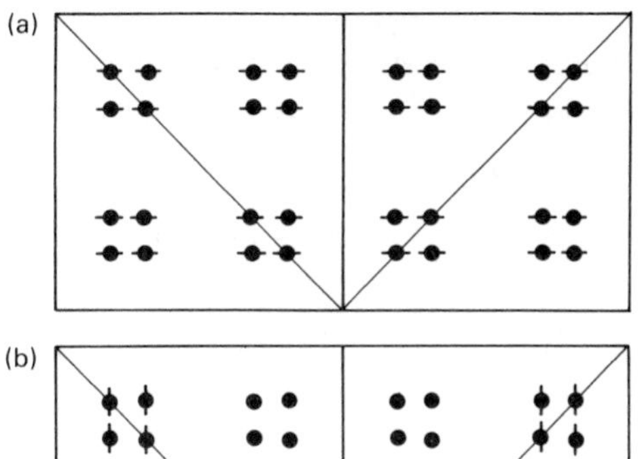

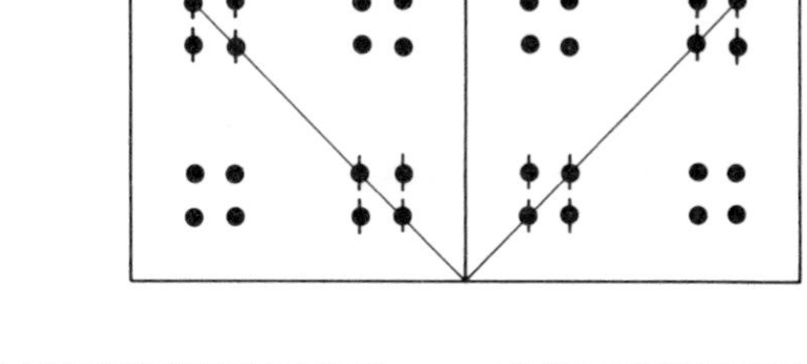

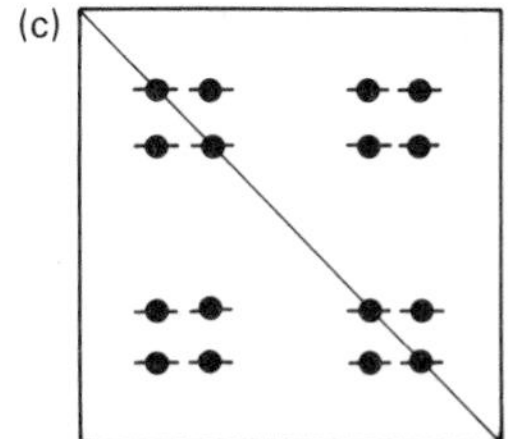

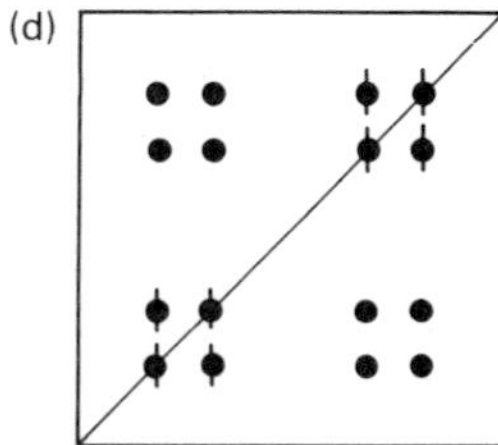

Fig. P11. Typical two-dimensional spectra recorded using; (a) complex transform in both dimensions; (b) real transform in t_1 (or complex transform with zeroed imaginary part); (c) Phase modulation giving echo selection; (d) phase-sensitive presentation. Key: phase-twist line, dispersion-mode line, absorption-mode line.

Finally, it should be mentioned that **flip-angle effects** are generally inaccessible in phase-sensitive experiments since the echo and **antiecho** components of the spectrum will possess different intensities, resulting in lineshape distortions after the hypercomplex Fourier transform.

FURTHER READING

For a critical assessment of techniques, see
Keeler, J. and Neuhaus, D. (1985). *J. Magn. Reson.* **63,** 454.

Phase shift See **phase**.

Phase-shifter See **spectrometer**.

Phase-twist lineshape See **phase-sensitive experiments**.

Polarization operators In analogy to **shift operators**, it is possible to define polarization operators. For spins $I = \frac{1}{2}$, these are given by;

P37 $$I^{\alpha} = \tfrac{1}{2}\mathbf{1} + I_z, \qquad I^{\beta} = \tfrac{1}{2}\mathbf{1} - I_z, \qquad I_z = \tfrac{1}{2}(I^{\alpha} - I^{\beta}).$$

Polarization operators are useful for the representation of non-equilibrium states in weakly coupled systems. For a two-spin system *IS*, for example, the density matrix is given by

$$\sigma = P_{\alpha\alpha}I^{\alpha}S^{\alpha} + P_{\alpha\beta}I^{\alpha}S^{\beta} + P_{\beta\alpha}I^{\beta}S^{\alpha} + P_{\beta\beta}I^{\beta}S^{\beta} \tag{P38}$$

where the *P*s are the populations.

From their definition, it follows that the polarization operators behave as follows (see also **angular momentum**):

$$\begin{aligned} I^{\alpha}|\alpha\rangle &= |\alpha\rangle, \qquad I^{\alpha}|\beta\rangle = 0, \\ I^{\beta}|\alpha\rangle &= 0, \qquad I^{\beta}|\beta\rangle = |\beta\rangle. \end{aligned} \tag{P39}$$

The transformation properties of polarization operators under r.f. pulses follow directly from (P37):

$$\begin{aligned} I^{\alpha} &\xrightarrow{\beta[I_x \cos\phi + I_y \sin\phi]} I^{\alpha}\cos^2(\beta/2) + I^{\beta}\sin^2(\beta/2) \\ &+ (\mathrm{i}/2)\sin\beta[I^{+}\exp\{-\mathrm{i}\phi\} - I^{-}\exp\{\mathrm{i}\phi\}], \\ I^{\beta} &\xrightarrow{\beta(I_x \cos\phi + I_y \sin\phi]} I^{\beta}\cos^2(\beta/2) + I^{\alpha}\sin^2(\beta/2) \\ &-(\mathrm{i}/2)\sin\beta[I^{+}\exp\{-\mathrm{i}\phi\} - I^{-}\exp\{\mathrm{i}\phi\}], \\ I^{\alpha} &\xrightarrow{\beta I_z} I^{\alpha}, \\ I^{\beta} &\xrightarrow{\beta I_z} I^{\beta}, \end{aligned} \tag{P40}$$

with flip-angle β and phase shift ϕ.

FURTHER READING

Polarization operators are described in more detail in

Weitekamp, D. P., Garbow, J. R. and Pines, A. (1982). *J. Chem. Phys.* **77,** 2870.

See also

Levitt, M. H. (1988) in *Pulse methods in* 1*D and* 2*D liquid phase NMR*. (ed. W. S. Brey), Grune and Swalton Inc., Orlando, Florida.

Polarization transfer See **cross-polarization.**

Populations See **partition function**.

Powder spectrum A randomly oriented or powder sample contains microcrystallites oriented at all possible angles with respect to the applied static magnetic field with equal probability. The NMR spectrum of such a sample is characteristically broad. It is often referred to as a powder spectrum (Fig. P12). The discontinuities in the theoretical spectrum of

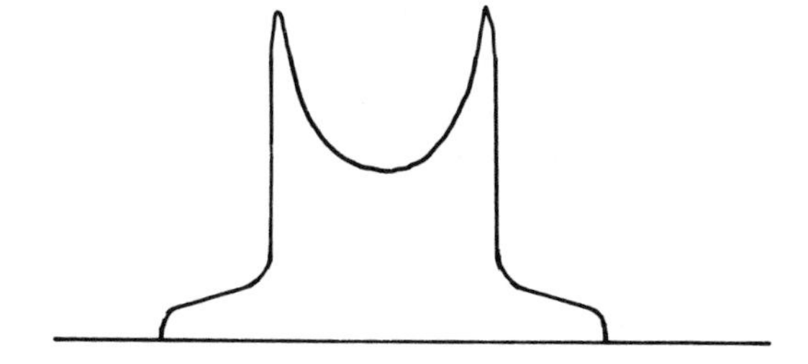

Fig. P12. A typical powder spectrum.

Fig. P12 are not observed experimentally, due to smoothing by residual broadening.

The 'powder spectrum' derives from the fact that molecular motion is restricted. In the liquid state, asymmetric lines are not seen. The difference between a liquid and a powder spectrum is that in a powder any given molecule is in a particular orientation. It remains in this orientation for a long time compared to the inverse of the anisotropy of the spectral absorption. In a liquid, all orientations are assumed by a given molecule in a short time with respect to the spectral anisotropy. The average over all orientation results in a resonance line at the average or isotropic value of the shielding **tensor** (the trace of the tensor):

$$\bar{\sigma} = \tfrac{1}{3}(\sigma_{xx} + \sigma_{yy} + \sigma_{zz}). \tag{P41}$$

In contrast, the powder pattern represents the different interactions experienced by each molecule as a result of its particular orientation in the magnetic field.

FURTHER READING

The theoretical details of powder spectra are dealt with in any good text on solid state NMR. See for example

Mehring, M. (1983). *High resolution NMR spectroscopy in solids,* (2nd edn). Springer-Verlag, Berlin.

Power spectrum See **absolute-value mode**.

Preamplifier See **amplifier**.

Precession See **Larmor precession**.

Probe The function of NMR probe is two fold. Firstly, it is the means by which r.f. power is transmitted to the sample in order to perturb the spin-state populations. Secondly, it is required to detect the minute e.m.f.'s generated by the rotating bulk magnetization of the spins. Since these functions are in many respects reciprocal, it is convenient to examine the detection process in more detail.

The most sensitive method of NMR detection to date relies on the principle of induction, i.e. a fluctuating magnetic field induces an e.m.f. in a loop of conductor through which the flux passes. The effect of perturbation of the nuclear spin system is to produce a bulk component of magnetization M per unit volume which precesses about the static field with a characteristic Larmor frequency

$$\omega_0 = \gamma B_0 \qquad \text{(P42)}$$

where γ is the **magnetogyric ratio** and B_0 is the strength of the static field. Since for a 90° pulse, the rotating field exists in the transverse ($x'-y'$) rotating frame, the aim is to produce a receiving coil (i.e. loop of conductor) in which the maximum e.m.f. is generated. In a reciprocal sense this implies that when used for transmission, the same coil should generate an homogeneous r.f. field (B_1 field) which is predominantly in the $x'-y'$ plane. If a superconducting magnetic is employed to generate B_0 (invariably the case in modern spectrometers) the situation is complicated by the fact that the axis of the sample is usually parallel to B_0. Thus, to transmit or receive a transverse field B_1, Helmholtz coils are required (Fig. P13). Typically, the induced e.m.f. in the receiver coils is 10^{-9}–10^{-5} V, which at the lower limit approaches the amplitude of the noise generated in the coil due to random thermal motion of electrons. The r.m.s. noise e.m.f. over a bandwidth Δv at the Larmor frequency of interest is given by

$$(\overline{N^2})^{\frac{1}{2}} = \sqrt{4k\ \mathrm{Tr}\ \Delta v} \qquad \text{(P43)}$$

where T is the absolute temperature, k is the Boltzmann constant, and r is the coil resistance. Equation (P43) therefore implies that for a given receiver bandwidth, r and T should be as small as possible and of course B_1 must be as large as possible if probe efficiency is to be high. Unfortunately, the requirements upon r and B_1 are generally in conflict. For example, B_1 can be doubled by doubling the number of turns on the coil, but since the radius of the wire has to be halved to fit in the same space, r increases fourfold. In addition there are a variety of other subtle effects such as the skin effect and proximity effects. The former derives from the fact that at high frequencies current flows only on the surface of

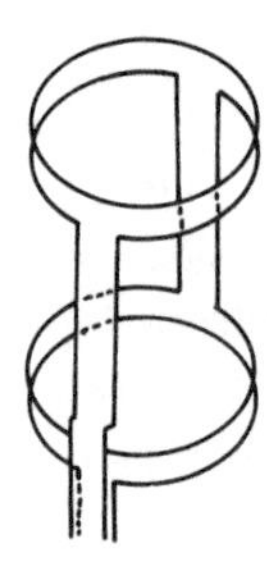

Fig. P13. Helmholtz coil arrangement used in NMR probes designed for superconducting magnets.

the conductor, which in turn is responsible for the latter, since for several closely spaced conductors, there will be regions of zero field and hence zero current. The net effect is an increase in effective resistance of the conductor. In practice, these effects are very difficult to calculate, and the best design for Helmholtz coils is often assessed experimentally.

FURTHER READING

Hoult, D. I. (1978). *Progr. NMR Spectr.* **12,** 41.

Product basis If we consider a two-spin $\frac{1}{2}$ system IS (see **spin system**), each spin can be characterized by the wave functions $|\beta\rangle$ and $|\alpha\rangle$, depending upon whether the spin is aligned parallel or against the applied static magnetic field. However, if we consider the system as a whole we are faced with the problem of finding a wavefunction for a system composed of four energy levels, rather than two (Fig. P14). We can in fact

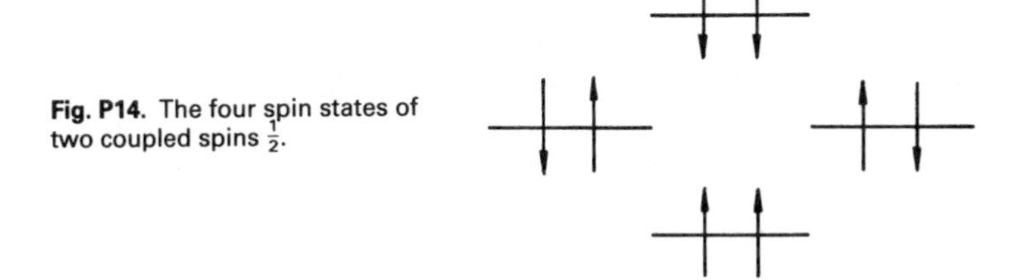

Fig. P14. The four spin states of two coupled spins $\frac{1}{2}$.

adequately describe this system in terms of the product basis. That is, each energy level is described by a wavefunction which is a simple product of the wavefunctions of the individual nuclei (Fig. P15). In the case of two uncoupled nuclei, or two weakly coupled nuclei (see **weak coupling**), this simple product basis is the **eigenbasis** of the **Hamiltonian**. In the case of **strong coupling** it is not, and more complicated wavefunctions are necessary. The justification for using the simple product basis in the case of uncoupled or weakly coupled nuclei can be made clear from the behaviour of the functions in Fig. P15 when inserted into the **Schrödinger equation**. Given the two nuclei I and S, the Hamiltonian

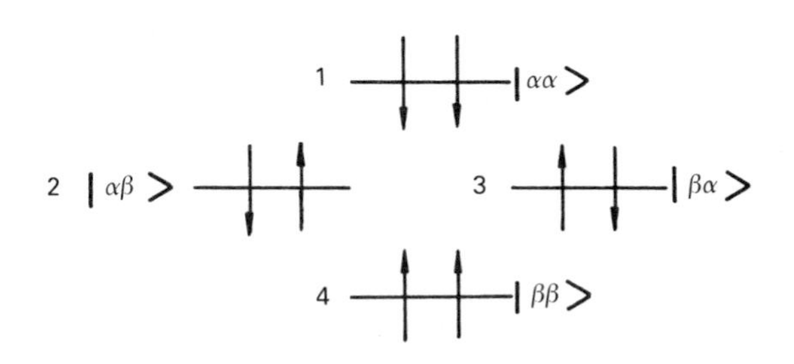

Fig. P15. The four product functions corresponding to the four spin states of two weakly coupled spins $\frac{1}{2}$.

operators for the individual nuclei would be $\mathcal{H}_I$ and $\mathcal{H}_S$ respectively. Thus, for the two-spin system, the corresponding Hamiltonian must be $\mathcal{H}_{IS} = \mathcal{H}_I + \mathcal{H}_S$. Now, if the corresponding energy of a particular state is given by E, then the correct choice of wavefunction for that state must obey the Schrödinger equation:

P44 $$H\,|\psi\rangle = E\,|\psi\rangle.$$

Considering the wavefunction $|\alpha\alpha\rangle$ which describes the highest energy state, the corresponding Schrödinger equation must be

P45 $$\mathcal{H}_I\,|\alpha\alpha\rangle + \mathcal{H}_S\,|\alpha\alpha\rangle = \mathcal{H}_{IS}\,|\alpha\alpha\rangle = E_I\,|\alpha\alpha\rangle + E_S\,|\alpha\alpha\rangle = (E_I + E_S)\,|\alpha\alpha\rangle$$

and thus the product function satisfies the Schrödinger equation. Note that this is only true if the operation $\mathcal{H}_I\,|\alpha\alpha\rangle$ has no effect upon the S spin, i.e. ψ_S is a constant of this operation. This is of course the case for uncoupled systems, and is an excellent approximation in the case of weak coupling.

Product functions See **product basis**.

Product operator formalism The **density matrix** formalism for the theoretical descriptions of NMR experiments becomes very cumbersome in systems with a large number of spins. In addition, very little insight is gained into the workings of the experiment during the calculation, since this approach deals with the state of the spin system, irrespective of the observable that will be finally detected.

An alternative approach is to express the density matrix as a linear combination of base operators, U_n;

P46 $$\sigma(t) = \sum_n c_n(t) U_n.$$

The calculation can be considerably simplified by judicious choice of the set $\{U_n\}$. For specific situations, **spherical tensor operators** and **single-transition operators** have been used. However, in the case of a loosely coupled spin $\frac{1}{2}$ system, the use of product operators is particularly useful. They provide physical insight, and at the same time afford computational convenience. The complete base set $\{U_n\}$ for an N-spin $\frac{1}{2}$ system consists of 4^N product operators. They are orthogonal but not normalized. For a two-spin system IS, the 16 product operators are:

$\frac{1}{2}\mathbf{1}$ where $\mathbf{1}$ is the unity operator or **identity**

P47 $$\begin{aligned}&I_x,\ I_y,\ I_z,\ S_x,\ S_y,\ S_z\\&2I_xS_x,\ 2I_xS_y,\ 2I_xS_z\\&2I_yS_x,\ 2I_yS_y,\ 2I_yS_z\\&2I_zS_x,\ 2I_zS_y,\ 2I_zS_z.\end{aligned}$$

Any density operator can be expressed as a linear combination of this set of base operators. The advantage in expanding the density operator into this linear combination is that the fate of each of the operator terms can be followed throughout the calculation and can be equated with a physical meaning. It must be emphasized that these operators do not possess any 'magical' properties. They are entirely equivalent to the corresponding density matrix at a given time during the experiment. This can be explicitly proven by expressing each of the 16 terms in (P47) in matrix form. For example, the equilibrium density matrix for a two-spin $\frac{1}{2}$ system is given by

P48
$$\sigma(0) = \tfrac{1}{4}\mathbf{1} + \tfrac{1}{4}\,.\,P\begin{bmatrix} -1 & 0 & 0 & 0 \\ 0 & 0 & 0 & 0 \\ 0 & 0 & 0 & 0 \\ 0 & 0 & 0 & +1 \end{bmatrix}$$

which is equivalent to the product operator expression

P49
$$\tfrac{1}{4}\mathbf{1} + \tfrac{1}{4}\,.\,P(I_z + S_z) = \tfrac{1}{4}\begin{bmatrix} 1 & 0 & 0 & 0 \\ 0 & 1 & 0 & 0 \\ 0 & 0 & 1 & 0 \\ 0 & 0 & 0 & 1 \end{bmatrix}$$
$$+\tfrac{1}{8}\,.\,P\begin{bmatrix} -1 & 0 & 0 & 0 \\ 0 & -1 & 0 & 0 \\ 0 & 0 & +1 & 0 \\ 0 & 0 & 0 & +1 \end{bmatrix} + \tfrac{1}{8}\,.\,P\begin{bmatrix} -1 & 0 & 0 & 0 \\ 0 & +1 & 0 & 0 \\ 0 & 0 & -1 & 0 \\ 0 & 0 & 0 & +1 \end{bmatrix}$$

where $P = \omega\hbar/kT$. In both formalisms it is common practice to drop the unity operator in all further calculations, since it does not contribute to the observable magnetization.

In exact analogy to the density matrix formalism, the effects of free precession and r.f. pulses are described by a sequence of transformations (see **unitary transformation**):

P50
$$\exp\{-\mathrm{i}\phi U_m\}U_n \exp\{\mathrm{i}\phi U_m\} = \sum_t C_{tn}(r, \phi)B_t$$

where ϕU_m corresponds directly to the relevant **Hamiltonian** and is as follows:

P51a $\omega_I \tau I_z$ for chemical shift precession,

P51b $\pi J_{IS}\tau 2I_z S_z$ for evolution under weak J-coupling.

P51c βI_k for r.f. pulses of flip-angle β and phase k.

This will become clearer later. Before proceeding to specific examples, it is convenient to describe the 16 operators of (P47) in terms of their physical interpretation. Since each operator is a complete matrix, rather than a matrix element, a given product operator represents an entire spin multiplet. Their physical interpretation is as follows:

I_z longitudinal magnetization of spin I,

I_x in-phase x magnetization of spin I,

I_y in-phase y magnetization of spin I,

$2I_xS_z$ x magnetization of spin I antiphase with respect to spin S,

$2I_yS_z$ y magnetization of spin I antiphase with respect to spin S,

$2I_xS_x$, $2I_yS_y$, $2I_xS_y$, $2I_yS_x$ two-spin coherence of spins I and S,

$2I_zS_z$ longitudinal two-spin order of spins I and S.

The term antiphase represents multiplets with individual components that have opposite phases. Each of the above physical interpretations can be derived by explicit generation of these in their matrix form followed by extraction of observable magnetization using the density matrix formalism. The value of the product operator formalism is that no explicit matrix manipulations are required, and this is thus a shorthand method by which calculations on NMR spin systems can be performed.

In product operator calculations throughout this book, a standard shorthand notation due to Sorensen *et al.* (1983) is used to signify a transformation such as that in (P50):

P52 $$\sigma(t) \xrightarrow{\mathcal{H}_1\tau} \sigma(t+\tau)$$

where $\mathcal{H}_1$ is the relevant Hamiltonian effective during the time τ, and the σ's are represented by product operators. To illustrate the algebra of product operators, we will analyse a simple pulse-and-collect experiment for a two-spin system IS, and compare this result with that calculated for an identical system, using the density matrix formalism (see **density matrix**). As usual we ignore relaxation. We begin with the two-spin system at thermal equilibrium. Without loss of generality, the relevant expression in the product operator formalism can be described by (cf. P49):

P53 $$\sigma(0) = I_z + S_z.$$

If, now, we apply an r.f. pulse of flip-angle 90° ($\pi/2$ radians) with phase along the x axis, the relevant transformation is given according to (P51c.)

P54 $$I_z + S_z \xrightarrow{\pi/2(I_x+S_x)} -I_y - S_y.$$

This result, in common with all transformations, can be derived from the

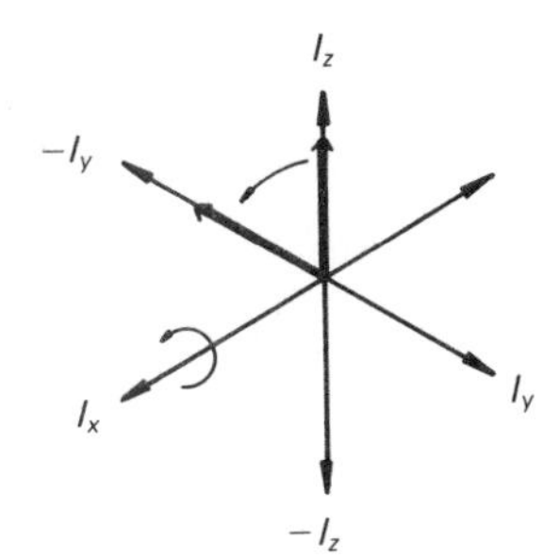

Fig. P16. Transformation of I_z under the influence of I_x.

cyclic commutation relations of the **angular momentum** operators. Conveniently, these transformations can be represented in terms of cartesian coordinates, leading to a pictorial illustration of the effects of the various Hamiltonians upon the spin system. In the case of an r.f. pulse along the x axis, the transformations are shown in Fig. P16. Here, the effect of a $\pi/2$ r.f. pulse upon a vector representing I_z demonstrates how (P54) is derived. Figure P16, together with other relevant transformations in pictorial form, is given in Appendix 1. Knowledge of these is sufficient to allow calculation of arbitrarily complex spin dynamics.

To continue the analysis, it is necessary to consider what happens when the terms $-I_y - S_y$ of (P54) evolve under chemical shift and spin coupling terms. Since the terms of the Hamiltonian corresponding to each of these commute, the evolutions can be considered in either order. Taking chemical shift evolution first, and using the pictorial representations in Appendix 1, we find

$$-I_y - S_y \xrightarrow{\omega_I \tau I_z} \xrightarrow{\omega_S \tau S_z} -I_y \cos \omega_I \tau + I_x \sin \omega_I \tau - S_y \cos \omega_S \tau + S_x \sin \omega_S \tau \quad \text{P55}$$

where the first transformation of course only operates on spin I, and the second on spin S. The trigonometric functions in equation P55 derive from the fact that terms in $-I_y$ modulate with a cosinusoidal dependence on $\omega_I \tau$ and $\omega_S \tau$ (they begin with unit intensity), and terms in I_x and S_x show a sinusoidal modulation (they begin with zero intensity). Each term on the right-hand side of (P55) now evolves under the scalar coupling

$$\begin{aligned} &-I_y \cos \omega_I \tau + I_x \sin \omega_I \tau - S_y \cos \omega_S \tau + S_x \sin \omega_S \tau \xrightarrow{\pi J_{IS} \tau 2 I_z S_z} \\ &-I_y \cos \omega_I \tau \cos \pi J_{IS} \tau + 2 I_x S_z \cos \omega_I \tau \sin \pi J_{IS} \tau \\ &+I_x \sin \omega_I \tau \cos \pi J_{IS} \tau + 2 I_y S_z \sin \omega_I \tau \sin \pi J_{IS} \tau \\ &-S_y \cos \omega_S \tau \cos \pi J_{IS} \tau + 2 S_x I_z \cos \omega_S \tau \sin \pi J_{IS} \tau \\ &+S_x \sin \omega_S \tau \cos \pi J_{IS} \tau + 2 S_y I_z \sin \omega_S \tau \sin \pi J_{IS} \tau. \end{aligned} \quad \text{P56}$$

In order to extract the observables, it is necessary to determine which terms on the right-hand side of (P56) can generate an e.m.f. in the receiver coils. In the density matrix formalism, the magnetization is extracted from the following formulae (see **density matrix**):

P57 $$\langle M_x \rangle = \mathrm{Tr}\{\sigma . F_x\}, \qquad \langle M_y \rangle = \mathrm{Tr}\{\sigma . F_y\}.$$

In the product operator formalism, the equivalent operation to (P57) is simply to note that only terms representing in phase magnetization can represent observables. Thus, we can write for the x and y components of the magnetization

P56 $$\begin{aligned} \langle M_x \rangle &= +I_x \sin \omega_I \tau \cos \pi J_{IS} \tau + S_x \sin \omega_S \tau \cos \pi J_{IS} \tau, \\ \langle M_y \rangle &= -I_y \cos \omega_I \tau \cos \pi J_{IS} \tau - S_y \cos \omega_S \tau \cos \pi J_{IS} \tau. \end{aligned}$$

Using the trigonometric identities given in Appendix 2, (P58) can be written

P59 $$\begin{aligned} \langle M_x \rangle &= \tfrac{1}{2} I_x [\sin(\omega_I \tau + \pi J_{IS} \tau) + \sin(\omega_I \tau - \pi J_{IS} \tau)] \\ &\quad + \tfrac{1}{2} S_x [\sin(\omega_S \tau + \pi J_{IS} \tau) + \sin(\omega_S \tau - \pi J_{IS} \tau)], \\ \langle M_y \rangle &= -\tfrac{1}{2} I_y [\cos(\omega_I \tau + \pi J_{IS} \tau) + \cos(\omega_I \tau - \pi J_{IS} \tau)] \\ &\quad - \tfrac{1}{2} S_y [\cos(\omega_S \tau + \pi J_{IS} \tau) + \cos(\omega_S \tau - \pi J_{IS} \tau)]. \end{aligned}$$

We can now describe the resulting NMR spectrum by performing a mental **Fourier transform** upon (P57). With regard to $\langle M_x \rangle$, we find four resonance lines with frequencies $\omega_I + \pi J_{IS}$, $\omega_I - \pi J_{IS}$, $\omega_S + \pi J_{IS}$, $\omega_S - \pi J_{IS}$. Since these terms have a sinusoidal dependence upon the evolution time τ, they will result in four dispersion-mode lineshapes. Each individual multiplet component will have the same phase since the four sinusoidal components have the same sign. (Remember that two dispersion-mode lineshapes can also be antiphase with respect to each other!). By an entirely analogous argument, $\langle M_y \rangle$ consists of four absorption-mode lines which have the same phase relation with respect to each other. In theory, these should be represented with negative intensity since $-I_y$ terms are involved. This arises from the sign convention which has been adopted in the literature, but this is unimportant since it is the relative phases which are meaningful. The resulting spectrum is thus equivalent to that calculated using the density matrix formalism.

The above analysis illustrates the more important transformations which have been used freely throughout this work. However, a few additional rules are required for the analysis of specialized techniques involving multiple-quantum coherence. The latter are described in the product operator formalism by terms such as $2I_xS_x$, $2I_xS_y$, $2I_yS_x$, $2I_yS_y$. None of these terms describes pure multiple-quantum coherence, but consist of superposition of zero-quantum and double-quantum coherence. This is proven by expansion of each angular momentum operator into raising and lowering operators, followed by explicit multiplication: (see **shift**

operators)

P60
$$2I_xS_x = \tfrac{1}{2}(I^+S^+ + I^+S^- + I^-S^+ + I^-S^-),$$
$$2I_yS_y = -\tfrac{1}{2}(I^+S^+ - I^+S^- - I^-S^+ + I^-S^-),$$
$$2I_xS_y = 1/2\mathrm{i}(I^+S^+ - I^+S^- + I^-S^+ - I^-S^-),$$
$$2I_yS_x = 1/2\mathrm{i}(I^+S^+ + I^+S^- - I^-S^+ - I^-S^-).$$

Pure zero-quantum and double-quantum coherence can be obtained from the linear combinations:

P61
$$\tfrac{1}{2}(2I_xS_x - 2I_yS_y) = \tfrac{1}{2}(I^+S^+ + I^-S^-) = 2\mathrm{QT}_x,$$
$$\tfrac{1}{2}(2I_xS_y + 2I_yS_x) = 1/2\mathrm{i}(I^+S^+ - I^-S^-) = 2\mathrm{QT}_y,$$
$$\tfrac{1}{2}(2I_xS_x + 2I_yS_y) = \tfrac{1}{2}(I^+S^- + I^-S^+) = \mathrm{ZQT}_x,$$
$$\tfrac{1}{2}(2I_yS_x - 2I_xS_y) = 1/2\mathrm{i}(I^+S^- - I^-S^+) = \mathrm{ZQT}_y.$$

The precession of double-quantum and zero-quantum coherence depends upon the sum and difference of the chemical shifts, respectively:

P62
$$2\mathrm{QT}_x \xrightarrow{(\omega_I I_z + \omega_S S_z)\tau} 2\mathrm{QT}_x \cos(\omega_I + \omega_S)\tau + 2\mathrm{QT}_y \sin(\omega_I + \omega_S)\tau,$$
$$\mathrm{ZQT}_x \xrightarrow{(\omega_I I_z + \omega_S S_z)\tau} \mathrm{ZQT}_x \cos(\omega_I - \omega_S)\tau + \mathrm{ZQT}_y \sin(\omega_I - \omega_S)\tau.$$

The evolution is unaffected by couplings between nuclei actively involved in the transition:

P63
$$2I_xS_x \xrightarrow{\pi J_{IS}\tau 2I_zS_z} 2I_xS_x$$

but multiple-quantum coherence evolves under coupling to 'passive' spins, i.e. those not actively involved in the transition. Obviously this can only occur in spin systems containing more than two spins.

The rules described above are sufficient for an understanding of most theoretical manipulations contained in this work. Notable exceptions are calculations involving **strong coupling**, which are more easily performed using the density matrix formalism. In addition, the product operator formalism is of enormous value in a variety of other situations in NMR, and it is not possible to give an exhaustive list here. For a detailed description of the product operator formalism, the reader is referred to the paper cited below.

FURTHER READING

Sorensen, O. W., Eich, G. W., Levitt, M. H., Bodenhausen, G., and Ernst, R. R. (1983). *Prog. NMR Spectr.* **16,** 163.

Progressive connectivity See **connectivity networks**.

Projection operator A projection operator projects an arbitrary function $|\psi\rangle$ onto the function $|n\rangle$, which may be represented in **Hilbert space** by

P64 $$P_n = \frac{|n\rangle\langle n|}{\langle n|n\rangle}$$

where P_n is represented in **bra-ket notation**. If $|\psi\rangle$ is expanded into a linear combination of orthogonal functions $|i\rangle$,

P65 $$|\psi\rangle = \sum_i C_i\,|i\rangle$$

then the projection is given by

P66 $$P_n\,|\psi\rangle = \frac{|n\rangle\langle n|}{\langle n|n\rangle}\sum_i C_i\,|i\rangle$$

P67 $$= \sum_i C_i\,|n\rangle\,\frac{\langle n|i\rangle}{\langle n|n\rangle} = C_n\,|n\rangle.$$

Equation (P67) is derived by noting that $\langle n|i\rangle$ is zero unless $i = n$, since n is expanded in a linear combination of orthogonal functions. The only function which survives is thus $C_n\,|n\rangle$, which is just the component of $|n\rangle$ within $|\psi\rangle$.

FURTHER READING

Friedrichs, K. O. (1973). *Spectral theory of operators in Hilbert space.* Springer-Verlag, New York.

Propagator In the **density matrix** formalism for the description of pulse NMR experiments, we are interested in the time evolution of the density matrix under the appropriate **Hamiltonian** corresponding to r.f. pulses or free precession periods. Integration of the **Liouville–von Neumann equation** in the case of a time-independent Hamiltonian $\mathcal{H}$ gives the following expression for the density matrix $\sigma_{(t)}$ at time t:

P68 $$\sigma(t) = \exp\{-\mathrm{i}\mathcal{H}t\}\,\sigma_{(0)}\exp\{\mathrm{i}\mathcal{H}t\}$$

where $\exp\{-\mathrm{i}\mathcal{H}t\}$ is known as a propagator. It is most often used in its **matrix representation** U, where (P68) becomes

P69 $$\sigma(t) = U\sigma_{(0)}U^{-1}.$$

Pseudo-echo transformation An inherent property of many two-dimensional NMR spectra is the generation of the phase-twist lineshape. While this undesirable feature can be circumnavigated in the majority of cases by use of phase-sensitive manipulation (see **phase-sensitive**

experiments), in certain experiments it is unavoidable. However, the dispersion-mode contributions to the phase-twist lineshape can be eliminated by an alternative (but less satisfactory) procedure known as pseudo-echo transformation or pseudo-echo weighting. This is achieved by rendering the signal envelope symmetrical about the centre of the detection periods, i.e.

$$S(t_1) = S(t_1^{\max} - t_1), \qquad S(t_2) = S(t_2^{\max} - t_2). \tag{P70}$$

After complex Fourier transformation, the dispersion component (i.e. the imaginary part) vanishes, since the sine transfomation of a symmetrical envelope is zero. Thus, in the absence of overlapping lines, a pure absorption signal is obtained by calculating the square root of the power spectrum, i.e. the **absolute-value mode**:

$$S(\omega_1, \omega_2) = \{[\mathrm{Re}\, S(\omega_1, \omega_2)]^2 + [\mathrm{Im}\, S(\omega_1, \omega_2)]^2\}^{\frac{1}{2}},$$

and for $\mathrm{Im} = 0$,

$$S(\omega_1, \omega_2) = \mathrm{Re}\, S(\omega_1, \omega_2). \tag{P71}$$

Usually, acquisition begins at $t_1, t_2 = 0$, and hence the envelope is not symmetrical, as it would be in the case of an echo. However, the envelope can be transformed into a pseudo-echo by a weighting function which transforms the time domain signal according to (P70). In practice either a Gaussian transformation or a sine–bell transformation is utilized. The disadvantage of pseudo-echo weighting is that the signal is strongly attenuated around $t_1 = t_2 \approx 0$, and this severe degradation of the signal to noise ratio sometimes occurs. For this reason phase-sensitive experiments are preferable.

***P*-type peak** See **antiecho**.

Pulse See **composite pulse**, **Gaussian pulse**, **hard pulse**, **Z-pulse**.

Pulse droop See **pulse width**.

Pulse sequence In modern Fourier transform NMR, it is commonplace to apply a train of r.f. pulses with which to perturb the spin system. While several such pulse sequences have been devised in the context of one-dimensional NMR (see **inversion recovery sequence**, **Carr–Purcell–Meiboom–Gill sequence**) a much larger number is found in two-dimensional NMR. A pulse sequence often begins with a 90° r.f. pulse of given phase to convert the equilibrium longitudinal magnetization into transverse magnetization (Fig. P17).

The following r.f. pulses depend entirely upon how the spin system is to be probed. A two-dimensional sequence (see **two-dimensional NMR**)

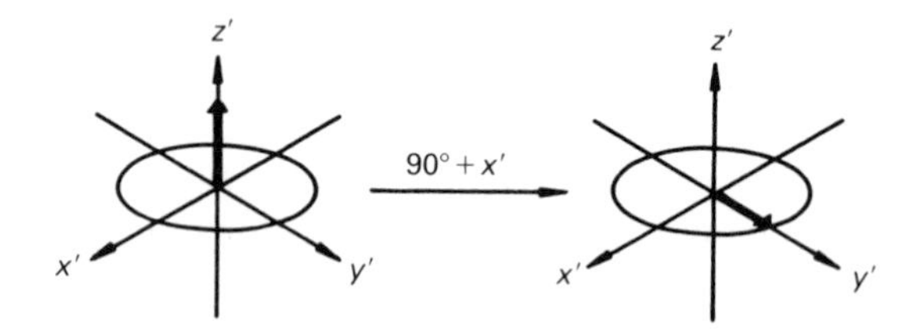

Fig. P17. A 90° r.f. pulse converts equilibrium magnetization into transverse magnetization.

invariably contains two time periods under which the spin system evolves under a given **Hamiltonian**. One of the simplest (yet most useful) sequences is the two-pulse sequence used in **correlated spectroscopy** (COSY) (Fig. P18).

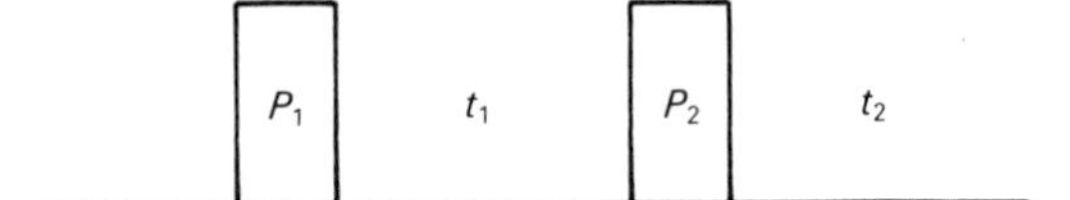

Fig. P18. Two-pulse sequence for acquisition of COSY spectra.

This sequence illustrates three important characteristics of all two-dimensional experiments. The spin system is always prepared in a suitable state during the preparation period. In the case of the COSY sequence the preparation consists simply in the creation of transverse magnetization. More elaborate schemes are possible. For example, the creation of **multiple-quantum coherence** is the key principle in experiments such as **double-quantum filtered correlated spectroscopy**. Irrespective of the manner by which the spin system is prepared, there follows an evolution period during which the spin system evolves under the Hamiltonian which is operative during this period. In the case of the COSY experiment, this consists of the Zeeman and spin coupling Hamiltonians; but the Hamiltonian during t_1 can be 'tailored' by the application of further r.f. pulses. Finally, the spin system evolves during t_2 under the influence of the Hamiltonian operative during that period. This Hamiltonian may be different from that which operates during t_1. The response of the spin system to r.f. pulses is detected during t_2 in the conventional manner, and thus t_2 can be thought of as the detection period in one-dimensional NMR.

For further details on the use of pulse sequences in NMR, refer to the relevant subheadings for each experiment.

Pulse width In a standard pulse-and-collect **Fourier transform** NMR experiment, equilibrium longitudinal magnetization is perturbed by the application of an r.f. pulse. For example, an r.f. pulse applied along the x axis of the **rotating frame** causes the classical bulk magnetization vector (see **classical formalism**) to be rotated in the y'–z' plane. The angle through which the magnetization vector is rotated (θ), depends upon the **magnetogyric ratio** of the perturbed nuclei (γ), the strength of the applied field (B_1) and the length of time for which the pulse is applied, t_p;

P72 $$\theta = \gamma B_1 t_p.$$

The value of t_p is normally measured in μs and is otherwise known as the pulse width. In practical terms, the pulse width should be as small as possible, in order to ensure that the spin system is perturbed equally over the spectral **sweep-width** of the nuclei under investigation (see **Fourier transform**).

In general, NMR spectrometers employ a rectangular pulse shape, primarily since it is easy to generate. However, in many situations this pulse shape is not ideal. For example, in selective excitation experiments the **Gaussian pulse** shape has distinct advantages. In these cases the definition of pulse width is more difficult.

From inspection of (P72), it is clear that for a given value of t_p, $\theta = 90°$. Under these conditions a rectangular r.f. pulse of width t_p is known as a 90° or $\pi/2$ pulse, for obvious reasons. In principle, a 180° pulse should thus be equivalent to a r.f. pulse with twice the width of a 90° pulse. While in well-designed spectrometers this is the case, in poorly designed spectrometers the phenomenon of pulse droop causes a lengthening of the 180° pulse (Fig. P19). Pulse droop arises from a time-dependent fall in the strength of B_1, which is in turn derived from a fall in power output from the spectrometer transmitter. In practice, most spectrometers are designed such that the transmitter power falls drastically for long pulses, in order to protect the probe against inadvertent application of a very long pulse (seconds). However, it should certainly be possible to obtain continuous power output over tens of μs.

An additional difficulty is encountered if the B_1 field is very inhomogeneous. In such cases different parts of the sample will experience different values of θ. This is most noticeable when a 180° pulse is applied to the sample. In theory, no signal should be observed, since the magnetization will be along the $-z$ axis for a perfect 180° pulse. In practice, however, a finite signal is observed, since regions of sample experience an effective B_1 which is slightly greater or slightly less than

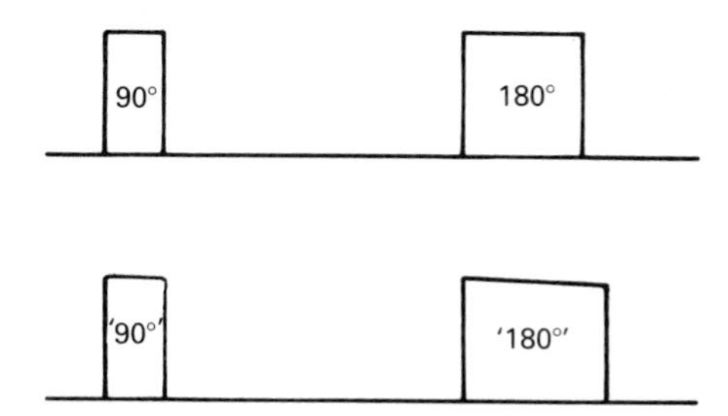

Fig. P19. (a) Ideally, a 180° pulse is twice the width of a 90° pulse. (b) In poorly designed spectrometers, a 180° pulse is more than twice the length of a 90° pulse due to pulse droop.

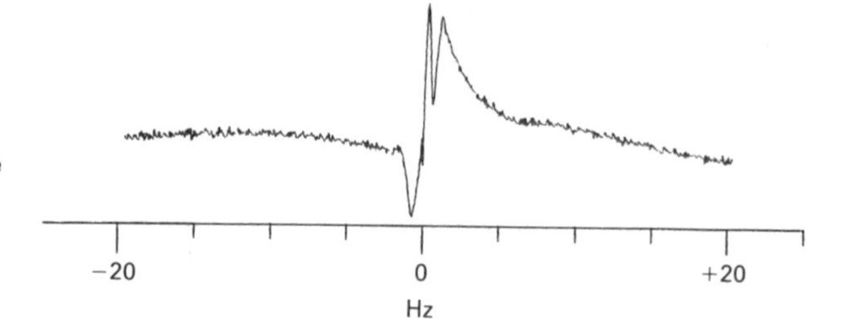

Fig. P20. The response of a sample of H_2O to a 180° pulse. This spectrum was recorded while the sample was stationary in the magnet.

that which corresponds to a perfect 180° pulse (Fig. P20). See also **off-resonance effects**.

Pure state In quantum mechanics, we are often concerned with phenomena in which a maximum of information is available about the system under consideration. A system which is in a state from which the maximum of information may be derived is termed a pure state. It is characterized by an experiment that gives a result which is predictable with certainty when the system is in that state (and only that state). A pure state can thus be identified by specifying that experiment which describes it uniquely.

When it is not convenient to identify a pure state by specifying the relevant experiment, the state may be identified as a linear combination (superposition) of eigenstates of a suitable complete set of operators. The representation of a pure state by either of these means is usually called a wavefunction, ψ.

In NMR, we are invariably concerned with states which are described by a superposition of pure states. For example, consider the simple case of an ensemble of spins $\frac{1}{2}$ in a static magnetic field. Each spin has two definite orientations in the field ('up' or 'down') which are described by the wavefunctions $|\beta\rangle$ and $|\alpha\rangle$. The state $|\psi\rangle$ of an individual spin may always be represented as a linear superposition of these states:

$$|\psi\rangle = C_\alpha\,|\alpha\rangle + C_\beta\,|\beta\rangle. \qquad \text{P73}$$

However, the state of the spin ensemble is a state with less than maximal information, and it is necessary to examine the statistical behaviour in order to predict the results of observations. In NMR this is achieved by describing the spin system in terms of the **density matrix**.

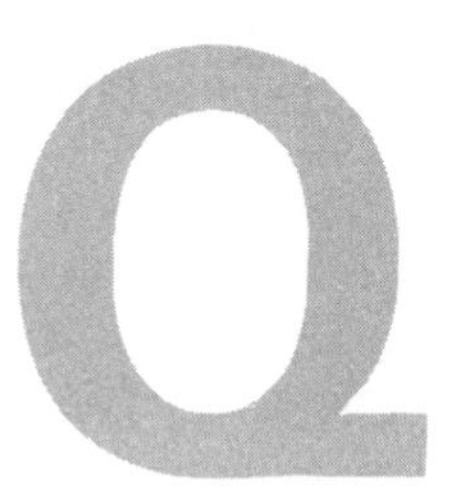

Quadrature detection In the **classical formalism** for the description of NMR experiments, the detectable magnetization is represented by a vector which precesses in the rotating x'–y' frame (see **rotating frame**). A detector aligned along the x' axis will be insensitive to the sense of rotation of the vector, i.e. the sign of the frequency with respect to the transmitter **offset** is not determined (Fig. Q1). One method by which this may be overcome is to arrange for a second detector aligned along the y' axis. It is now possible to discriminate between the signs of the frequencies (Fig. Q2). This approach is known as quadrature detection. However, provision of two pairs of coils into an already crowded **probe** is a difficult and unnecessary complication. An equivalent situation can be derived by purely electronic means. A block diagram of a quadrature detection system is shown in Fig. Q3. The signal is split into two equal parts using a splitter. Each is then fed into a **phase-sensitive detector**, one of which is fed with a reference which is 90° out of phase with respect to the other. After filtration, the resulting signals are digitized. The workings of this system are most easily derived by the application of some trigonometry. Consider the case of a vector precessing in the rotating frame with a frequency offset $+\Delta\omega$ from the transmitter carrier. The signal $f(t)$ induced in the receiver coils is a function of the offset,

$$f(t) = \cos \Delta\omega t. \tag{Q1}$$

Using the identity $\cos(x) = \frac{1}{2}(\exp(\mathrm{i}x) + \exp(-\mathrm{i}x))$, we can express (Q1) as follows:

$$f(t) = \tfrac{1}{2}(\exp\{\mathrm{i}\,\Delta\omega t\} + \exp\{-\mathrm{i}\,\Delta\omega t\}). \tag{Q2}$$

If we were to **Fourier transform** this response, we would obtain

$$f(\omega) = \tfrac{1}{2}(\mathrm{Abs}(+\Delta\omega) + \mathrm{i}\,\mathrm{Dis}(+\Delta\omega) + \mathrm{Abs}(-\Delta\omega) + \mathrm{i}\,\mathrm{Dis}(-\Delta\omega)), \tag{Q3}$$

giving resonance lines at $\pm\Delta\omega$; the sign of the precession frequency is not determined. However, using the quadrature detector, the output from the unshifted channel will be $\cos(\Delta\omega t)$, and from the phase shifted channel will be (in complex notation) $\mathrm{i}\sin(\Delta\omega t)$. The detected signal is therefore

$$f(t) = \cos(\Delta\omega t) + \mathrm{i}\sin(\Delta\omega t). \tag{Q4}$$

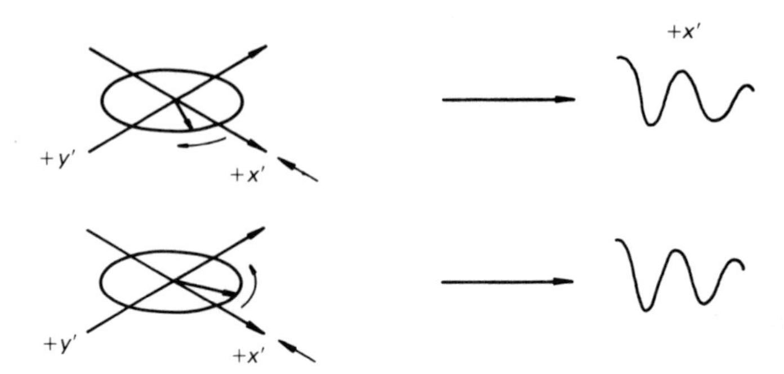

Fig. Q1. A single detector aligned along the x' axis of the rotating frame is insensitive to the sense of rotation of a magnetization vector in the transverse plane.

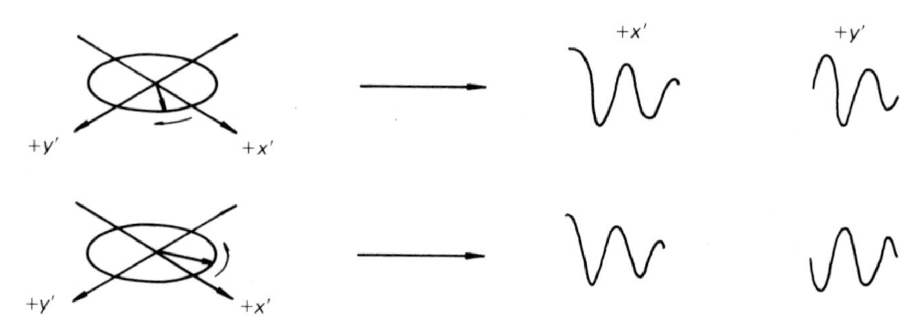

Fig. Q2. Two orthogonal detectors allow the sense of precession of transverse magnetization to be determined.

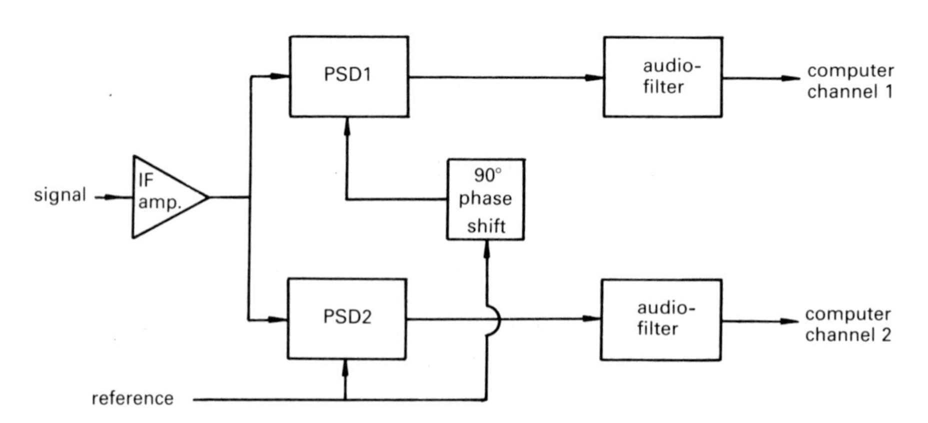

Fig. Q3. Block diagram of a typical quadrature detection system.

Using the additional identity $\sin(x) = -1/2\mathrm{i}[\exp\{\mathrm{i}x\} - \exp\{-\mathrm{i}x\}]$, (Q4) becomes

Q5
$$f(t) = \tfrac{1}{2}(\exp\{\mathrm{i}\,\Delta\omega t\} + \exp\{-\mathrm{i}\,\Delta\omega t\}) + \tfrac{1}{2}(\exp\{\mathrm{i}\,\Delta\omega t\} - \exp\{-\mathrm{i}\,\Delta\omega t\}) = \exp\{\mathrm{i}\,\Delta\omega t\}.$$

Fourier transformation of (Q5) gives

Q6
$$f(\omega) = \mathrm{Abs}(+\Delta\omega t) + \mathrm{i}\,\mathrm{Dis}(+\Delta\omega t).$$

The sign of the precession frequency has now been determined, and the absorption (Abs) and dispersion (Dis) components are the real and imaginary parts of the spectrum respectively. See also **CYCLOPS**.

FURTHER READING

Hoult, D. I. (1978). *Progr. NMR Spectr.* **12,** 41.

Quadrature image see **image response**.

Quadrupole relaxation In nuclear spins with $I > \frac{1}{2}$, couplings termed quadrupolar interactions exist, and may be interpreted as nuclear interactions with electric field gradients. The quadrupolar **Hamiltonian** is given by

Q7
$$\mathcal{H}_Q = \sum_{k=1}^{n} \mathbf{I}_k \mathbf{Q}_k \mathbf{I}_k,$$

with the quadrupole coupling tensor $\mathbf{Q}_k$. As the molecule reorients, the components of $\mathbf{Q}_k$ become random functions of time and provide a **relaxation** mechanism for quadrupolar nuclei ($I > \frac{1}{2}$). In the **extreme narrowing** limit, the relaxation rates are given by

Q8
$$\frac{1}{T_1} = \frac{1}{T_2} = \frac{3}{40}\frac{2I+3}{I^2(2I-1)}\left(1 + \frac{\eta^2}{3}\right)\left(\frac{e^2Qq}{\hbar}\right)^2 \tau_c$$

where η is the asymmetry parameter and $(e^2Qq/\hbar)$ is the quadrupole coupling constant. The relaxation rate is seen to depend upon τ_c and the quadrupolar coupling constant. The quadrupolar interaction is usually dominated for nuclei with spin $I > \frac{1}{2}$ (unless $e^2qQ/\hbar = 0$ due to molecular symmetry). Note that the interaction is entirely intramolecular (Q7).

FURTHER READING

Abragam, A. (1961). *The principles of nuclear magnetism,* Chapter 8. Clarendon Press, Oxford.

Quantization See **angular momentum**.

Quantum number See **angular momentum**.

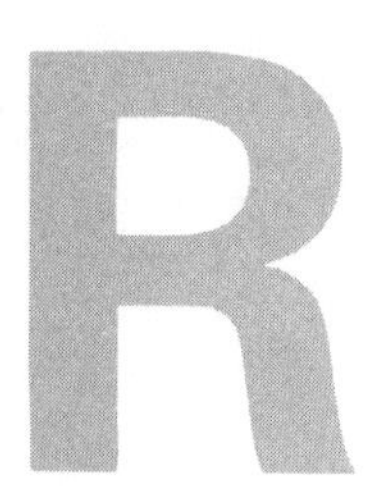

Raising operator See **shift operator**.

Real part See **complex number**.

Receiver See **spectrometer**.

Reference frequency See **phase-sensitive detector**.

Regressive connectivity See **connectivity networks**.

Relaxation The phenomenologically formulated **Bloch equations** predict that the population difference (n) between two spin states decays exponentially to equilibrium due to **spin–lattice relaxation**, which is characterized by a time constant T_1:

R1
$$\frac{dn}{dt} = -\frac{n}{T_1}.$$

The spin–lattice relaxation process is responsible for the establishment of thermal equilibrium between two spin states after the application of the static field B_0 (Fig. R1).

The term spin–lattice relaxation derives from the fact that the relaxation process involves a non-radiative energy transfer to the 'lattice' degrees of freedom of the system. In the presence of a static magnetic field B_0 along the $+z$ direction, the z component of the **magnetization** will thus obey the equation

R2
$$\frac{dM_z}{dt} = -\frac{(M_z - M_0)}{T_1}$$

where M_0 is the equilibrium value of the magnetization. This equation tells us that if we flip the bulk magnetization vector (see **classical formalism**) into the $-z$ direction with a 180° r.f. pulse, then it will eventually lie along the equilibrium $+z$ direction. The time dependence of this motion is characterized by T_1 (Fig. R2). This situation is clearly equivalent to Fig. *R*1, where the net excess of spins against the field direction eventually decay to the equilibrium situation where a net excess is aligned along the

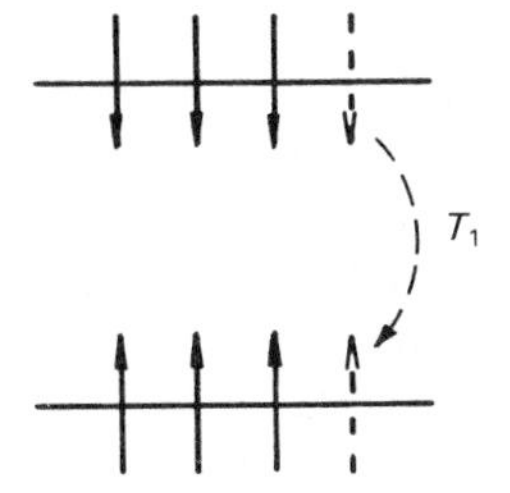

Fig. R1. T_1 relaxation is the process where thermal equilibrium is established between two spin states in a magnetic field in response to a perturbation.

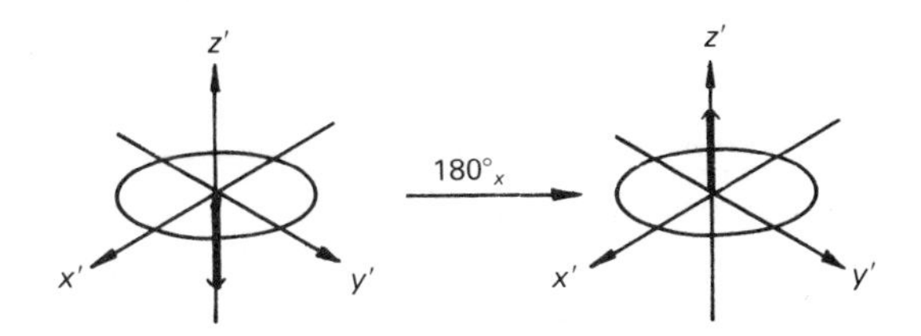

Fig. R2. Time dependence of the magnetization after application of a 180° pulse.

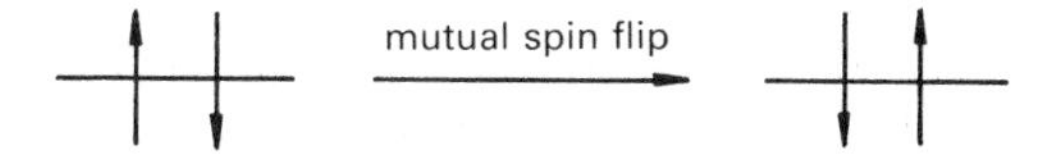

Fig. R3. T_2 processes involve a mutual exchange of spin energy which is an 'entropic' process.

field direction (see **Boltzmann distribution**). Before discussing the mechanisms by which T_1 relaxation occurs, it is necessary to consider the behaviour of the M_x and M_y components of the magnetization. Since these components in general have a decay time different from T_1, it is necessary to introduce another time constant T_2, corresponding to the **spin–spin relaxation** time. Often T_1 and T_2 are different because relaxation along the M_z direction (longitudinal relaxation) and the M_x and M_y directions (transverse relaxation) depend upon different processes within the spin system. In view of this distinction T_1 is sometimes called the longitudinal relaxation time, and T_2 is sometimes known as the transverse relaxation time. The important point is that whereas changes in M_z (T_1 processes) involve the exchange of Zeeman energy with the 'lattice', changes in M_x and M_y (T_2 processes) do not alter the total Zeeman energy of the nuclear spins. Rather, T_2 processes involve a mutual exchange of spin energy (Fig. R3), hence the term spin–spin relaxation. The net effect of this energy transfer is to cause a loss of phase coherence in the x–y plane, which is of course equivalent to a decay of the bulk magnetization vector in this plane. In thermodynamic terms, it is convenient to regard T_1 as an enthalpic process, whereas T_2 is an entropic process.

Both T_1 and T_2 relaxation is caused by time-dependent magnetic or electric fields at the nucleus which are derived from the random thermal motions present in the sample. Thus, unlike other forms of spectroscopy, the probability of spontaneous decay of an excited state is vanishingly small in NMR. In the case of the proton, fluctuating local magnetic fields may derive from translational motion of other nuclei, from unpaired electrons, or from spin rotation in which the molecular rotation generates magnetic fields at the nucleus. Also, changes in chemical shielding can modulate the total effective field. Quadrupolar nuclei are further affected by local changes in the electrostatic field gradient due to rotational or vibrational motion. In order for any of these events to cause relaxation, there must be a time-dependent interaction which acts directly on the spins. An essential requirement for relaxation is that the molecular motion in question must have a suitable time scale. That is, interactions which cause fluctuations at or near the Larmor frequency will be most effective in causing relaxation. This excludes phenomena such as electronic motions and molecular vibration. Conversely, rotational and diffusional motions are very important sources of relaxation in liquids. These processes affect both T_1 and T_2. Additionally, random forces which modulate the spin energy levels at very low frequencies (without inducing transitions) contribute to T_2 but not to T_1. Finally, under certain circumstances, slow rotational or torsional motions and chemical exchange processes can also be important relaxation mechanisms. In the light of the above discussion it is clear that in order to calculate T_1 and T_2 values for a spin system, a theoretical framework is required that accounts for the frequency distributions of the relevant motions. Furthermore, if we make the reasonable assumption that relaxation is related to the amplitude of the thermal motion, it is necessary to account for this parameter also. However, at first sight the latter requirement would seem to be difficult. For example, the dipole–dipole interaction is the most important relaxation mechanism for protons in liquids, and yet the average value of the **dipolar coupling** in liquids is zero. Nevertheless at any given instant in time, the dipolar field is not zero. One measure of the strength of this field is the mean square average. Thus, if $f(t)$ is some random force with a mean value of zero, its mean square average is given by $\overline{f^*(t)f(t)}$, where * represents the complex conjugate (see **complex number**). Although the mean of $f(t)$ is zero, the mean square average value is not. The mean square average is simply a measure of the strength of the force. To find the frequency variation (spectrum) we can sample the force during a given time interval $-T$ and $+T$, and convert from the time domain t to the frequency domain ω by calculating the **Fourier transform**:

R3 $$f_T(\omega) = \int_{-T}^{+T} f(t) \exp\{i\omega t\} \, dt.$$

Thus, if $f(t)$ represents the oscillatory motion in the sample, then $f_T(\omega)$ represents its spectrum. We are now interested in the total energy at frequency ω during the period $-T$ to $+T$. This is represented by the **power spectrum**, $|f_T(\omega)|^2$. If T is allowed to increase to infinity, then the available power would follow suit. However, the quantity

R4 $$J(\omega) = \lim_{T\to\infty} \frac{1}{2T} \overline{f_T^*(\omega) f_T(\omega)}$$

will tend to a definite value. Note the similarly of $\overline{f^*(t) f(t)}$ (time domain) with $\overline{f_T^*(\omega) f_T(\omega)}$ (frequency domain). The quantity $J(\omega)$ is a spectral density function which is a measure of the power at frequency ω. There is a close relationship between $J(\omega)$ and the **autocorrelation function** ($\rho(t)$) of $f(t)$. The autocorrelation function is the time average of the product of $f(t)$ and $f^*(t+\tau)$,

R5 $$\rho(\tau) = \overline{f^*(t+\tau) f(t)}$$

which is a measure of the correlation between the value of a function with itself at times differing by τ. The autocorrelation function thus measures the persistence of the fluctuations. $\rho(\tau)$ is large for short times, and rapidly decay to zero as τ increases. Frequently the decay is exponential, with a time constant τ_c, and $\rho(\tau)$ thus becomes

R6 $$\rho(\tau) = \overline{f^*(t) f(t)} \exp\{-|\tau|/\tau_c\},$$

where τ_c is called the **correlation time**. An important property of the autocorrelation function is that its Fourier transform is the power spectrum of the original function, i.e.

R7 $$J(\omega) = \int_{-\infty}^{+\infty} \rho(\tau) \exp\{i\omega\tau\}\, d\tau$$

and if $\rho(\tau)$ is given by (R6), then

R8 $$J(\omega) = \frac{2\tau_c}{1+\omega^2\tau_c^2} \overline{f^*(t) f(t)}.$$

Spectral density functions such as (R8) are fundamental to the theoretical description of relaxation. They allow the motional characteristics of the system (defined by τ_c) to be expressed in terms of the power at frequency ω. Note that (R8) is formulated on the assumption that $\rho(\tau)$ decays exponentially. The precise form of the various relaxation equations can be found under **spin–lattice relaxation** (T_1) and **spin–spin relaxation** (T_2). See also **anisotropic chemical shift relaxation**, **cross-relaxation, quadrupole relaxation**, **scalar coupling relaxation**, **spin–rotation relaxation**, **rotating frame spin–lattice relaxation**.

FURTHER READING

A simple introduction to relaxation can be found in
Farrar, T. C. and Becker, E. D. (1971). *Pulse and Fourier transform NMR*. Academic Press, New York.

RELAY See **relayed correlation spectroscopy**.

Relayed correlation spectroscopy (RELAY) is related to **correlated spectroscopy** (COSY), being a simple extension of it. In its simplest form, the homonuclear RELAY experiment consists of four r.f. pulses (Fig. R4). The first two r.f. pulses, separated by the variable delay t_1, are entirely analogous to the COSY experiment. The RELAY experiment differs from COSY in the extension of the pulse sequence with a free precession period 2τ, followed by a third 90° pulse. A 180° pulse in the middle of the 2τ period serves to refocus chemical shifts. The purpose of the additional delay and r.f., pulses is to allow relayed coherence transfer between two spins which are not directly scalar coupled, but are coupled through a common partner, i.e. **spin systems** of the type I–S–M, where $J_{IM}=0$. The efficiency of this relayed transfer depends upon the magnitudes of the coupling constants J_{IS} and J_{SM}, and upon the value of τ. To extract the relevant transfer function, it is convenient to analyse the RELAY experiment for the three-spin system I–S–M using the **product operator formalism**. The density matrix after the second r.f. pulse is identical to (C57) (see **correlated spectroscopy**). Now, consider the term corresponding to transverse S magnetization (the seventh term in C57):

$$2I_zS_y \sin \omega_I t_1 \sin \pi J_{IS} t_1. \tag{R9}$$

This term can be subject to relayed transfer from I to M via S. During the 2τ interval, the effective **Hamiltonian** contains no chemical shift terms since they are refocused by the 180° pulse (in the limit of weak coupling). The term in (R9) thus evolves exclusively under the scalar coupling Hamiltonian during the 2τ period:

$$2I_zS_y \sin \omega_I t_1 \sin \pi J_{IS} t_1 \xrightarrow{\pi J_{IS} 2\tau 2I_zS_z} \xrightarrow{\pi J_{SM} 2\tau 2S_zM_z}$$

$$\begin{aligned}[&2I_zS_y \cos \pi J_{IS}2\tau \cos \pi J_{SM}2\tau - 4I_zS_xM_z \cos \pi J_{IS}2\tau \sin \pi J_{SM}2\tau \\ &-S_x \sin \pi J_{IS}2\tau \cos \pi J_{SM}2\tau \\ &-2S_yM_z \sin \pi J_{IS}2\tau \sin \pi J_{SM}2\tau] \sin \omega_I t_1 \sin \pi J_{IS} t_1.\end{aligned} \tag{R10}$$

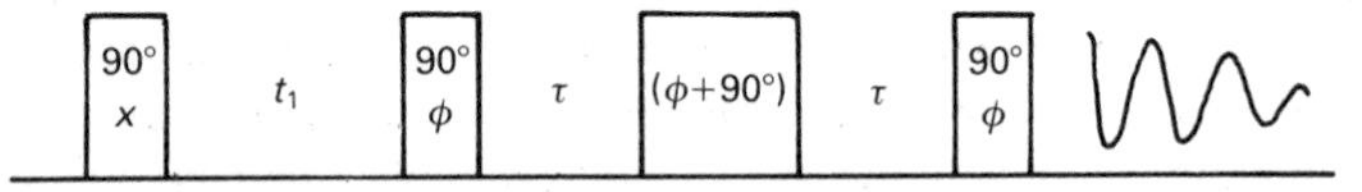

Fig. R4. The four-pulse sequence for acquisition of relayed correlation spectra.

In order for coherence to be transferred from I to M, the transverse S magnetization in (R9) must evolve to be in phase with respect to J_{IS} and antiphase with respect to J_{SM}. Only the last term in (R10) corresponds with these requirements at the end of the 2τ interval. The final 90° pulse converts this term into transverse M magnetization.

R11

$$-2S_yM_z \sin \pi J_{IS}2\tau \sin \pi J_{SM}2\tau \sin \omega_I t_1 \sin \pi J_{IS}t_1 \xrightarrow{(\pi/2)(I_x+S_x+M_x)}$$
$$2S_zM_y \sin \pi J_{IS}2\tau \sin \pi J_{SM}2\tau \sin \omega_I t_1 \sin \pi J_{IS}t_1.$$

The term on the right-hand side of (R11) describes a crosspeak at $\omega_1 = \omega_I$ and $\omega_2 = \omega_m$ with antiphase doublet structure in both dimensions. This can be formally proven by allowing the relevant term to evolve during t_2. Each individual resonance line of the multiplet can then be extracted as described under correlated spectroscopy (COSY).

The transfer function for the transfer of coherence between I and M can be obtained from (R11). It is given by $\sin \pi J_{IS}2\tau \sin \pi J_{SM}2\tau$. Thus, it is clear that the correct value of τ must be chosen, since for some values the transfer function could be zero! The optimum value is of course equal to unity. This in turn requires both $\pi J_{IS}2\tau$ and $\pi J_{SM}2\tau$ to equal $\pi/2$ radians ($\sin(\pi/2) = \sin 90° = 1$). Unless $J_{IS} = J_{SM}$, then optimum transfer cannot be achieved. Since this is rarely the case, then a compromise value of τ must be chosen. In practice, **relaxation** is also of importance in the determination of the correct τ value if the relevant J values are small. In these cases τ may be quite long, and since the spin system will start to relax during 2τ, the calculated optimum value on the basis of the above calculations (where relaxation is ignored) would be too large.

In principle, the RELAY sequence can be extended with additional relay steps. This is achieved simply by adding additional τ–180°–τ–90° steps after the last pulse. In this manner two-step or even multi-step relayed coherence transfer is possible. However, the transfer function becomes more complicated as the number of relay steps is increased. For example, coherence can be transferred from spin I to X in the **spin system** $ISMQX$ using a three-step relay sequence such as that shown in Fig. R5. Assuming next-neighbour couplings are zero, the transfer function for this transfer is given by $\sin(\pi J_{IS}2\tau_1)\sin(\pi J_{SM}2\tau_1)$ $\sin(\pi J_{SM}2\tau_2)\sin(\pi J_{MQ}2\tau_2)\sin(\pi J_{MQ}2\tau_3)\sin(\pi J_{QX}2\tau_3)$. Here again the coherence transfer efficiency is not 100% unless all couplings are equal.

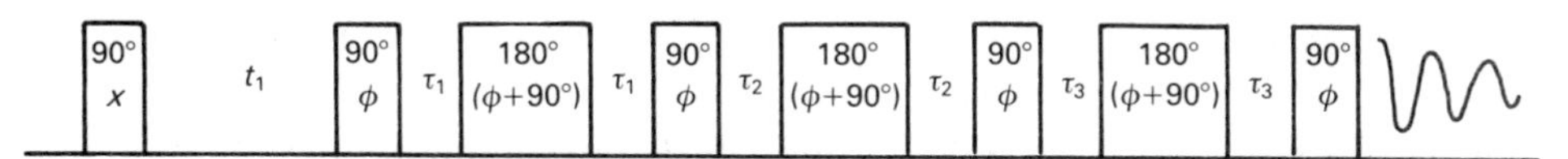

Fig. R5. The eight-pulse sequence for acquisition of three-step relayed correlation spectra.

An added complication in the RELAY experiment exists when next-neighbour couplings are not zero. In the above analyses this has been assumed to be the case. If for example a one-step relay is performed upon the three-spin system *ISM*, with $IM \neq 0$, then the spin system evolves under a Hamiltonian which consists of the additional term $\pi J_{IM} 2\tau 2I_z M_z$. The effect of this term is to generate cosine terms in the transfer function, which complicates the optimization of the experiment.

The RELAY experiment is of great value in biomolecular NMR. In application to the resonance assignment of proteins, its prime use is in the correlation of N–H proton resonances with α, β, and γ CH protons. These assignments are often difficult to obtain using conventional COSY. In addition, it is particularly useful in the assignment of the ring protons of carbohydrates. Here, next-neighbor couplings are negligibly small, and a three-step RELAY experiment in this application gives a transfer function which is very closely approximated by the above. It is therefore possible to optimise the experiment for the coupling network of a given monosaccharide.

FURTHER READING

Relayed correlation spectroscopy was first described by

Eich, G. W., Bodenhausen, G. and Ernst, R. R. (1982). *J. Am. Chem. Soc.* **104,** 3731.

For applications to proteins see

King, G. and Wright, P. E. (1983). *J. Magn. Reson.* **54,** 328

Wagner, G. (1983). *J. Magn. Reson.* **55,** 151.

Wagner, G. (1984). *J. Magn. Reson.* **57,** 497.

For an application to carbohydrates see

Homans, S. W., Dwek, R. A., Fernandes, D. L., and Rademacher, T. W. (1984). *Proc. Natl. Acad. Sci.* USA, **81,** 6286.

For an application of heteronuclear RELAY, see

Bolton, P. H., and Bodenhausen, G. (1982). *Chem. Phys. Lett.* **89,** 139.

Resolution See **digital resolution**.

Ring current shift Ring current shifts are a class of conformation-dependent shifts observed in ^{1}H NMR spectra of proteins and tRNAs. They are natural probes of structure. In proteins, ring current shifts originate from the aromatic ring of histidine, phenylalanine, tyrosine, and tryptophan residues. In addition, the heme in the cytochromes, myoglobin, and haemoglobin can also generate ring current shifts, which in these cases is particularly large. Ring current effects arise from the circulation of delocalized π electrons around the aromatic ring. This sets up a local magnetic field in exactly the same manner as a current-carrying conductor. This local field may either oppose or add to the applied static

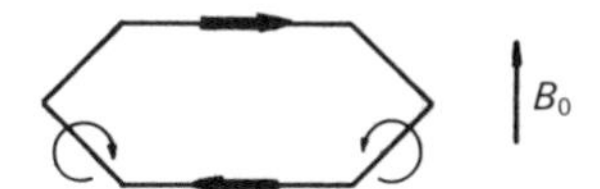

Fig. R6. Circulation of delocalized π electrons in an aromatic ring set up local magnetic fields in analogy to a current carrying conductor.

field (Fig. R6). Protons which are less than about 0.7 nm from the ring centre (more in the case of haem) experience a chemical shift which may be upfield or downfield depending upon the location of the proton with respect to the plane of the ring (Fig. R7). Above the plane of the ring, the ring current flux lines oppose B_0, and thus the shift is upfield (shielding). In the plane of the ring the ring current flux reinforces B_0, and the shift is downfield (deshielding). The flux due to the ring current has two main consequences. Firstly, the aromatic ring protons of histidine, phenylalanine, tyrosine, and tryptophan lie in the plane of the ring and are thus heavily deshielded, which leads to characteristic resonance positions in the 'aromatic' region of the spectrum (see **chemical shift**) ~ 6.5–8.2 ppm. Secondly, protons derived from other residues may be held in proximity to the aromatic ring due to the tertiary structure of the protein. This usually creates large upfield shifts, since the hydrophobic interaction is energetically most favourable when the protons are above the centre of the ring. These resonances are often observed upfield of 1 ppm. In general these are methyl signals, but sometimes single-proton resonances may occur here also.

If the magnitude of the ring current shift with respect to the spatial position of a given proton could be quantified, then in principle conformational information may be obtained. To this end three main approaches have been used. These are the classical dipolar model of Pople (1956), the semiclassical current-loop model (Johnson and Bovey 1958) and the quantum mechanical model of Haigh and Mallion (1972). In biological applications, the three models give almost indistinguishable shift predictions. As an example of the theoretical aspects, the Johnson–Bovey model is perhaps the most useful. The Johnson–Bovey equation evaluates the magnetic flux produced by two current loops parallel to the plane of the ring at a distance q above and below it. These loops

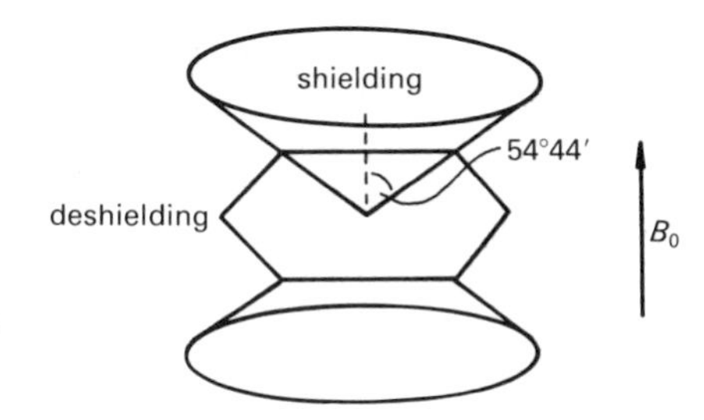

Fig. R7. Regions of shielding (−) and deshielding (+) in the vicinity of an aromatic ring due to ring currents.

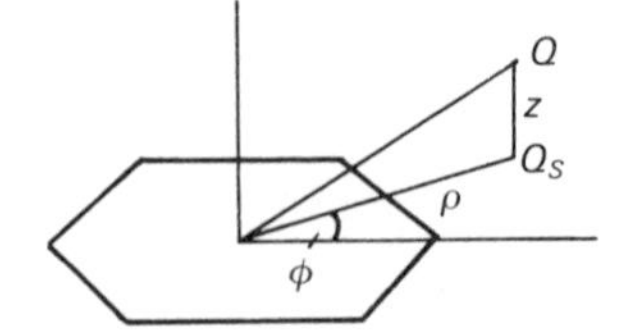

Fig. R8. Parameters of the Johnson–Bovey theory of ring current shifts. See text for details.

represent the six delocalized π electrons. The Johnson–Bovey equation in its original form is given by

R12
$$\delta_{\mathrm{RCS}} \times 10^{-6} = \frac{ne^2}{6\pi mc^2}\left\{\frac{1}{a[(1+\rho)^2+Z^2]^{\frac{1}{2}}}\left[K + \frac{1-\rho^2-Z^2}{(1-\rho)^2+Z^2}E\right]\right\},$$

where δ_{RCS} is the ring current shift, n is the number of π electrons, a is the ring radius, e is the electronic charge, m is electronic mass, c the speed of light in a vacuum, and ρ and Z are the cylindrical coordinates of the proton relative to the ring centre (Fig. R8).

The coefficients K and E are the first and second elliptic integrals, which are functions of ρ, Z, and q.

FURTHER READING

Haigh, C. W. and Mallion, R. B. (1972). *Org. Magn. Reson.* **4,** 203.
Johnson, C. E. and Bovey, F. A. (1958). *J. Chem. Phys.* **29,** 1012.
Pople, J. A. (1956). *J. Chem. Phys.* **24,** 1111.

For a review of applications of ring current calculations, see
Perkins, S. J. (1982). *Biol. Magn. Reson.* **4,** 193.

ROESY See **rotating frame Overhauser effect spectroscopy**.

Rotary echoes Rotary echoes can be thought of as the 'B_1' analogue of **spin echoes**. If an r.f. field B_1 is applied to a nuclear spin system at thermal equilibrium along the x' axis of the **rotating frame**, then according to the **classical formalism**, the z magnetization will be rotated around the y'–z' plane. In the presence of an inhomogeneous B_1 field the magnetization vectors from nuclei in various parts of the sample fan out as they precess in the y'–z' plane. If the **phase** of the B_1 field is now switched by 180° at a time τ, the magnetization vectors will essentially reverse in time, resulting in the formation of a rotary echo along the z' axis at a time 2τ. This echo is entirely analogous to the conventional spin echo in the transverse (X'–Y') plane. The decay of the envelope of the echo maxima decreases exponentially with a time constant $T_2\rho$ (T_2 in the rotating frame):

R13
$$\frac{1}{T_2\rho} = \frac{1}{2}\left(\frac{1}{T_1}+\frac{1}{T_2}\right).$$

In certain experiments involving **spin locking** (see e.g. **homonuclear Hartmann–Hahn spectroscopy**) the formation of rotary echoes is a disadvantage and it is necessary to arrange for their destruction.

Rotating frame The **classical formalism** describes nuclear resonance in terms of the precession of magnetization vectors about the applied static magnetic field B_0. The frequency of this precession is defined as $\omega = \gamma B_0$, where ω is the **Larmor precession** frequency and γ is the **magnetogyric ratio** (Fig. R9). In order to visualize the effect of r.f. pulses and free precession periods, it is inconvenient to work with this vector model as it stands. It is far easier to understand the workings of more complex pulse sequences (see e.g. **Carr–Purcell–Meiboom–Gill sequence**) if the bulk magnetization vector can be made stationary at equilibrium. One mechanism by which this can be achieved is to view the system in terms of the rotating frame of coordinates. In this representation, the normal (laboratory) cartesian axes x, y, z are replaced by axes x', y', z' which are presumed to rotate at the Larmor frequency of the spins. This representation is known as the rotating frame of coordinates. In this frame the bulk magnetization vector appears stationary. Initial difficulty in the comprehension of this situation might be alleviated by consideration of a simple analogy. Imagine a small coin placed upon a rotating gramophone record. To a stationary observer the coin appears to be moving in a circular motion at the same rate as the record. If, however, the observer were able to stand on the record, the coin would appear to be stationary. Imaginary x', y', z' axes drawn on the record would thus represent the rotating frame of coordinates.

The concept of the rotating frame is enormously useful, since it simplifies the treatment of otherwise complex gyration of the bulk magnetization vector. Of course, it is not possible to impose the new axes upon the system under consideration without making allowances for its presence. This can be achieved by making a mental note of the fact that a vector which is stationary in the x'–y' plane is actually inducing an e.m.f. in the receiver coils with a frequency ω rad s^{-1}. However, since

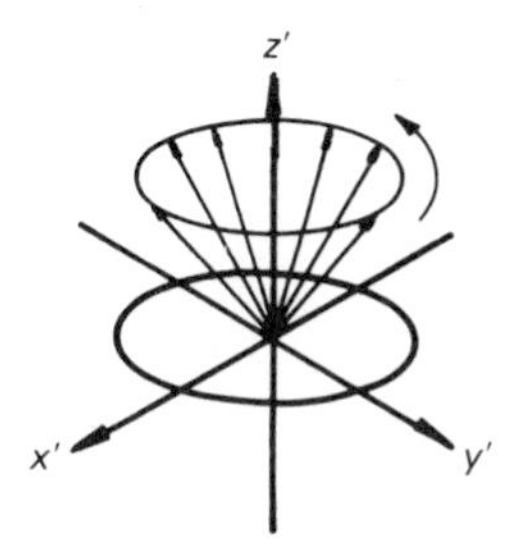

Fig. R9. Precession of magnetization vectors about a static magnetic field B_0.

the **phase-sensitive detectors** in the receiver detect the difference between the received frequency and the reference which is usually the same as ω, then the spectrometer effectively detects the signal in the rotating frame.

On a more theoretical basis, the imposition of the rotating frame of coordinates is a visualization of an interaction representation defined by $U = \exp\{-i\mathcal{H}_Z t\}$, where $\mathcal{H}_Z$ is the Zeeman **Hamiltonian**. Hamiltonians which are static in the laboratory frame then become time dependent in the rotating frame. The NMR signal after phase-sensitive detection is directly proportional to the **expectation values** in the rotating frame of the $x(I_x)$ or $y(I_y)$ component **angular momentum** operators.

Rotating frame imaging See **imaging**.

Rotating frame Overhauser effect spectroscopy (ROESY) In analogy to **nuclear Overhauser effect spectroscopy** (NOESY), there exists a technique known as rotating frame Overhauser effect spectroscopy (ROESY). The rotating frame Overhauser effect depends upon **rotating frame spin–lattice relaxation** ($T_{1\rho}$) rather than conventional T_1 processes.

The pulse sequence for acquisition of ROESY spectra is shown in Fig. R10. At first sight it appears identical to that used for the acquisition of **homonuclear Hartmann–Hahn** (HOHAHA) spectra. However, the r.f. power used to achieve spin locking is significantly smaller in ROESY. In addition, it is usual to place the transmitter **carrier** at the low-field end of the spectrum. The combined low power and transmitter offset prevents the appearance of HOHAHA crosspeaks in the ROESY spectrum by diasabling the **Hartmann–Hahn condition**. This is very important since HOHAHA crosspeaks are opposite in sign to ROESY peaks and are usually much larger, and hence these may easily obscure a genuine transverse NOE. In addition relayed effects can be observed, such as HOHAHA–ROESY or ROESY–HOHAHA transfer which can lead to completely erroneous conclusions when ROESY is used as a conformational probe. For these reasons it is essential to examine the offset dependence of crosspeak intensities to rule out the possibility of contributions from coherence transfer.

At the time of writing the theoretical aspects of ROESY have not been fully elucidated. It would appear that quantitation of crosspeak

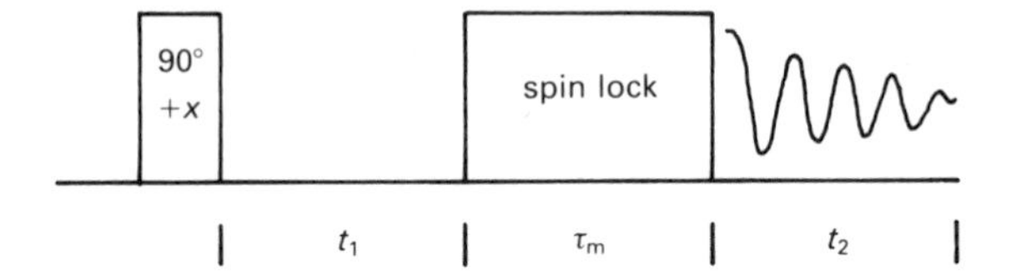

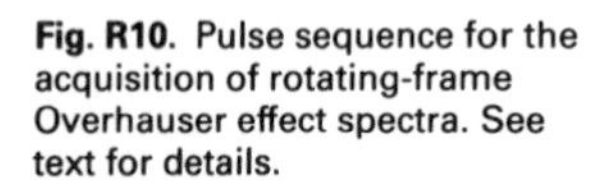
Fig. R10. Pulse sequence for the acquisition of rotating-frame Overhauser effect spectra. See text for details.

intensities in terms of internuclear distances (cf. NOESY) is complicated by offset effects and B_1 field inhomogeneity. Despite these drawbacks, a qualitative interpretation of ROESY spectra can be extremely useful.

An important aspect of the technique is that crosspeak intensity increases monotonically with correlation time. This can be rationalized by noting that the Overhauser effect is taking place in the presence of a weak r.f. field rather than a large static magnetic field. The weak r.f. field guarantees the '**extreme narrowing** limit' ($\omega\tau_c \ll 1$) for all values of τ_c and ω of practical interest. Unlike NOESY, therefore, crosspeak intensities will not tend to zero when $\omega\tau_c \approx 1$, which often appears to be the case at high fields for small peptides, nucleic acids, and carbohydrates. Use of the ROESY technique in these cases at least allows qualitative distance information to be obtained. A second advantage when working in the extreme narrowing limit is that NOEs generated in a linear chain of spins alternate in sign. Thus it is possible to determine whether a weak ROE crosspeak derives from transfer via an intermediate spin (limited **spin diffusion**, the so-called 'three-spin effect') or is an authentic long-range ROE. Similarly, it is possible to distinguish between authentic ROE crosspeaks and those due to chemical exchange from the opposite signs of crosspeak intensities. In conventional NOESY spectra of macromolecules in the spin-diffusion limit, all crosspeaks are of the same sign regardless of the presence of 'three-spin effects' or chemical exchange.

FURTHER READING

The original rotating frame Overhauser effect experiment was described under the acronym CAMELSPIN by

Bothner-By, A. A., Stephens, R. L., Lee, J., Warren, C. D., and Jeanloz, R. W. (1984). *J. Am. Chem. Soc.* **106,** 811.

ROESY was originally described by

Bax, A. and Davis, D. G. (1985). *J. Magn. Reson.* **63,** 207.

Separation of three-spin and direct effects is described in

Bax, A., Sklenar, V., and Summers, M. (1986). *J. Magn. Reson* **70,** 327.

Rotating frame spin–lattice relaxation ($T_1\rho$) Under **spin-locking** conditions, B_1 plays the role of the static field in the rotating frame, so relaxation in the direction of B_1 (i.e. along the x' or y' axis, depending on the phase (x' or y') of the spin-lock field) is analogous to spin–lattice relaxation. For this reason, such processes are characterized by a time $T_1\rho$, usually called T_1 in the rotating frame. Since in the absence of B_1, relaxation along x' or y' is characterized by T_2 then clearly $T_1\rho$ must be related to T_2. In fact $T_1\rho = T_2$ for the majority of liquids.

An important consequence of $T_1\rho$ phenomena is the existence of a rotating frame Overhauser effect (see **rotating frame Overhauser effect spectroscopy**). The measurement of $T_1\rho$ *per se* is important in the determination of scalar spin–spin coupling between two nuclei *IS*, when the relaxation of either *I* or *S* is so fast that the coupling is unobservable (see **scalar coupling**). By studying $T_1\rho$ of either *I* or *S* as a function of B_1, both *J* and T_1 can be measured in (S6).

In solids $T_1\rho$ is very different from T_2, since in solids the local magnetic field at a nucleus is strongly dominated by static magnetic dipolar fields derived from $\mathscr{H}_d$ (see **Hamiltonian**) that originate from other nearby nuclei. The effective field in the rotating frame is thus dominated by $\mathscr{H}_d$.

Rotation operator In NMR it is often necessary to predict in theoretical terms the result of a given NMR experiment. To represent the behaviour of a spin system in response to a series of r.f. pulses and free precession periods (delays), we use the spin **density matrix**. Integration of the **Liouville–von Neumann** equation tells us that the state of the density matrix at time t_1 ($\sigma(t_1)$) is related to the density matrix at some earlier time t ($\sigma(t)$) by

R14 $$\sigma(t_1) = \exp\{-\mathrm{i}\mathscr{H}t\}\sigma(t)\exp\{\mathrm{i}\mathscr{H}t\}$$

where $\mathscr{H}$ is the Hamiltonian (assumed time independent) under which the spin system evolves. Equation (R14) formally describes a rotation of the density matrix. The effect of an r.f. pulse may be described by a similar rotation. The **exponential operators** $\exp\{-\mathrm{i}\mathscr{H}t\}$ and $\exp\{\mathrm{i}\mathscr{H}t\}$ are thus known as rotation operators. They are usually expressed explicitly in their **matrix representations**. The product of the matrices ($\exp\{-\mathrm{i}\mathscr{H}t\}$) and ($\exp\{\mathrm{i}\mathscr{H}t\}$) gives unity, since the second matrix is the inverse of the first. In fact (R14) is reminiscent of the transformation of a given operator into a different base, e.g.

R15 $$\mathscr{H}_{(\text{eigenbase})} = U\mathscr{H}_{(\text{product base})}U^{-1}$$

as found in calculations involving **strong coupling**. Several rotation operators in their matrix forms are given in Appendix 4.

S

Saturation Consider two spin states $\frac{1}{2}$, to which correspond two non-degenerate energy levels in a static magnetic field B_0. The **Boltzman distribution** equation shows that at thermal equilibrium a net excess of spins will populate the lowest energy level (Fig. S1). If we label the energy levels with the states $|\alpha\rangle$ and $|\beta\rangle$, we can define two transition probabilities $P_{\alpha\to\beta}$ and $P_{\beta\to\alpha}$, corresponding to transitions from state $|\alpha\rangle$ to $|\beta\rangle$ and from $|\beta\rangle$ to $|\alpha\rangle$ respectively. If we define the number of spins in state $|\alpha\rangle$ as N_α and the number of spins in state $|\beta\rangle$ as N_β, then the rate of change of population of state $|\beta\rangle$ is given by

$$\begin{aligned}\dot{N}_\beta &= -N_\beta P_{\beta\to\alpha} + N_\alpha P_{\alpha\to\beta} \\ &= P(N_\alpha - N_\beta)\end{aligned} \tag{S1}$$

where since the transition probabilities for upward and downward transitions are equal, $P_{\beta\to\alpha} = P_{\alpha\to\beta} = P$. If the population difference is defined by $\delta = N_\beta - N_\alpha$, then

$$N_\beta = \tfrac{1}{2}(N + \delta), \qquad N_\alpha = \tfrac{1}{2}(N - \delta) \tag{S2}$$

where $N = N_\alpha + N_\beta$. If (S2) is substituted in (S1), we obtain

$$\dot{N}_\beta = (\tfrac{1}{2})\dot{\delta} = -P\delta, \tag{S3}$$

i.e. $\dot{\delta} = -2P\delta$.

The solution of (S3) is simply

$$\delta = \delta_0 \exp\{-2P\} \tag{S4}$$

where δ_0 is the difference at $t = 0$. Equation (S4) shows that the application of an r.f. field (at the Larmor frequency of the spins) will result in exponential decay of the population difference δ, and eventually δ will equal zero. Since the amplitude of the e.m.f. induced in the receiver coils is proportional to the population difference, then clearly if we apply an r.f. field for long enough the resonance line will disappear. This phenomenon is known as saturation. In some cases saturation may be deliberately imposed by selective irradiation in experiments such as nuclear Overhauser effect **difference spectroscopy**. In general however, e.g. in pulse-and-collect spectroscopy, saturation must be avoided if

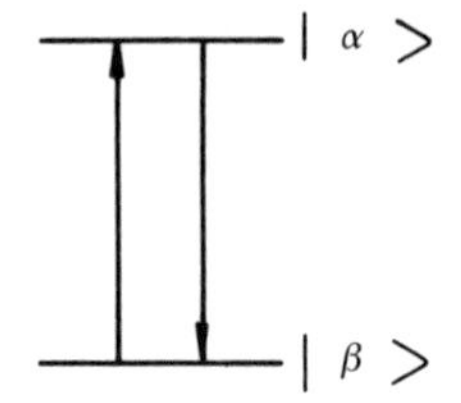

Fig. S1. The two spin states and transitions of a single spin $\frac{1}{2}$.

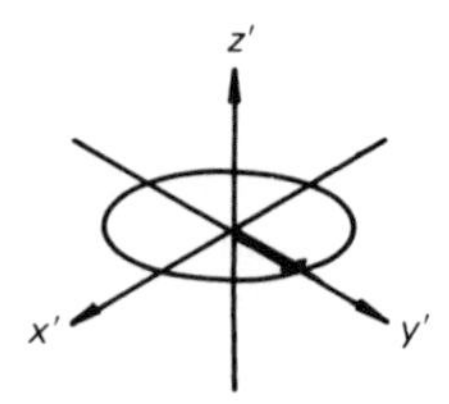

Fig. S2. Transverse magnetization is created along the y' axis after the application of a 90° pulse along the x' axis of the rotating frame. No net z' magnetization is generated.

maximum sensitivity is to be realized. Since **spin–lattice relaxation** is the mechanism by which the population difference is restored, it follows that it is necessary to wait for a time equal to several T_1 values between the application of r.f. pulses. A value of $5T_1$s is commonly employed, although this is rarely possible in the case of two-dimensional spectroscopy, and a degree of saturation is inevitable due to the severe time requirements of most two-dimensional methods.

A common misconception is often found when attempting to relate saturation to the **classical formalism** for the description of NMR experiments. Since saturation corresponds to equal spin state populations, it is tempting to equate this with the situation after the application of a 90° pulse, when no magnetization is to be found along the $+z'$ or $-z'$ axes (Fig. S2). The important point is that there is **phase coherence** after the application of the 90° pulse. Conversely, saturation creates an equalization of spin state populations, but creates no phase coherence (Fig. S3).

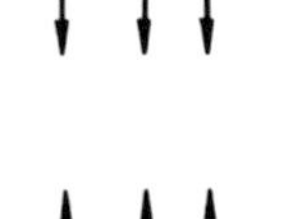

Fig. S3. Saturation causes an equalization of spin state populations, but no phase coherence is created.

Scalar coupling See **spin coupling**.

Scalar coupling relaxation The scalar (spin–spin) coupling **Hamiltonian** is given by

S5 $$\mathcal{H}_J = \gamma^2\hbar^2 \sum_{i<k} \mathbf{I}_i \, . \, \mathbf{J}_{ik} \, . \, \mathbf{I}_k .$$

The local field experienced by nucleus I_i may fluctuate in time in one of two ways: either I_k is time dependent, or J_{ik} is time dependent. In either case a relaxation mechanism exists in terms of spin I_i.

If the **spin–lattice relaxation** time T_1^k of spin I_k is short in comparison with $1/J$, where J is the spin coupling constant expressed in rad s^{-1}, then the local field produced at nucleus I_i by I_k fluctuates with a correlation time $\tau_k = T_1^k$, Under these conditions the relaxation rates of spin I_i are given by

S6 $$\frac{1}{T_1^i} = \frac{2J^2}{3} S(S+1) \times \frac{\tau_k}{1+(\omega_i - \omega_k)^2\tau_k^2}$$

S7 $$\frac{1}{T_2^i} = \frac{J^2}{3} S(S+1) \left\{ \tau_k + \frac{\tau_k}{1+(\omega_i - \omega_k)^2\tau_k^2} \right\}$$

where S is the spin of nucleus I_k, and ω_i and ω_k are the **Larmor precession** frequencies of the spins. This relaxation mechanism is often described as scalar relaxation of the second kind.

Scalar relaxation due to the time dependence of J_{ik} is often described as scalar relaxation of the first kind, and arises in chemically exchanging systems. If the exchange rate is much larger than either the spin–spin coupling (J) or $1/T_1^i$ or $1/T_1^k$, and if the nuclei are coupled for a time much greater than the time they are uncoupled, then this system reduces to scalar relaxation of the second kind, where τ_k now becomes the exchange rate. If the exchange rate is of the order of the spin coupling, more detailed analysis is required, as described by Allerhand and Gutowsky (1966). Although the dipolar Hamiltonian $\mathcal{H}_d$ is generally much larger than $\mathcal{H}_J$, in liquids the magnitude of τ_k or the exchange rate τ_E can be in the range where $(\omega_i - \omega_k)\tau \approx 1$. Under these circumstances scalar interactions may represent the dominant relaxation mechanism.

FURTHER READING

Allerhand, A. and Gutowsky, H. S. (1964). *J. Chem. Phys.* **41,** 2115 and **42,** 1587.

Schrödinger and Heisenberg representation In the **density matrix** formalism, as introduced under that heading, we followed the time evolution of the density matrix $\sigma(t)$ under the influence of the relevant **Hamiltonians**. The **expectation value** of any operator $\hat{o}$ corresponding to an observable was then shown to be computable from an expression of the form

S8 $$\langle \delta \rangle = \mathrm{Tr}\{\hat{o} \,.\, \sigma(t)\}.$$

Equation (S8) is expressed in the Schrödinger representation where the time dependence of the spin system is associated with $\sigma(t)$, while the operator is time independent. However, it is occassionally more useful to examine the problem in the Heisenberg representation, where the time dependence is on the operator o. Under these circumstance (S8) becomes

S9 $$\langle\delta\rangle = \mathrm{Tr}\{\hat{o}(t)\sigma(o)\}$$

and the form of $\hat{o}(t)$ is calculated from the solution of the equation

S10 $$\frac{\mathrm{d}\hat{o}(t)}{\mathrm{d}t} = -\mathrm{i}[\hat{o}(t), \mathscr{H}(t)]$$

where at $t=0$, $\hat{o}(0)=\hat{o}$. With regard to the calculations which are considered in this volume, each representation can be considered equivalent. In general we use the Schrödinger representation.

Schrödinger equation At the atomic level the relationship between the energy, E, of a particle and its wavefunction ψ is given by the Schrödinger equation. When written in its time-independent form, the Schrödinger equation corresponds with the mathematical eigenvalue equation

S11 $$\mathscr{H}\psi = E\psi.$$

In this equation $\mathscr{H}$ is the **Hamiltonian** operator for the system, which contains a variety of terms including spin–spin interactions, interaction with the static magnetic field, and perturbation terms. The energy E, in units of $\hbar$, corresponds to the observable for a given Hamiltonian. In NMR we may use the Schrödinger equation to calculate the energy levels of a spin system in a magnetic field. This is quite straightforward, and requires a knowledge of the behaviour of **angular momentum** operators. As a example consider the weakly coupled (see **weak coupling**) two-spin system IS. The energy levels, of which there are four, may be described in terms of the **product basis** (Fig. S4). In order to calculate the energies of these four states we shall insert the relevant values for the wavefunction ψ (i.e. $|\alpha\alpha\rangle$, $|\alpha\beta\rangle$, $|\beta\alpha\rangle$, $|\beta\beta\rangle$) into (S11) in turn. However, we

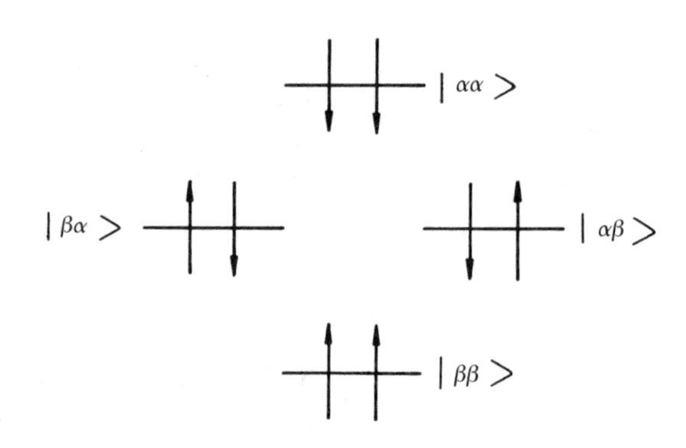

Fig. S4. The four energy levels and product-base wavefunctions of a weakly coupled two-spin system.

also require an expression for the relevant Hamiltonian. In the liquid state this can simply be expressed in terms of the interaction of each spin with the static magnetic field, and the scalar spin coupling between the nuclei. these are sometimes called the Zeeman and scalar coupling Hamiltonians respectively:

S12 $$\mathcal{H} = \mathcal{H}_Z + \mathcal{H}_J.$$

At this point the reader may experience some difficulty with the notion that $\mathcal{H}_Z$ and $\mathcal{H}_J$ are phenomenologically formulated. That is, the particular forms of $\mathcal{H}_Z$ and $\mathcal{H}_J$ which are employed are found to predict the experimental results accurately. However, on reflection it is clear that Newtonian mechanics is based upon similar principles. The Hamiltonian relevant to the present problem is given by

S13 $$\mathcal{H} = \mathcal{H}_Z + \mathcal{H}_J = \omega_I I_z + \omega_S S_z + J_{IS} I_z S_z$$

where I_z and S_z are the z-component angular momentum operators of spins I and S respectively, ω_I and ω_S are the Larmor precession frequencies, and J_{IS} is the scalar spin-coupling constant. Equation (S11) can then be reformulated to the present problem. Thus, for state 1, with the corresponding wavefunction $|\alpha\alpha\rangle$, we find

S14 $$(\omega_I I_z + \omega_S S_z + J_{IS} I_z S_z)\,|\alpha\alpha\rangle = E\,|\alpha\alpha\rangle.$$

Using the rules for the operation of I_z and S_z upon $|\alpha\rangle$ and $|\beta\rangle$ (see **angular momentum**), we can evaluate (S14), remembering that I_z acts only on spin I, S_z upon spin S, and I_zS_z upon both. Each step is clearly seen if the equation is decomposed further:

S15 $$\omega_I I_z\,|\alpha\alpha\rangle + \omega_S S_z\,|\alpha\alpha\rangle + J_{IS} I_z S_z\,|\alpha\alpha\rangle = E\,|\alpha\alpha\rangle$$

and using the angular momentum rules we find

S16 $$\begin{aligned} \omega_I I_z\,|\underline{\alpha}\alpha\rangle &= \tfrac{1}{2}\omega_I\,|\alpha\alpha\rangle \\ \omega_S S_z\,|\alpha\underline{\alpha}\rangle &= \tfrac{1}{2}\omega_S\,|\alpha\alpha\rangle \\ J_{IS} I_z S_z\,|\underline{\alpha\alpha}\rangle &= \tfrac{1}{4}J_{IS}\,|\alpha\alpha\rangle \end{aligned}$$

where the underlined component of the wavefunction is that which is operated upon. The complete equation may therefore be written

S17 $$(\omega_I I_z + \omega_S S_z + J_{IS} I_z S_z)\,|\alpha\alpha\rangle = (\tfrac{1}{2}(\omega_I + \omega_S) + \tfrac{1}{4}J_{IS})\,|\alpha\alpha\rangle$$

and by comparison with (S11), the energy of state 1 (or simply state $|\alpha\alpha\rangle$) is given by

S18 $$E_1 = \tfrac{1}{2}(\omega_I + \omega_S) + \tfrac{1}{4}J_{IS}.$$

An analogous series of calculations allows us to compute the energies for the remaining three states. In summary,

$$E_1 = \tfrac{1}{2}(\omega_I + \omega_S) + \tfrac{1}{4}J_{IS}$$
$$E_2 = \tfrac{1}{2}(\omega_I + \omega_S) - \tfrac{1}{4}J_{IS}$$
$$E_3 = \tfrac{1}{2}(-\omega_I + \omega_S) - \tfrac{1}{4}J_{IS} \quad \text{S19}$$
$$E_4 = \tfrac{1}{2}(-\omega_I - \omega_S) + \tfrac{1}{4}J_{IS}$$

and the frequencies of the resonance lines are given by the energy differences of those states corresponding to a single-quantum transition:

$$E_1 - E_2 = +\omega_S + \tfrac{1}{2}J_{IS}$$
$$E_2 - E_4 = +\omega_I - \tfrac{1}{2}J_{IS}$$
$$E_3 - E_4 = +\omega_S - \tfrac{1}{2}J_{IS} \quad \text{S20}$$
$$E_1 - E_3 = +\omega_I + \tfrac{1}{2}J_{IS}$$

The signs of the energies are dependent upon the interpretation of the Hamiltonian, i.e. whether $E_1 > E_2$, etc., or the reverse. In either case, the transition energies in (S20) lead to a correct result given by two doublets at ω_I and ω_S with a splitting of J_{IS}.

SECSY See **spin echo correlated spectroscopy**.

Secular determinant See **variational method**.

Selective excitation See **Gaussian pulse, delays alternating with nutation for tailored excitation**.

Selective population transfer (SPT) Selective population transfer arises from the 'reshuffling' of spin populations after the selective perturbation of a single NMR transition. Consider a weakly coupled two-spin $\frac{1}{2}$ system IS (Fig. S5). At thermal equilibrium, the populations of states and their

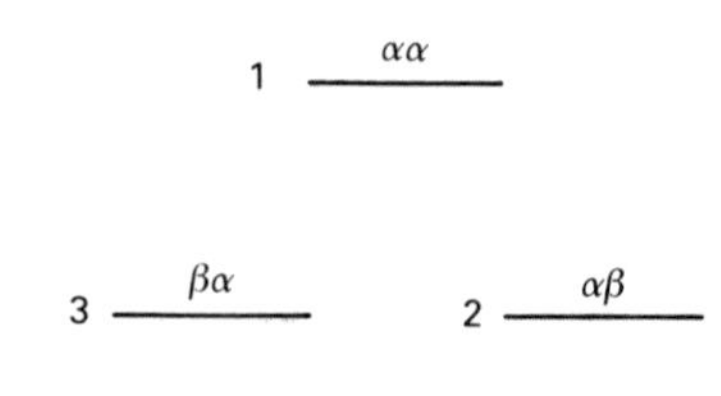

Fig. S5. Energy levels of a weakly coupled two-spin system.

differences is as follows:

S21

$$
\begin{array}{ll}
(1)\ P^0 - \delta & (3) - (1) = +\delta \\
(2)\ P^0 & (4) - (2) = +\delta \\
(3)\ P^0 & (2) - (1) = +\delta \\
(4)\ P^0 + \delta & (4) - (3) = +\delta
\end{array}
$$

Now consider what happens when a selective 180° pulse is applied to an I spin transition, e.g. (1) – (3). The new populations and their differences will be

S22

$$
\begin{array}{ll}
(1)\ P^0 & (3) - (1) = -\delta \\
(2)\ P^0 & (4) - (2) = +\delta \\
(3)\ P^0 & (2) - (1) = +\delta \\
(4)\ P_0 + \delta & (4) - (3) = +\delta
\end{array}
$$

It can be seen that the intensities of the S spin transition resonance lines are perturbed (Fig. S6). This effect is due to selective population transfer (SPT). These SPT effects have been used to gain a sensitivity advantage in the assignment of protons directly attached to a ^{13}C nucleus. However, modern two-dimensional methods have all but replaced the SPT experiment. In certain circumstances, such as in one-dimensional NOE experiments, SPT effects are undesirable, and it is necessary to ensure that an entire multiplet is completely inverted or saturated to avoid them. It is readily seen from the above that inversion of both I spin transitions ((3) – (1) and (2) – (4)) restores the S spin intensities to their values in the absence of irradiation (Fig. S6).

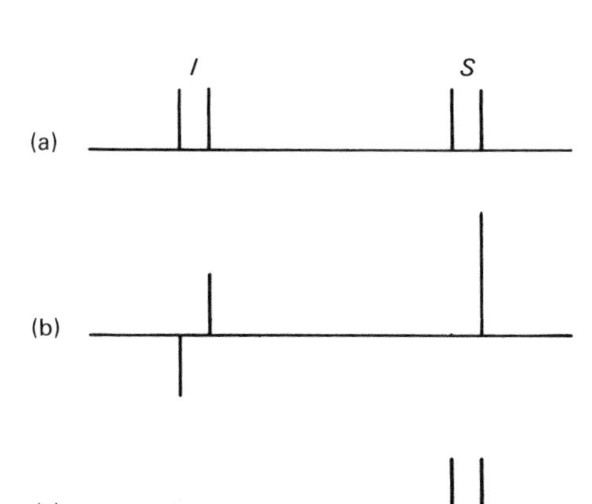

Fig. S6. (a) Stick spectrum of two weakly coupled spins; (b) Same spectrum after inversion of an I spin transition by a selective 180° pulse; (c) Spectrum after inversion of both I spin transitions.

FURTHER READING

For some interesting applications of SPT effects to heteronuclear polarization transfer, see:

Sorensen, S., Hansen, R. S., and Jakobsen, H. J. (1974). *J. Magn. Reson.* **14,** 243.

Jakobsen, H. J., Linde, S. A., and Sorensen, S. (1974). *J. Magn. Reson.* **15,** 385.

Shielding constant See **chemical shift**.

Shift See **chemical shift, ring current shift**.

Shift operators The shift operators, otherwise known as raising and lowering operators, are defined by the equations

S23
$$I^+ = I_x + \mathrm{i}I_y$$
$$I^- = I_x - \mathrm{i}I_y$$

where I_x and I_y are the x and y component **angular momentum** operators. The effects of I^+ and I^- can easily be derived from the properties of I_x and I_y:

S24
$$I_x\,|\alpha\rangle = \tfrac{1}{2}\,|\beta\rangle$$
$$I_x\,|\beta\rangle = \tfrac{1}{2}\,|\alpha\rangle$$
$$I_y\,|\alpha\rangle = \tfrac{1}{2}\mathrm{i}\,|\beta\rangle$$
$$I_y\,|\beta\rangle = -\tfrac{1}{2}\mathrm{i}\,|\alpha\rangle.$$

Thus, for example,

S25
$$I^+\,|\alpha\rangle = I_x\,|\alpha\rangle + \mathrm{i}I_y\,|\alpha\rangle$$
$$= \tfrac{1}{2}\,|\beta\rangle + \tfrac{1}{2}\mathrm{i}^2\,|\beta\rangle = 0,$$

whereas

S26
$$I^+\,|\beta\rangle = I_x\,|\beta\rangle + \mathrm{i}I_y\,|\beta\rangle$$
$$= \tfrac{1}{2}\,|\alpha\rangle - \tfrac{1}{2}\mathrm{i}^2\,|\alpha\rangle = |\alpha\rangle.$$

A similar procedure for I^- gives the four expressions for the shift operators:

S27
$$I^+\,|\alpha\rangle = 0$$
$$I^+\,|\beta\rangle = |\alpha\rangle$$
$$I^-\,|\alpha\rangle = |\beta\rangle$$
$$I^-\,|\beta\rangle = 0$$

and the ability of I^+ to convert a state with a magnetic quantum number

m to $m+1$ gives rise to the term raising operator. The opposite gives rise to the term lowering operator.

Raising and lowering operators are of particular value in the description of multiple-quantum coherence. For example, pure triple-quantum coherence in a three-spin system *ISM* may be described in terms of operator products:

S28 $$\mathrm{TQT}_x = \tfrac{1}{4}(4I_xS_xM_x - 4I_xS_yM_y - 4I_yS_xM_y - 4I_yS_yM_x)$$

which is more compact when written in terms of shift operators:

S29 $$\mathrm{TQT}_x = \tfrac{1}{2}(I^+S^+M^+ + I^-S^-M^-).$$

Equation (S29) gives a more 'pictorial' appearance to triple-quantum coherence, since it conveys the idea of mutual flipping of all three spins.

Shift probe See **paramagnetic centre**.

Sidebands See **spinning sidebands**.

Signal averaging One of the advantages of **Fourier transform** NMR is the possibility to record data by signal averaging. In a simple pulse-and-collect experiment, the response to the r.f. perturbation is recorded as a function of time. This response is known as the **free induction decay** (FID) . It is digitized (see **analogue-to-digital converter**) and stored in memory prior to Fourier transformation. In signal averaging, this process is repeated a number of times, resulting in the gradual accumulation of a number of FIDs in the same memory locations, which results in their addition. The purpose of this procedure is to obtain an overall increase in the signal-to-noise ratio of the resulting spectrum. Since NMR is a relatively insensitive technique by spectroscopic standards, studies on biomolecules which are generally of low concentration (often 1 mM or less) require a certain degree of signal averaging. In addition, techniques such as **CYCLOPS**, and the mandatory phase cycles found in two-dimensional NMR, require a finite number of transients to be collected during an experiment.

The mechanism by which signal averaging improves the signal-to-noise ratio is not hard to understand. The desired signal is derived from a state of phase coherence in the sample, which in turn is created by the r.f. pulse. Addition of FIDs therefore results in the coherent addition of the wanted signals. In contrast, the **noise**, which is derived mainly from thermal e.m.f.'s generated in the sample and probe, is a random function which is not phase coherent. Addition of FIDs will therefore not result in coherent addition of the noise. In fact, the signal-to-noise ratio of the spectrum increases by the square root of the number of transients collected. Thus, in order to double the signal-to-noise ratio, we must collect four times as many transients.

From the above it might be thought that an arbitrarily low sample concentration might give a spectrum with workable signal-to-noise ratio simply by acquiring a suitable number of transients. To some extent this is true, but the square root function is equivalent to the law of diminishing returns. Thus to increase the signal-to-noise ratio tenfold requires a hundredfold increase in the number of transients. We cannot simply repeat the pulse-and-collect sequence more rapidly in order to reduce the time requirement, since, if an insufficient delay is left between the application of successive r.f. pulses, the ensemble spin system will eventually reach **saturation**. In general we must wait for several T_1's (see **spin–lattice relaxation**) between r.f. pulses. This can impose a severe limitation upon samples with long T_1's, and in the solid state requires a different experimental regime (see **cross-polarization**) in order to improve the effective sensitivity (signal-to-noise ratio per unit time).

FURTHER READING

Ernst, R. R., Bodenhausen, G., and Wokaun, A. (1987). *Principles of NMR in one and two dimensions*, p. 148ff. Clarendon Press, Oxford.

Signum function See **Hilbert transform**.

Sine–bell function See **convolution**.

Sine transform See **Fourier transform**.

Single-transition operator The expansion of the density matrix into a complete set of single-transition operators is found to be useful for the description of selective excitation of a single transition in a complex spin system.

The single-transition operators I_x^{rs}, I_y^{rs}, I_z^{rs}, I^{+rs}, and I^{-rs} refer to the transition between states $|r\rangle$ and $|s\rangle$. All other states are disregarded. The operators associated with the transition between $|r\rangle$ and $|s\rangle$ are defined as follows:

$$\langle \mathrm{i}\,|I_x^{rs}|\,j\rangle = \tfrac{1}{2}(\delta_{ir}\delta_{js} + \delta_{is}\delta_{jr})$$

S30 $$\langle \mathrm{i}\,|I_y^{rs}|\,j\rangle = \mathrm{i}/2(-\delta_{ir}\delta_{js} + \delta_{is}\delta_{jr})$$

$$\langle \mathrm{i}\,|I_z^{rs}|\,j\rangle = \tfrac{1}{2}(\delta_{ir}\delta_{jr} - \delta_{is}\delta_{js})$$

where $\delta_{nm} = 1$ if $n = m$, and is zero otherwise. Single transition operators are defined in the **eigenbasis** of the **Hamiltonian**, in contrast to **shift operators** and **polarization operators**, which are defined in the **product**

basis. In the weak coupling approximation, these bases are identical, and we can therefore make the following equivalences for a two-spin $\frac{1}{2}$ system in terms of shift and polarization operators:

S31

$$
\begin{aligned}
I_x^{1,2} &= I_1^{\alpha} I_{2x}, & I_y^{1,2} &= I_1^{\alpha} I_{2y}, \\
I_x^{3,4} &= I_1^{\beta} I_{2x}, & I_y^{3,4} &= I_1^{\beta} I_{2y}, \\
I_x^{1,3} &= I_{1x} I_2^{\alpha}, & I_y^{1,3} &= I_{1y} I_2^{\alpha}, \\
I_x^{2,4} &= I_{1x} I_2^{\beta}, & I_y^{2,4} &= I_{1y} I_2^{\beta}, \\
I_x^{1,4} &= \tfrac{1}{2}(I_k^+ I_l^+ + I_k^- I_l^-), & I_y^{1,4} &= \mathrm{i}/2(-I_k^+ I_l^+ + I_k^- I_l^-), \\
I_x^{2,3} &= \tfrac{1}{2}(I_k^+ I_l^- + I_k^- I_l^+), & I_y^{2,3} &= \mathrm{i}/2(-I_k^+ I_l^- + I_k^- I_l^+).
\end{aligned}
$$

where $|1\rangle = |\alpha\alpha\rangle$, $|2\rangle = |\alpha\beta\rangle$, $|3\rangle = |\beta\alpha\rangle$, $|4\rangle = |\beta\beta\rangle$.

The transformations of single-transition operators can be described in three-dimensional space. If the coherence and the selective r.f. pulse correspond to the same transition between $|r\rangle$ and $|s\rangle$, we find

S32

$$I_\beta^{rs} \xrightarrow{\phi I_\alpha^{rs}} I_\beta^{rs} \cos\phi + I_\gamma^{rs} \sin\phi$$

with α, β, $\gamma = x, y, z$. If the pulse is applied to a different transition which is connected via a common eigenstate, the relevant transformation is

S33

$$I_x^{st} \xrightarrow{\phi I_x^{rs}} I_x^{st} \cos(\phi/2) + I_y^{rt} \sin(\phi/2).$$

In other words, the angle of rotation appears to be halved whenever the latter condition exists. This implies that coherence is completely transferred for $\phi = \pi$, which is of course the case since the eigenstates will be flipped with respect to each other (i.e. $|\alpha\alpha\rangle \leftrightarrow |\alpha\beta\rangle$).

FURTHER READING

Ernst, R. R., Bodenhausen, G., and Wokaun, A. (1987). *Principles of NMR in one and two dimensions*. pp. 38–40. Clarendon Press, Oxford.

Slow exchange See **chemical exchange**.

Soft pulse See **Gaussian pulse**.

Solid state NMR The NMR spectrum of a solid typically consists of a number of relatively broad lines. However, this property is not due to any inherent lack of resolution at a given field strength. Rather, the larger linewidths of solid state NMR spectra reflect incomplete **averaging** of

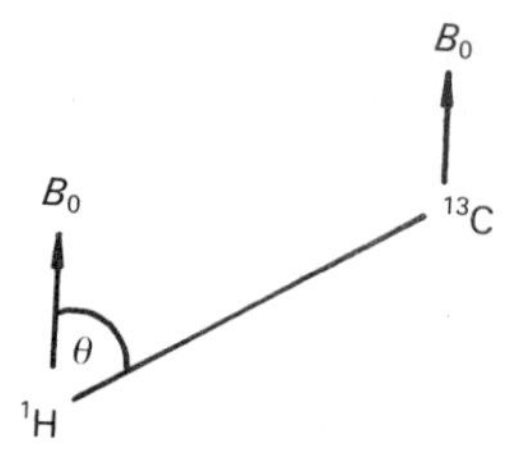

Fig. S7. Illustration of the orientation of an internuclear vector with respect to the applied field.

several components of the total spin **Hamiltonian**. In contrast, NMR spectra of liquids are very sharp due to averaging of all interactions except chemical shifts and scalar couplings, and other anisotropic interactions are lost. The value of solid state NMR is that these interactions can be observed and exploited.

The main interaction between nuclear spins is dipole–dipole coupling between their magnetic moments. These interactions are described theoretically in terms of the dipolar coupling Hamiltonian, and depend upon the orientation of the internuclear vector with respect to the applied field. By reference to Fig. S7, we can simplify the form of the dipolar Hamiltonian as follows:

$$\mathscr{H} = \sum_{i<j} K r_{ij}^{-3}(3\cos^2\theta_{ij} - 1) \text{ (other terms)} \qquad \text{S34}$$

where K collects together a variety of constants. Thus each dipolar interaction produces a splitting, which is orientation dependent. In a crystal powder or amorphous solid, all orientations occur, resulting in inhomogeneous broadening. This broadening may be of the order of 20 kHz.

A second source of line broadening in solids is due to **chemical shift anisotropy**. This arises from asymmetry in the electron density surrounding a given nucleus. In liquids an average chemical shift is observed due to averaging over all orientations on a timescale short in comparison with the measurement time. In solids, a complex lineshape results from a sum of all possible chemical shifts.

In practical circumstances, 'high-resolution' solid state NMR spectra can be obtained using a combination of dipolar decoupling and **magic-angle spinning** (MAS). The effect of dipolar decoupling is similar to that observed in NMR spectra of liquids under conditions of scalar **spin decoupling**, and is in fact achieved in an analogous manner. The effect of MAS has no true counterpart in liquid state NMR, but the overall purpose of this procedure is to remove the effects of chemical shift anisotropy. Interestingly, MAS was originally devised in order to suppress dipolar couplings, but is only effective when the strength of these couplings is less than attainable spinning speeds. In practical situations, dipolar decoupling in **spin space** using efficient composite pulse trains (see **composite pulse** and **average Hamiltonian theory**) is found to be more useful.

Under ideal conditions, the residual linewidth following dipolar decoupling and MAS will be determined by the magnitude of T_2 (see **spin–spin coupling**). In solids, T_2 is very small since the zero frequency spectral density function $J(0)$ (see **relaxation**) is large due to restricted motion. The inherent linewidth is therefore much larger than that found in the liquid state, and may be measured in tens of Hz. A second consequence of very rapid spin–spin relaxation is that the pulse trains commonly employed in liquid state NMR for the investigation of phenomena such as multiple-quantum coherence cannot be employed in solids since the signal decays before the pulse sequence is completed. Therefore elegant schemes (see **order-selective excitation**) involving time-reversal sequences are required such that the overall effect of the pulse sequence approaches the **unity operator**. A final difference between solid state and liquid state NMR which is worthy of note is the magnitude of T_1. **Spin–lattice relaxation** is very inefficient in solid state NMR due to the restricted motion, and therefore T_1 is very large (tens of seconds). Therefore by analogy with pulse-and-collect NMR of liquids, a low sensitivity per unit time results from the extremely long (5 times T_1) interpulse delays needed to re-establish thermal equilibrium (see **spin temperature**). This is overcome by using a technique known as **cross-polarization**. Solid state NMR is just beginning to find applications to biological systems. A prime difficulty with the technique is the large amounts of solid material which are required. In addition, it is generally necessary to isotopically enrich the sample with either ^{13}C or ^{15}N, and therefore such experiments become extremely expensive. Nevertheless, the unique information content of solid state NMR spectra presents a favourable argument for increased use of this technique in studying biological systems in the future.

FURTHER READING

Many good texts exist in solid-state NMR, See for example:

Gerstein, B. C. and Dybrowki, C. R. (1985). *Transient techniques in NMR of solids.* Academic Press, London.

Mehring, M. (1983). *High resolution NMR spectroscopy in solids.* (2nd edn). Springer-Verlag, Berlin.

Slichter, C. P. (1978). *Principles of magnetic resonance.* (2nd edn.). Springer-Verlag, Berlin.

For an introductory review of solid-state NMR, see:

Schaefer, J., and Stejskal, E. (1979). In *Topics in Carbon*-13 *NMR spectroscopy* **3,** Chapter 4.

Solomon–Bloembergen equations See **spin–lattice relaxation**, **spin–spin relaxation**.

Solvent suppression In biological NMR spectroscopy, there are many instances where it may be desirable to record both one- and two-dimensional spectra in the presence of a high concentration of solvent H_2O (typically 90% H_2O/10% D_2O). In these circumstances it is necessary to suppress the strong H_2O resonance so that the dynamic range of the receiver and or the analogue-to-digital converter is not exceeded.

Perhaps the simplest means by which the strong H_2O resonance (or indeed any solvent resonance) may be suppressed is by **saturation**, i.e. the application of a weak r.f. field at the **Larmor precession** frequency of the solvent. However, this technique is not ideal since protons which are in **chemical exchange** with the solvent (NHs, OHs) may also be partially saturated due to saturation transfer. A second technique employs an **inversion recovery sequence** which exploits the differences in T_1 relaxation between the solvent (long T_1) and the macromolecule (short T_1). The sequence is adjusted such that the solvent resonance lies at the null point (i.e. no effective Z magnetization before the 90° pulse) whereas the resonances derived from the macromolecule have fully relaxed. However, B_1 field inhomogeneity often drastically impairs the efficacy of this technique. For these reasons a great deal of effort has been expended in the application of composite pulse techniques for solvent suppression. Some of the more important examples are described below.

1. THE JUMP-AND-RETURN SEQUENCE

This sequence consists of two 90° pulses of opposite **phase** separated by an adjustable delay (Fig. S8(a)). It derives its name from the fact that the effective flip-angle is zero at the transmitter position: magnetization is flipped into the x–y plane, experiences no precession during the delay, and is returned to the $+z$ axis by the second 90° pulse. Resonance lines which are **offset** from the transmitter position precess during the delay and are not returned fully along the $+z$ axis by the second pulse. Since the precession is proportional to the offset, the flip-angle is variable off-resonance, and is adjusted by both the offset and the interpulse delay.

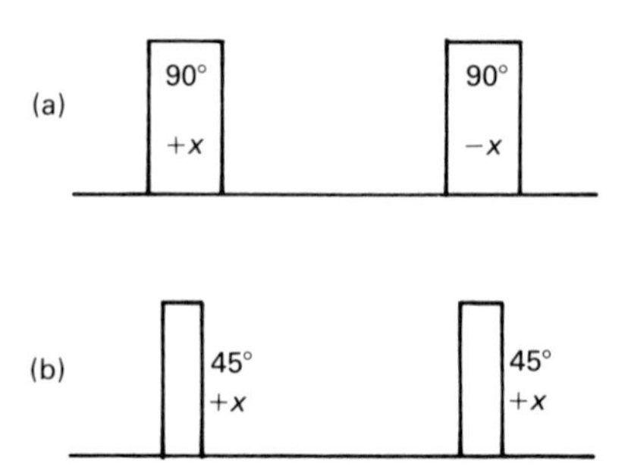

Fig. S8. Pulse sequences for solvent suppression. (a) the 'jump and return' sequence; (b) The 11 sequence.

It is clear that a 180° phase difference must exist about the on-resonance condition since the magnetization vectors precess in opposite directions about the on-resonance condition, and the spectrum must therefore be phased separately for each segment.

2. THE 1–1 SEQUENCE

This is similar to the jump-and-return sequence, and consists of two 45° pulses of identical phase separated by a delay (Fig. S8(*b*)). This sequence produces a region of maximum suppression at a position offset from that of the transmitter. This offset is adjusted by varying the interpulse delay, and the flip-angle for a given resonance is dependent upon the offset from the transmitter. Two suppression maxima are found symmetrically disposed about the transmitter frequency. The phase distortions introduced by this sequence are rather more severe than those introduced by the jump-and-return technique.

3. 'BINOMIAL' COMPOSITE PULSES

Recently, a series of composite pulses has been described which are particularly efficient in their application to solvent suppression. These have been devised on the criterion that a broad flat region of near-zero excitation is required around the solvent frequency, combined with efficient excitation of relatively distant resonances. In this way small static field inhomogeneities and errors in the transmitter position are tolerable.

A suitable frequency-domain function which satisfies these criteria is $f(\nu) = \sin^n(\pi\nu t)$ where n is positive integer. All derivatives of $f(\nu)$ to the $(n-1)$th inclusive are zero at $\nu = 0$. The **Fourier transform** of $f(\nu)$ $(f(t))$ is given by

S35 $$f(t) \alpha \sum_{k=0}^{k=n} (-1)^k \binom{n}{k} \delta(t + \{k - n/2\}\tau).$$

Assuming the approximate Fourier relationship between this time-domain function and its frequency-domain partner $f(\nu)$, a suitable time-domain function can be obtained from (S35). This is $n+1$ equally-spaced delta functions with alternating signs, and amplitudes given by the binomial coefficients $\binom{n}{k}$. Suitable composite pulses are therefore $1\bar{1}, 1\bar{2}1, 1\bar{3}3\bar{1} \ldots$, where the numbers indicate relative pulse widths (the sum equalling the required flip-angle) and the overbars indicate phase inversion. Interpulse spacings are all equal (τ). The first member of the binomial series $(1\bar{1})$ is seen to be identical in form to the jump-and-return sequence above. The sequence $1\bar{3}3\bar{1}$ provides performance better by an order of magnitude.

FURTHER READING

Hore, P. J. (1983). *J. Magn. Reson.* **54,** 539.

Spectral density functions See **relaxation**.

Spectrometer A block diagram of a typical NMR spectrometer designed for liquid state studies is shown in Fig. S9. At the heart of the system is the NMR **probe** which is situated within the spectrometer magnet. The NMR sample is in turn located within the probe.

In order to perturb the spin system with r.f. energy, the spectrometer contains sophisticated pulse programmer and transmitter units, which allow for the application of complex pulse sequences (see **pulse sequence**) to the sample of interest. The r.f. source is a very stable crystal oscillator or synthesizer unit which runs continuously, and all frequencies in the spectrometer are ideally derived from it. The continuous-wave

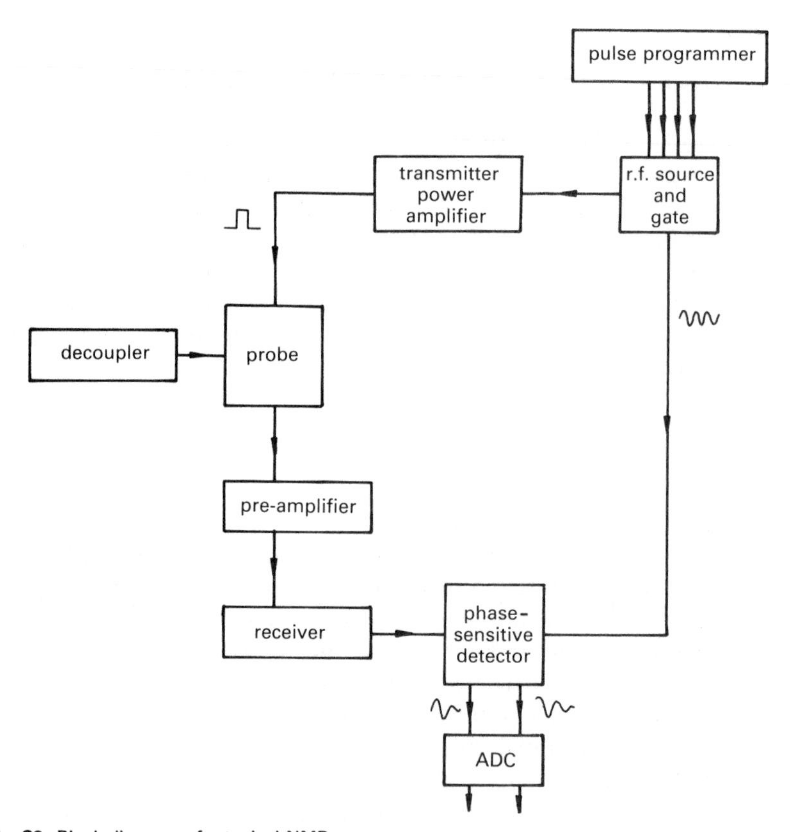

Fig. S9. Block diagram of a typical NMR spectrometer.

signal derived from the source is controlled in amplitude and **phase** by the gate unit. The pulse programmer controls these parameters indirectly by switching the phase of the r.f. by 0, 90°, 180°, 270° depending on the required pulse phase and switches the r.f. on and off for a period determined by the required pulse width. All of these parameters are programmed into the pulse programmer by the operator prior to the start of the experiment. In addition, most modern spectrometers are equipped with a dedicated phase shifter, which allows the pulse phase to be adjusted in increments smaller than 90°. This is usually achieved either by incorporating an electronic 'delay line' into the signal path in order to achieve a variable phase, or alternatively, the transmitter frequency is 'jumped' for a finite period of time, which effectively amounts to a phase shift when the transmitter frequency is returned to its initial value. Irrespective of the precise phase-shift hardware, the low-level signal from the gate unit is amplified in a high-power amplifier to levels involving several tens of W. In the case of simple rectangular pulse envelopes, a non-linear amplifier may be used, but if pulse-shaping circuitry is to be included in the transmitter signal path (see e.g. **Gaussian pulse**), then a **linear amplifier** is required. The transmitter amplifier must be correctly matched into the probe in order that the available transmitter power is dissipated into the sample. This is achieved by use of tuned circuits within the probe.

In order to perform double-resonance experiments, a high-power decoupler is necessary. This may consist of a simple signal source, high-power amplifier, and simple gate unit, or more usually the decoupler signal path is often very similar to that found in the transmitter. In some spectrometers the decoupler and transmitter paths are designed symmetrically for ease of use. In any case, it is necessary to arrange for the decoupler and transmitter frequencies to be phase coherent, since without this requirement their relative phases are meaningless. Phase coherence is easily achieved using the same signal source for transmitter and decoupler. The decoupler irradiating frequency can then be varied using a simple synthesizer system.

The response of the nuclear spin system is detected by the receiver circuitry which is gated on after completion of the transmitter pulse train. The low-level signal derived from the probe is increased to a more manageable level by the preamplifier (see **amplifier**), and may be converted to a lower intermediate frequency for further amplification. However, in simpler spectrometers the signal is detected directly following preamplification, with further gain at **audio-frequency**. Detection is invariably achieved using a **phase-sensitive detector**. For this purpose a reference frequency is required which is derived from the transmitter r.f. source, so that the requirements for phase coherence can be met. Receiver phase shifts can be generated simply by the inclusion of an electronic delay in the receiver reference frequency path. The signals derived from the phase-sensitive detector are passed finally to the **analogue-to-digital converter** where they are digitized and passed into computer memory.

In addition to the main circuitry shown in Fig. S9, a second, much simpler spectrometer circuit is required in order to ensure that the r.f. source and the r.f. field are matched in long-term stability. The special circuitry required for this purpose is described under **lock**.

Spherical tensor operators The **product operator formalism** is of particular value for the description of NMR experiments since it gives a simple physical insight into the workings of such experiments. However, in some cases it is convenient to employ an alternative formalism which utilizes spherical tensor operators. The use of the spherical tensor basis set is advantageous because every operator product is associated uniquely with a particular coherence level or coherence order of the spin system. The cartesian components of the **angular momentum** operators (product operators) can be transformed to the spherical tensor components using the following relations:

$$\begin{aligned} I_{+1} &= -(I_x + \mathrm{i}I_y)/\sqrt{2} = (-1/\sqrt{2})I^+ \\ I_0 &= I_z \\ I_{-1} &= (I_x - \mathrm{i}I_y)/\sqrt{2} = (1/\sqrt{2})I^- \end{aligned} \quad \text{S36}$$

where I^+ and I^- are **shift operators**. When these spherical tensor operators are combined to form operator products the coherence level associated with a particular product is just the sum of the indices of the component nuclear spin operators. For a two-spin system IS we can thus define 16 operator products (in analogy with cartesian product operators), which can be classified according to the coherence levels to which they correspond:

$$\begin{aligned} 0;&\quad \mathbf{1}/2,\ I_0,\ S_0,\ 2I_0S_0,\ 2I_{+1}S_{-1},\ 2I_{-1}S_{+1} \\ \pm 1;&\quad I_{+1},\ I_{-1},\ S_{+1},\ S_{-1},\ 2I_+S_0,\ 2I_-S_0,\ 2I_0S_+,\ 2I_0S_- \\ \pm 2;&\quad 2I_+S_+,\ 2I_-S_-. \end{aligned} \quad \text{S37}$$

By use of spherical tensor notation, it is easier to see how a particular coherence transfer pathway can be selected. The evolution of product operators in the spherical basis is described in analogy to cartesian product operators:

Chemical shift

$$I_p \xrightarrow{\omega_I \tau I_z} I_p \exp(-\mathrm{i}p\omega_I\tau), \qquad p = 0, \pm 1. \quad \text{S38}$$

Spin coupling

S39 $$I_{\pm 1} \xrightarrow{\pi J_{IS}\tau 2I_zS_z} I_{\pm 1}\cos(\pi J_{IS}\tau) \mp 2\mathrm{i}I_{\pm 1}S_0\sin(\pi J_{IS}\tau)$$

S40 $$2I_{\pm 1}S_0 \xrightarrow{\pi J_{IS}\tau 2I_zS_z} 2I_{\pm 1}S_0\cos(\pi J_{IS}\tau) \mp \mathrm{i}I_{\pm 1}\sin(\pi J_{IS}\tau)$$

S41 $$2I_{\pm 1}S_{\pm 1} \xrightarrow{\pi J_{IS}\tau 2I_zS_z} 2I_{\pm 1}S_{\pm 1}.$$

Note that free precession under either chemical shift or spin coupling does not change the coherence level.

r.f. pulses with flip angle β and phase shift ϕ;

S42 $$\begin{aligned} I_{\pm 1} \xrightarrow{-\phi I_z} \xrightarrow{\beta I_x} \xrightarrow{\phi I_z} & I_{\pm 1}(\cos\beta + 1)/2 \\ & + I_0(-\mathrm{i}\sin\beta/\sqrt{2})\exp(\pm \mathrm{i}\phi) \\ & + I_{\mp 1}[(\cos\beta - 1)/2]\exp(\pm 2\mathrm{i}\phi) \end{aligned}$$

S43 $$\begin{aligned} I_0 \xrightarrow{-\phi I_z} \xrightarrow{\beta I_x} \xrightarrow{\phi I_z} & I_{+1}(-\mathrm{i}\sin\beta/\sqrt{2})\exp(-\mathrm{i}\phi) \\ & + I_0\cos\beta + I_{-1}(-\mathrm{i}\sin\beta/\sqrt{2})\exp(+\mathrm{i}\phi). \end{aligned}$$

Note that pulses cause a change in coherence level.

In using the spherical tensor basis for the selection of coherence transfer pathways, it is conventional to view a quadrature signal (see **quadrature detection**) in which the real part is proportional to I_y and the imaginary part is proportional to I_x, as a pure absorption signal. Thus $\mathrm{i}I_{-1} = (I_y + \mathrm{i}I_x)/\sqrt{2}$ is a pure absorption signal, but $I_{+1} = -(I_x + \mathrm{i}I_y)/\sqrt{2}$ is a pure dispersion signal, and is the quadrature image.

As an example of the use of the formalism, consider the analysis of COSY for a two-spin system IS. At equilibrium, the state of the system is described in spherical tensor notation by

S44 $$\sigma(0) = I_0 + S_0.$$

The application of a $\pi/2$ r.f. pulse with a phase shift of ϕ gives

S45 $$\begin{aligned} I_0 + S_0 \xrightarrow{\pi/2(I\phi + S\phi)} & -(\mathrm{i}/\sqrt{2})I_{+1}\exp(-\mathrm{i}\phi) - (\mathrm{i}/\sqrt{2})I_{-1}\exp(+\mathrm{i}\phi) \\ & -(\mathrm{i}/\sqrt{2})S_{+1}\exp(-\mathrm{i}\phi) - (\mathrm{i}/\sqrt{2})S_{-1}\exp(+\mathrm{i}\phi) \\ & = \sigma(1). \end{aligned}$$

Note that the $\exp(\pm\mathrm{i}\phi)$ phase factors label the coherence level $I_{\mp 1}$ and $S_{\mp 1}$ operators, so that the fates of the latter can be followed through the

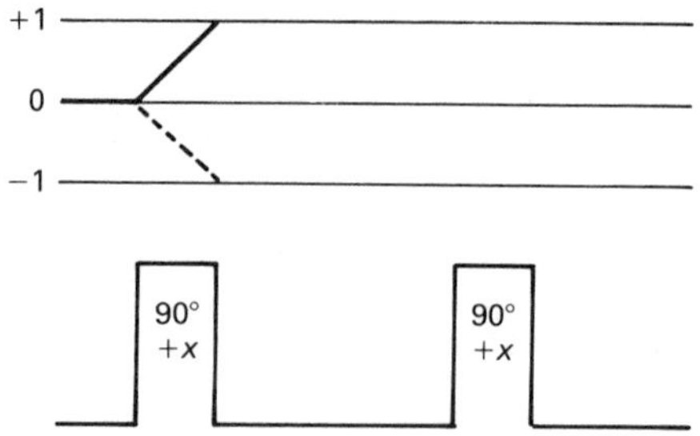

Fig. S10. Coherence transfer pathways after application of the first pulse in a COSY experiment.

sequence. This can be made clearer with a coherence pathway diagram (Fig. S10).

If the system is allowed to evolve under chemical shift and spin coupling terms for a period t_1, we find for the state of the system at the end of this period

$$\sigma(1) \xrightarrow{\omega_I I_z + \omega_S S_z}$$

$$- (\mathrm{i}/\sqrt{2})I_{+1} \exp(-\mathrm{i}\phi) \exp(-\mathrm{i}\omega_I t_1) - (\mathrm{i}/\sqrt{2})I_{-1} \exp(+\mathrm{i}\phi) \exp(\mathrm{i}\omega_I t_1)$$
$$- (\mathrm{i}/\sqrt{2})S_{+1} \exp(-\mathrm{i}\phi) \exp(-\mathrm{i}\omega_S t_1) \tag{S46}$$
$$- (\mathrm{i}/\sqrt{2})S_{-1} \exp(+\mathrm{i}\phi) \exp(\mathrm{i}\omega_S t_1) \xrightarrow{2\pi J_{IS} t_1 I_z S_z}$$

$$\begin{aligned}
&-(\mathrm{i}/\sqrt{2})I_{+1} \exp(-\mathrm{i}\phi) \exp(-\mathrm{i}\omega_I t_1) \cos \pi J_{IS} t_1 \\
&- (2/\sqrt{2})I_{+1}S_0 \exp(-\mathrm{i}\phi) \exp(-\mathrm{i}\omega_I t_1) \sin \pi J_{IS} t_1 \\
&- (\mathrm{i}/\sqrt{2})\mathrm{I}_{-1} \exp(+\mathrm{i}\phi) \exp(\mathrm{i}\omega_I t_1) \cos \pi J_{IS} t_1 \\
&+ (2/\sqrt{2})I_{-1}S_0 \exp(+\mathrm{i}\phi) \exp(\mathrm{i}\omega_I t_1) \sin \pi J_{IS} t_1 \\
&- (\mathrm{i}/\sqrt{2})\mathrm{S}_{+1} \exp(-\mathrm{i}\phi) \exp(-\mathrm{i}\omega_S t_1) \cos \pi J_{IS} t_1 \\
&- (2/\sqrt{2})S_{+1}I_0 \exp(-\mathrm{i}\phi) \exp(-\mathrm{i}\omega_S t_1) \sin \pi J_{IS} t_1 \\
&- (\mathrm{i}/\sqrt{2})\mathrm{S}_{-1} \exp(+\mathrm{i}\phi) \exp(\mathrm{i}\omega_S t_1) \cos \pi J_{IS} t_1 \\
&+ (2/\sqrt{2})S_{-1}I_0 \exp(+\mathrm{i}\phi) \exp(\mathrm{i}\omega_S t_1) \sin \pi J_{IS} t_1 = \sigma(2).
\end{aligned} \tag{S47}$$

Each term in (S47) corresponds with either a +1 or a −1 coherence level. We can thus extend the coherence level diagram as shown in Fig. S11.

The application of the second $\pi/2$ pulse of phase ψ, followed by free precession during t_2 under spin coupling and chemical shift terms, can be evaluated in an analogous manner to (S45), (S46) and (S47). We find at the end of this time that −2, −1, 0, +1 and +2 coherences are generated. However, only the −1 coherences are important since these are the only terms which will be recorded using a quadrature detector. The final coherence pathway diagram thus corresponds with Fig. S12.

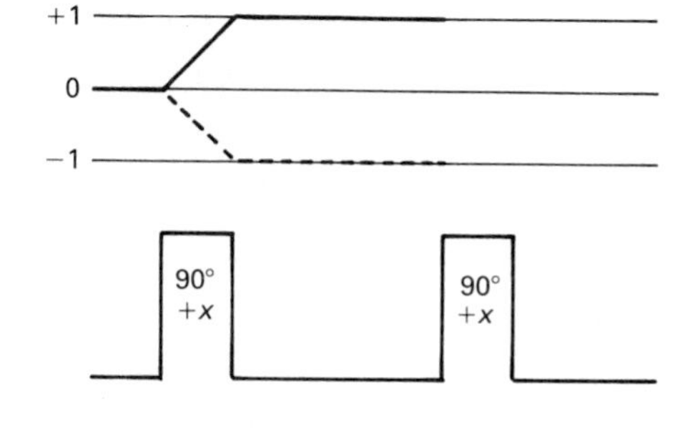

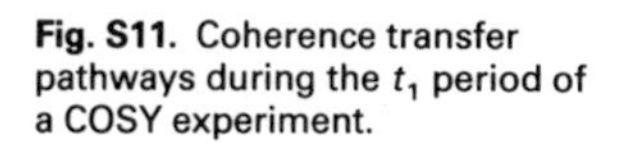
Fig. S11. Coherence transfer pathways during the t_1 period of a COSY experiment.

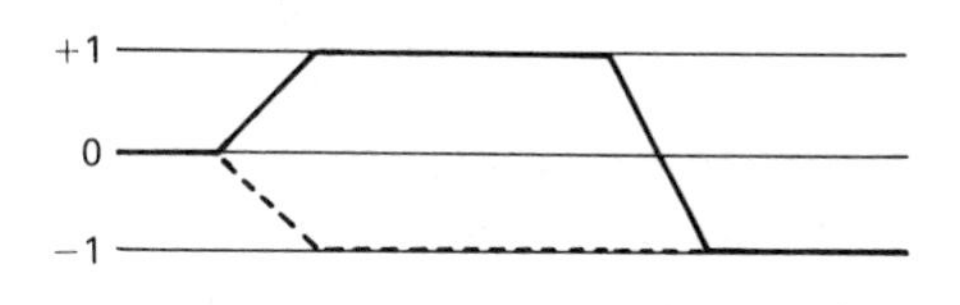

Fig. S12. Coherence transfer pathways after the second pulse in a COSY experiment.

The state of the system at the end of the t_2 period is too bulky to show in full, but after a little trigonometry the -1 coherence terms for spin I are given by (ignoring the numerical factors which are all equal):

$$\begin{aligned}
\sigma(4)(I_{-1}\text{ only}) = &+ I_{-1}\exp(\mathrm{i}\phi)\exp[\mathrm{i}(\omega_I + \pi J_{IS})t_1]\exp[\mathrm{i}(\omega_I + \pi J_{IS})t_2] \\
&+ I_{-1}\exp(\mathrm{i}\phi)\exp[\mathrm{i}(\omega_I + \pi J_{IS})t_1]\exp[\mathrm{i}(\omega_I - \pi J_{IS})t_2] \\
&+ I_{-1}\exp(\mathrm{i}\phi)\exp[\mathrm{i}(\omega_I - \pi J_{IS})t_1]\exp[\mathrm{i}(\omega_I + \pi J_{IS})t_2] \\
&+ I_{-1}\exp(\mathrm{i}\phi)\exp[\mathrm{i}(\omega_I - \pi J_{IS})t_1]\exp[\mathrm{i}(\omega_I - \pi J_{IS})t_2] \\
&+ I_{-1}\exp(\mathrm{i}\phi)\exp[\mathrm{i}(\omega_S + \pi J_{IS})t_1]\exp[\mathrm{i}(\omega_I + \pi J_{IS})t_2] \\
&+ I_{-1}\exp(\mathrm{i}\phi)\exp[\mathrm{i}(\omega_S + \pi J_{IS})t_1]\exp[\mathrm{i}(\omega_I - \pi J_{IS})t_2] \\
&+ I_{-1}\exp(\mathrm{i}\phi)\exp[\mathrm{i}(\omega_S - \pi J_{IS})t_1]\exp[\mathrm{i}(\omega_I + \pi J_{IS})t_2] \\
&+ I_{-1}\exp(\mathrm{i}\phi)\exp[\mathrm{i}(\omega_S - \pi J_{IS})t_1]\exp[\mathrm{i}(\omega_I - \pi J_{IS})t_2] \\
&+ I_{-1}\exp(2\mathrm{i}\psi)\exp(-\mathrm{i}\phi)\exp[\mathrm{i}(-\omega_I + \pi J_{IS})t_1] \\
&\times \exp[\mathrm{i}(\omega_I + \pi J_{IS})t_2] \\
&+ I_{-1}\exp(2\mathrm{i}\psi)\exp(-\mathrm{i}\phi)\exp[\mathrm{i}(-\omega_I + \pi J_{IS})t_1] \\
&\times \exp[\mathrm{i}(\omega_I - \pi J_{IS})t_2] \\
&+ I_{-1}\exp(2\mathrm{i}\psi)\exp(-\mathrm{i}\phi)\exp[\mathrm{i}(-\omega_I - \pi J_{IS})t_1] \\
&\times \exp[\mathrm{i}(\omega_I + \pi J_{IS})t_2] \\
&+ I_{-1}\exp(2\mathrm{i}\psi)\exp(-\mathrm{i}\phi)\exp[\mathrm{i}(-\omega_I - \pi J_{IS})t_1]
\end{aligned}$$

S48

$$\times \exp[i(\omega_I - \pi J_{IS})t_2]$$
$$+ I_{-1} \exp(2i\psi) \exp(-i\phi) \exp[i(-\omega_S + \pi J_{IS})t_1]$$
$$\times \exp[i(\omega_I + \pi J_{IS})t_2]$$
$$+ I_{-1} \exp(2i\psi) \exp(-i\phi) \exp[i(-\omega_S + \pi J_{IS})t_1]$$
$$\times \exp[i(\omega_I - \pi J_{IS})t_2]$$
$$+ I_{-1} \exp(2i\psi) \exp(-i\phi) \exp[i(-\omega_S - \pi J_{IS})t_1]$$
$$\times \exp[i(\omega_I + \pi J_{IS})t_2]$$
$$+ I_{-1} \exp(2i\psi) \exp(-i\phi) \exp[i(-\omega_S - \pi J_{IS})t_1]$$
$$\times \exp[i(\omega_I - \pi J_{IS})t_2]$$

The final density operator contains terms with phase factor $\exp(+i\phi)$, which correspond to magnetization which began as -1 coherence after the first pulse, and terms with phase factor $\exp(-i\phi)\exp(+2i\psi)$, which correspond to magnetization which existed as $+1$ coherence during t_1, and has been converted to -1 coherence by the second pulse. Both these signals which correspond to the antiecho and coherence transfer echo (P-type and N-type peaks), will reach the detector. In order to separate these, i.e. to achieve quadrature detection in the f_1 domain, we employ a **phase cycling** procedure (see **phase modulation**). The analysis we have just performed allows us to easily design the appropriate cycle. To select N-type peaks, it is necessary to arrange for the phase factor $\exp(+i\phi)$ to be zero when combined with the receiver phase $\exp(-i\phi_R)$. Thus, for the jth transient of a series of k transients per t_1 increment, the receiver phase is chosen so that

S49 $$\sum_{j=1}^{k} \exp(-i\phi_j)\exp(+2i\psi_j)\exp(-i\phi_{Rj}) = K$$

S50 $$\sum_{j=1}^{k} \exp(+i\phi_j)\exp(-i\phi_{Rj}) = 0$$

from which the following phase cycle is found to be appropriate.

ϕ	ψ	ϕ_R
x	x	x
x	y	$-x$
x	$-x$	x
x	$-y$	$-x$

This is identical to the sequence described for the phase-modulated COSY experiment.

FURTHER READING

Ernst, R. R., Bodenhausen, G., and Wokaun, A. A. (1987). *Principles of NMR in one and two dimensions*. Clarendon Press, Oxford.

Nakashima, T. T. and McClung, R. (1986). *J. Magn. Reson.* **70,** 187.

Spin See **angular momentum**.

Spin coupling Strictly, there is a variety of mechanisms which might be termed spin coupling. However, in NMR of liquids (see **averaging**), the term spin coupling invariably refers to scalar coupling between spins, which is characterized by the coupling constant J. A complete theoretical treatment for a two-spin system with a finite spin coupling between them ($J > 0$) predicts that the NMR spectrum is composed of a pair of doublets (see e.g. **density matrix**), one for each spin. We can understand this in simple qualitative terms by the following argument. In the absence of spin coupling, the NMR spectrum is composed of two singlets, which will appear at different Larmor frequencies if we assume that the nuclei (labelled I and S) are magnetically inequivalent (Fig. S13). Now if these nuclei are scalar coupled, which is usually the case if there is a through-bond connectivity between them, then the spin state of one nucleus is sensed by the other. For example, if I and S are both protons, then for a given spin state of I, there will be two spin states of S ($+\frac{1}{2}$ and $-\frac{1}{2}$). This results in a splitting of the resonance line of S into two lines (a doublet). The reverse argument explains why the resonance line of I is also now a doublet (Fig. S14). The splitting arises because the nuclear spin is coupled via the bonding electrons to the coupled nucleus, which experiences two different microenvironments, and thus resonates at two slightly different frequencies. A quantum mechanical treatment (see

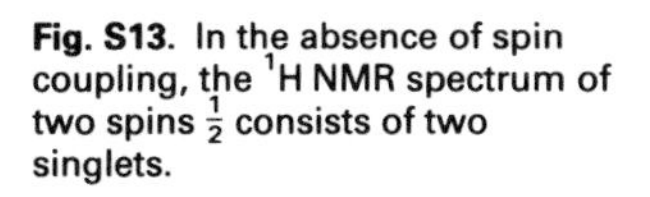

Fig. S13. In the absence of spin coupling, the ^1H NMR spectrum of two spins $\frac{1}{2}$ consists of two singlets.

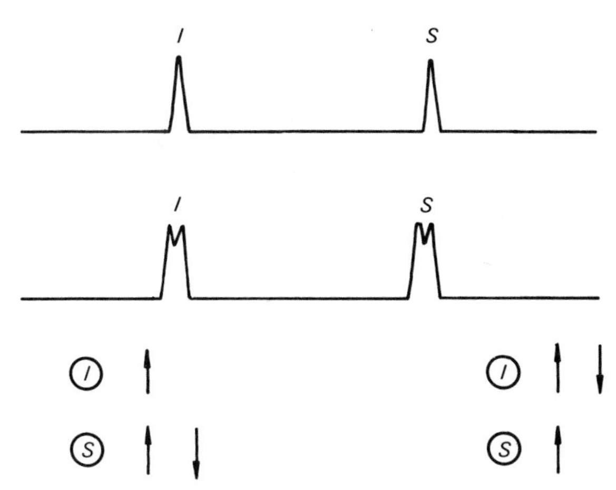

Fig. S14. The ^1H NMR spectrum of two weakly coupled spins $\frac{1}{2}$ consists of two doublets. Each nucleus senses the two spin states of the other.

density matrix) demonstrates that this frequency difference is equal to J, the scalar spin coupling constant. The value of J is independent of the applied magnetic field, and is thus measured in Hz. The magnitude of J depends upon the number and types of bond through which the nuclei are coupled. For example, geminal protons have a coupling around −12 Hz, whereas protons separated by three bonds have couplings in the region 2–9 Hz, depending upon the dihedral angle between them (see **Karplus equation**). On the other hand, couplings between ^{13}C and protons can be as much as 150 Hz.

If one of the nuclei has a spin $>\frac{1}{2}$, then the nucleus to which it is coupled becomes split into more than two lines. For example, a nucleus of spin 1 would split a proton into three lines of equal intensity, since there are now three spin states ($\frac{1}{2}$, 0, $-\frac{1}{2}$). Additional splittings also occur if more than one nucleus is responsible for the splitting. As an example consider the ^{1}H NMR spectrum of ethanol CH_3CH_2OH (Fig. S15). The methyl group is split into a triplet, with resonance lines in a 1:2:1 intensity ratio. This arises from the fact that each methyl proton is split by each CH_2 proton. Since each CH_2 proton has two possible spin states, there are four possible combinations which are sensed by the methyl protons (Fig. S15). Two of these combinations have the same effect upon the methyl protons, and so two lines of the theoretical quartet overlap to

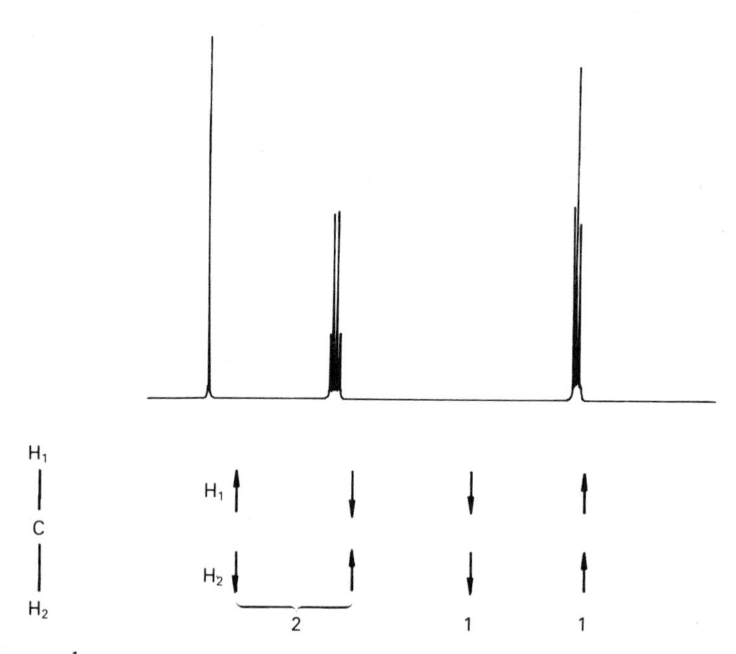

Fig. S15. The ^{1}H NMR spectrum of ethanol, showing how the methyl triplet derives from the four possible spin states of the methylene group.

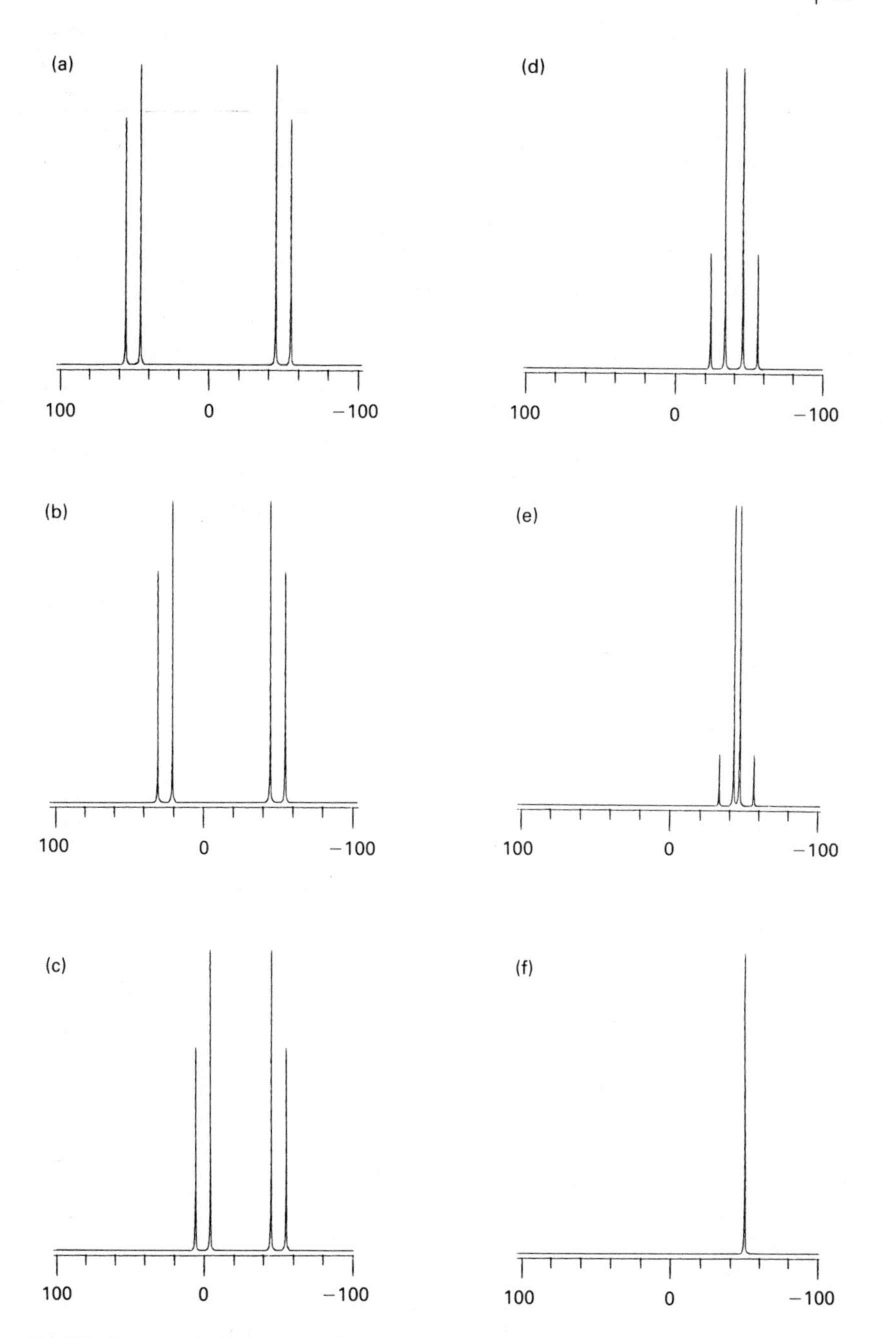

Fig. S16. Spectral simulations for two coupled spins with $J = 10$ Hz. The chemical shift difference between the spins is (a) 100 Hz, (b) 75 Hz, (c) 50 Hz, (d) 20 Hz, (e) 10 Hz, and (f) 0 Hz.

give a triplet with the 1:2:1 intensity ratio. Note that the methyl protons do not split each other, since they are magnetically equivalent due to free rotation about the C–C bond. A similar argument, when applied to the splitting of the CH_2 protons by the three methyl protons gives a quartet with a 1:3:3:1 intensity ratio. In the general case, the intensities are scaled according to Pascal's triangle.

Thus far, we have made an assumption in the discussion which is called the **high-field approximation**. We have assumed that the chemical shifts between resonances of the coupled nuceli are much greater than the J couplings. This is also called the **weak coupling** approximation, and the nuclei are described as weakly coupled. However, when the value of J is of the order of the chemical shift difference, then the intensities of the multiplets change. For example, the NMR spectrum of the two-spin system IS changes with the shift difference between the nuclei as shown in Fig. S16. In the limit that the shift difference is zero, a singlet is observed of double intensity, again demonstrating that equivalent nuclei do not split each other. The situation where the value of J is comparable to the shift difference is known as **strong coupling**. In practice, almost all multiplets in ^{1}H NMR spectra show partial strong coupling behaviour, in that multiplet intensities are invariably slightly skewed. However, in the majority of situations it is convenient (i.e. simpler) to treat the system using the weak coupling approximation.

A rigorous treatment of strong coupling can be found under that heading. However, it is instructive here to consider the difference between weak and strong coupling in the qualitative sense. In the case of weak coupling, the rotation of a spin is effectively isolated from its neighbours. Thus, if one spin is flipped by a pulse, there is no tendency for neighbouring spins to flip in sympathy. In contrast, if one spin in a strongly coupled system is flipped, there is a finite probability that other spins will flip also, this probability increasing as the strength of the coupling increases. Finally, it should be understood that the strength of the coupling is measured in terms of the relative magnitudes of J and the shift difference between the spins. The actual value of J does not change with the coupling strength.

Spin decoupling A system comprising two homonuclear or heteronuclear spins I and S between which a scalar (or dipolar) coupling exists can be effectively decoupled by a variety of methods. Highly efficient **composite pulse** schemes have been devised for broadband homonuclear or heteronuclear decoupling, and these are described under **broadband decoupling**. Here we consider the effects of a simple continuous-wave irradiation of strength $\gamma B_2 \gg 2\pi J$ at the **Larmor precession** frequency of one of the spins (I). In practical situations in biological NMR spectroscopy, this method is a simple and effective procedure to identify coupled spins (see **difference spectroscopy** and **gated decoupling**).

A simple physical picture of the effects of irradiating one of the spins can be had by noting that the r.f. field causes rapid I spin transitions, and since the probability of an upward transition is equal to that for a downward transition, the I spin multiplet rapidly becomes saturated (see **saturation**). Under these conditions, the effect of the I spin state upon the S spin (see **spin coupling**) is averaged out. In theoretical terms, the spin system evolves during the evolution period under an effective **Hamiltonian** which comprises only the Zeeman term for spin S. This can be illustrated by use of **average Hamiltonian theory**.

The complete Hamiltonian for a weakly coupled two-spin system IS is given by

S51 $$\mathcal{H} = \mathcal{H}_Z^I + \mathcal{H}_Z^S + \mathcal{H}_J^{IS}$$

where

S52 $$\begin{aligned} \mathcal{H}_Z^I &= \omega_I I_z \\ \mathcal{H}_Z^S &= \omega_S S_z \\ \mathcal{H}_J^{IS} &= 2\pi J_{IS} I_z S_z \end{aligned}$$

and ω_I, ω_S, J_{IS} are the Larmor precession frequencies and the spin coupling constant between spins I and S in obvious notation. Under conditions of continuous irradiation of spin I, it is convenient to transform into a frame rotating with respect to spin I. For this purpose we define a transformed Hamiltonian:

S53 $$\mathcal{H}^{\mathrm{T}} = \mathcal{H} - \omega_2 I_z$$

where ω_2 is the frequency of the applied irradiation ($\omega_2 = \omega_I$ for on-resonance decoupling). To zero order, the effective or average Hamiltonian is given by

S54 $$\bar{H}^0 = \frac{1}{t_c}\int_0^{t_c} \tilde{\mathcal{H}}^{\mathrm{T}}(t_1)\, \mathrm{d}t_1$$

where t_c is the cycle time

S55 $$t_c = 2\pi/(\gamma B_2)$$

and $\tilde{\mathcal{H}}^{\mathrm{T}}$ is the interaction representation of $\mathcal{H}^{\mathrm{T}}$:

S56 $$\tilde{\mathcal{H}}^{\mathrm{T}} = \exp\{-\mathrm{i}\gamma B_2 I_x t\}\, \mathcal{H}^{\mathrm{T}} \exp\{\mathrm{i}\gamma B_2 I_x t\}.$$

From (S54), the average Hamiltonian is given by

S57 $$\bar{\mathcal{H}}^0 = \mathcal{H}_Z^S.$$

Provided $\gamma B_2 \gg 2\pi J_{IS}$ and $\gamma B_2 \gg |\omega_I - \omega_2|$, higher-order terms of the

Magnus expansion are negligible, and I spin terms, coupling terms and the perturbing r.f. field are excluded from the effective Hamiltonian.

Spin diffusion Spin diffusion is a T_1 phenomenon (see **spin–lattice relaxation**) which is frequently observed in NMR of macromolecules. The decay rate of the longitudinal magnetization of a spin I to an ensemble of spins S can be written in generalized form as

S58 $$\frac{\mathrm{d}\langle I_z \rangle}{\mathrm{d}t} = -\rho_I(\langle I_z \rangle - I_0) - \sum_S \sigma_{IS}(\langle S_z \rangle - S_0).$$

Explicit expressions for ρ and σ are given under the heading spin–lattice relaxation. In the limit of 'slow' motion, 'slow' meaning $\omega\tau_c \gg 1$, σ becomes much greater than ρ. Then the rate of transfer of spin energy between nuclei (invariably protons) becomes much larger than the rate of transfer of energy to the lattice. This results in longitudinal relaxation rates of protons within the molecule which all tend to the same value:

S59 $$\frac{1}{T_1} = \frac{1}{N}\sum_S \rho_s$$

where T_1 is now an average value, and N is the number of protons. Since the **nuclear Overhauser effect** is dependent upon σ, in the presence of spin diffusion it is clear that this parameter will no longer be specific for proximal spins. In the extreme case, an homogeneous negative NOE will be observed throughout the whole spectrum. In practice, spin-diffusion is evident in the generation of three-spin effects (relayed NOEs) in either one-dimensional NOE difference or two-dimensional **nuclear Overhauser effect** (NOESY) **spectroscopy**. Under these conditions there is no simple relationship between the magnitude of the NOE and the internuclear distance, and for this reason NOESY spectra should only be interpreted in the initial rate approximation.

FURTHER READING

A detailed discussion of spin-diffusion in proteins is found in:

Kalk, A. and Berendsen, H. J. C. (1975). *J. Magn. Reson.* **24,** 343.

Spin echo All NMR experiments depend upon the generation of **phase coherence**. For various reasons, the phase coherence of the nuclear **magnetization** is gradually lost during the detection period and the detected signal dies away. However, a certain class of experiment exists, in which the phase coherence is refocused at some time after the initial perturbation, resulting in the formation of **spin echoes**. One of the simplest experiments consists of the Carr–Purcell sequence (Fig. S17). Transverse magnetization created by the first pulse decays during the τ

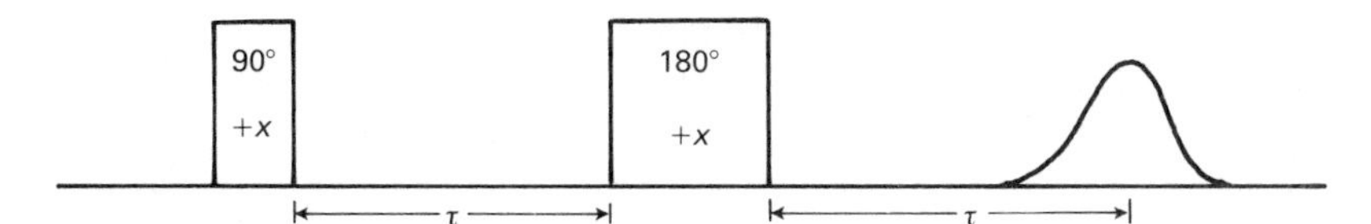

Fig. S17. The Carr–Purcell sequence for the generation of spin echoes.

period due to the loss in phase coherence of the individual spin vectors. The 180° pulse which is applied at the end of the τ period along the $+y$ axis flips the relative orientations of the individual spin vectors as shown in Fig. S18.

After the last 180° pulse, the spin vectors rephase during the τ period, creating a spin echo at the end of it. The phase coherence which is thus recreated may be detected at this time. The detection of a spin echo has a variety of uses. Since the effects of magnetic field inhomogeneity are refocused, collection of the spin echo avoids this undesirable artefact in the measurement of T_2 (see **Carr–Purcell–Meiboom–Gill sequence**). Also, the Carr–Purcell sequence may be used as a crude spin filter which allows for the selective detection of resonances with long T_2, since T_2 effects are not refocused in the spin echo. In fact spin echoes represent one of several echo phenomena which exist during NMR measurements in an inhomogeneous field. For example, see also **coherence transfer echo**, **rotary echo**.

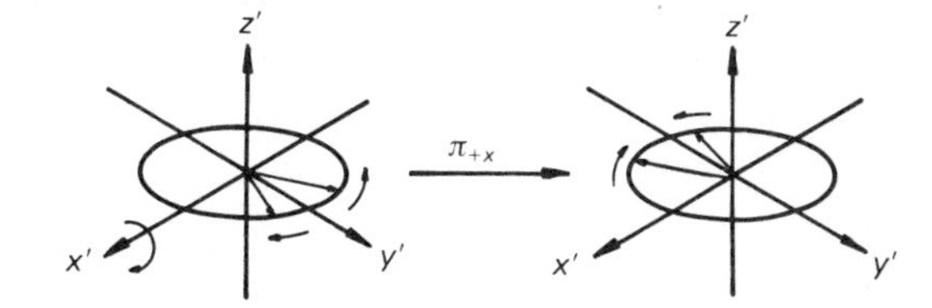

Fig. S18. A 180° pulse flips the orientations of dephasing spin vectors such that they rephase, thus creating a spin echo.

FURTHER READING

Farrar, T. C. and Becker, E. D. (1971). *Pulse and Fourier transform NMR.* Academic Press, New York.

Spin echo correlated spectroscopy (SECSY) The SECSY experiment is a variant of **correlated spectroscopy** (COSY). Effectively, the detection period is delayed after the mixing pulse, such that observation begins at the peak of the **coherence transfer echo**. This is achieved using the pulse sequence in Fig. S19. In the frequency domain, the effect of delayed acquisition leads to an ω_2-dependent shift of signals parallel to the ω_1 axis. This can be understood by redefining the evolution period of COSY

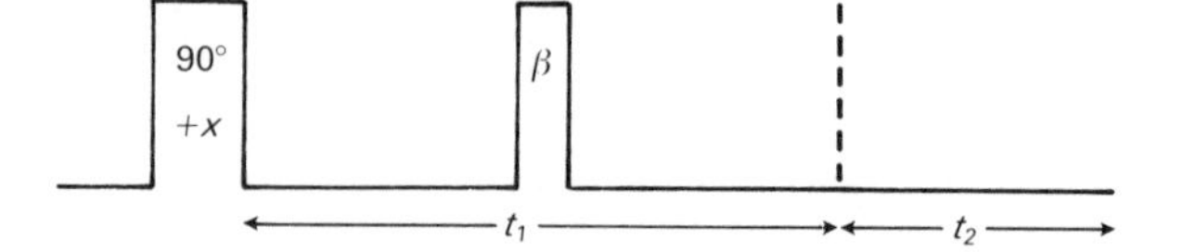

Fig. S19. Pulse sequence for the acquisition of homonuclear spin-echo correlated spectra.

to include part of the interval after the mixing period, as in Fig. S19. The detection period is thus delayed after the mixing pulse by δt_1:

S60 $$t_1' = (1 + \delta)t_1.$$

The peaks in the final spectrum then appear at frequencies ω_1':

S61 $$\omega_1' = \frac{1}{1+\delta}(\omega_1 + \delta\omega_2).$$

Thus in the pulse sequence of Fig. S19,

S62 $$\omega_1' = \tfrac{1}{2}(\omega_1 + \omega_2).$$

From (S62), it is seen that the separation between crosspeaks and diagonal peaks in the ω_1' dimension is halved in comparison with a conventional COSY spectrum (Fig. S20). The J-splittings are not scaled. Since detection occurs at the peak of an echo, the inhomogeneous contribution to the linewidth is eliminated in the absence of diffusion. This, together with an effective reduction in the size of the data matrix in the ω_1' dimension, would suggest obvious advantages over COSY. However, a serious disadvantage is the difficulty with which pure absorption-mode (see **phase-sensitive experiments**) spectra can be obtained. Although this is possible with the application of a **z-filter**, a reduction in sensitivity and more complex multiplet patterns result. In

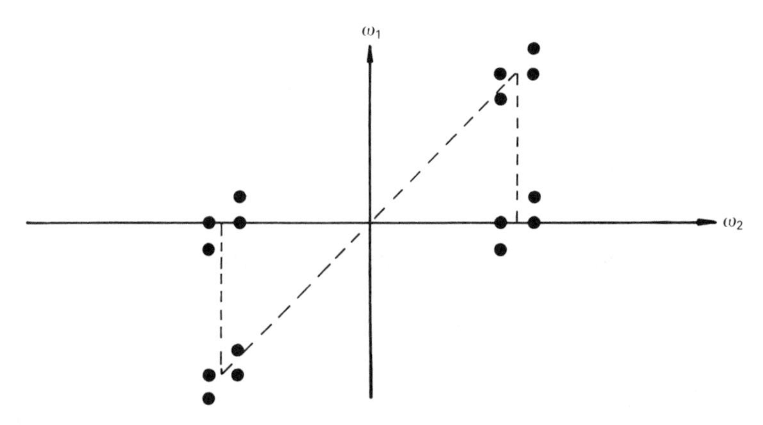

Fig. S20. Diagrammatic representation of a spin-echo correlated spectrum for a weakly coupled two-spin system.

addition, the inherent symmetry of conventional COSY-type experiments is often better suited for assignment purposes. Finally, in NMR studies on macromolecules, it is important to maximize the spectral dispersion in both dimensions. Thus, while SECSY was of value in the early days of two-dimensional NMR when the capacity of storage media was more limited, it has in recent times not enjoyed much favour.

FURTHER READING

See the original work of:

Nagayama, K., Kumar, A., Wuthrich, K., and Ernst, R. R. (1980). *J. Magn. Reson.* **40,** 321.

Spin–lattice relaxation, T_1 Spin–lattice relaxation is a process whereby non-radiative energy transfer takes place from an 'excited' spin to the 'lattice' degrees of freedom of the system. The basic principle underlying this relaxation mechanism is described under **relaxation**. More formally, expressions can be derived for the spin–lattice relaxation rate by consideration of transition probabilities between states. These expressions will depend upon the precise mechanism responsible for the relaxation. We will consider as an example, spin–lattice relaxation in a two-spin $\frac{1}{2}$ system IS (see **spin system**), where a dipole–dipole interaction exists between the spins. Dipole–dipole relaxation is actually the most important relaxation mechanism for spins $\frac{1}{2}$ in solution. For simplicity we will assume that the spins are not scalar (J) coupled. If $|\psi_i\rangle$ and $|\psi_j\rangle$ are two eigenstates of the **Hamiltonian** with energies E_i and E_j, we can define a transition probability (per unit time) between these states. To first order, this is given by

$$W_{ij} = (-1/t)(1/\hbar^2)\left|\int_0^t \langle M_j|\mathcal{H}'(t')|M_i\rangle \exp\{-\mathrm{i}\omega_{ij}t'\}\,\mathrm{d}t'\right|^2$$

where

S63 $$\omega_{ij} = (E_j - E_i)/\hbar.$$

In the case of a randomly fluctuating perturbing dipolar **Hamiltonian**, and when these fluctuations are rapid (i.e. in liquids and gases), W is time independent. If we define the four states of the two-spin system as $|\alpha\alpha\rangle$, $|\alpha\beta\rangle$, $|\beta\alpha\rangle$ $|\beta\beta\rangle$, then the transition probabilities per unit time between states are defined in Fig. S21. To each state we can introduce the occupational numbers $N_{\alpha\alpha}$, $N_{\alpha\beta}$, $N_{\beta\alpha}$, $N_{\beta\beta}$ in obvious notation. From the definition of the W's in Fig. S21 it follows that

$$\frac{\mathrm{d}N_{\alpha\alpha}}{\mathrm{d}t} = -(W_S + W_2 + W_I)N_{\alpha\alpha} + W_S N_{\alpha\beta} + W_2 N_{\beta\beta} + W_I N_{\beta\alpha}$$

$$\frac{\mathrm{d}N_{\alpha\beta}}{\mathrm{d}t} = -(W_S + W_I + W_0)N_{\alpha\beta} + W_S N_{\alpha\alpha} + W_0 N_{\beta\alpha} + W_I N_{\beta\beta}$$

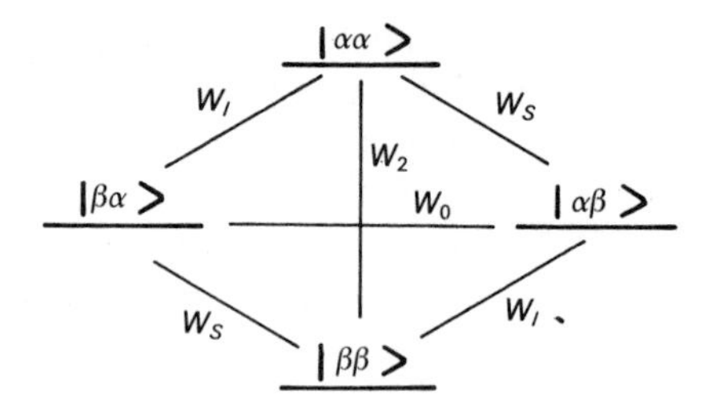

Fig. S21. Transition probabilities per unit time between eigenstates of the longitudinal components of spin operators.

S64

$$\frac{dN_{\beta\alpha}}{dt} = -(W_I + W_S + W_0)N_{\beta\alpha} + W_I N_{\alpha\alpha} + W_S N_{\beta\beta} + W_0 N_{\alpha\beta}$$

$$\frac{dN_{\beta\beta}}{dt} = -(W_I + W_S + W_2)N_{\beta\beta} + W_S N_{\beta\alpha} + W_I N_{\alpha\beta} + W_2 N_{\alpha\alpha}$$

where we ignore constant terms dependent upon the relevant Boltzman factor. Now the z-component magnetization for each of spins I and S is proportional to the difference in occupation numbers across the relevant transitions:

S65

$$\langle I_z \rangle \alpha (N_{\beta\beta} + N_{\beta\alpha}) - (N_{\alpha\beta} + N_{\alpha\alpha})$$

$$\langle S_z \rangle \alpha (N_{\beta\beta} + N_{\alpha\beta}) - (N_{\beta\alpha} + N_{\alpha\alpha}).$$

Inserting these values into (S64) gives

S66

$$\frac{d\langle I_z \rangle}{dt} = -(W_0 + 2W_I + W_2)(\langle I_z \rangle - I_0) - (W_2 - W_0)(\langle S_z \rangle - S_0)$$

$$\frac{d\langle S_z \rangle}{dt} = -(W_0 + 2W_S + W_2)(\langle S_z \rangle - S_0) - (W_2 - W_0)(\langle I_z \rangle - I_0),$$

where I_0 and S_0 are the equilibrium values of the magnetization of spins I and S. These equations are the **Bloch equations**, with the inclusion of a term representing the IS interaction. Frequently, these equations are written in a slightly different form:

S67

$$\frac{d\langle I_z \rangle}{dt} = -\rho_I(\langle I_z \rangle - I_0) - \sigma_{IS}(\langle S_z \rangle - S_0)$$

$$\frac{d\langle S_z \rangle}{dt} = -\rho_S(\langle S_z \rangle - S_0) - \sigma_{SI}(\langle I_z \rangle - I_0)$$

where

$$\rho_I = W_0 + 2W_I + W_2$$

$$\rho_S = W_0 + 2W_S + W_2$$

$$\sigma_{IS} = \sigma_{SI} = W_2 - W_0$$

The ρ's are commonly known as the direct relaxation rate constants, and the σ's are known as the cross-relaxation rate constants. Equations (S67) show that, in general, the decay of longitudinal magnetization is not a simple exponential, but is a linear combination of two exponentials (see below). If, however, $\omega_I = \omega_S$, then the observed quantity is $\langle I_z \rangle + \langle S_z \rangle$, and since $W_I = W_S$ the rate of decay of the magnetization will be

S68
$$\frac{d(\langle I_z \rangle) + \langle S_z \rangle)}{dt} = -2(W_I + W_2)(\langle I_z \rangle + \langle S_z \rangle - I_0 - S_0)$$

giving an exponential decay with a rate constant

S69
$$\frac{1}{T_1} = 2W_I + 2W_2 = \rho + \sigma.$$

Thus we can only strictly define T_1 according to (S69) when the Larmor frequencies of the coupled spins are identical. When this is not the case, a single T_1 value cannot be described since the relaxation is not a single exponential.

To proceed, it is necessary to derive explicit expressions for the transitions probabilities W_I, W_S, W_0 and W_2. This is achieved by evaluating (S63) by inserting of the relevant eigenstates, energies, and the dipolar Hamiltonian. Assuming that the **autocorrelation function** is exponential (see **relaxation**) with a time constant τ_c, i.e. the overall motion is isotropic, then the transition probabilities are

S70
$$W_I = \frac{3}{20}\frac{\gamma_I^2\gamma_S^2\hbar^2}{r^6}\cdot\frac{\tau_c}{1+\omega_I^2\tau_c^2}$$
$$W_S = \frac{\gamma_I^2\gamma_S^2\hbar^2}{r^6}\cdot\frac{\tau_c}{1+\omega_S^2\tau_c^2}$$
$$W_0 = \frac{1}{10}\frac{\gamma_I^2\gamma_S^2\hbar^2}{r^6}\cdot\frac{\tau_c}{1+(\omega_I-\omega_S)^2\tau_c^2}$$
$$W_2 = \frac{3}{5}\frac{\gamma_I^2\gamma_S^2\hbar^2}{r^6}\cdot\frac{\tau_c}{1+(\omega_I+\omega_S)^2\tau_c^2}$$

where τ_c is the correlation time for the internuclear vector of length r under the (assumed isotropic) motion. Thus, in the case of two spins with $\omega_I = \omega_S = \omega$, we find from (S69)

S71
$$\frac{1}{T_1} = \frac{6}{20}\frac{\gamma^4\hbar^2}{r^6}\left[\frac{\tau_c}{1+\omega^2\tau_c^2} + \frac{4\tau_c}{1+4\omega^2\tau_c^2}\right].$$

Note that (S71) contains two terms, one containing a frequency characteristic at ω, and the second carrying a frequency characteristic at 2ω. These are the spectral density functions $J(\omega)$ and $J(2\omega)$. Equation (S71), together with similar expressions for the **spin–spin relaxation** time T_2, are known as the Solomon–Bloembergen equations. In the case of **anisotropic motion**, these equations do not hold, and must be modified to take into account the different motional characteristics. In addition, the presence of motional cross-correlation can influence the form of these equations. Some may find difficulty with the notion that T_1 is only defined according to (S71) when $\omega_I = \omega_S$. There are many examples in the literature where 'T_1' values are reported for spin systems where $\omega_I \neq \omega_S$. We rationalize this anomaly by noting that for a large number of systems of practical interest, the decay of longitudinal magnetization (determined by, for example, the **inversion recovery sequence**) is very nearly exponential, and a 'T_1' can be defined. We can illustrate this with two examples. Consider an experiment where spin I is inverted by a 180° pulse, and spin S is undisturbed. The boundary conditions for the coupled differential equations (S67) are thus $\langle I_z \rangle = -I_0$, $\langle S_z \rangle = S_0$ at $t = 0$. Solution of these equations using the initial values gives at time t

S72 $$(I_0 - \langle I_z \rangle)/I_0 = 2C \exp\{-\lambda_1 t\} + 2(1 - C) \exp\{-\lambda_2 t\}$$

with

$$\lambda_1 = \tfrac{1}{2}(\rho_I + \rho_S) + \tfrac{1}{2}[(\rho_I - \rho_S)^2 + 4\sigma_{IS}^2]^{\frac{1}{2}}$$
$$\lambda_2 = \tfrac{1}{2}(\rho_I + \rho_S) - \tfrac{1}{2}[(\rho_I - \rho_S)^2 + 4\sigma_{IS}^2]^{\frac{1}{2}}$$
$$C = (\lambda_1 - \rho_S)/(\lambda_1 - \lambda_2).$$

Equations (S72) illustrate the double exponential relaxation behaviour described above. Plots of $\log(I_0 - \langle I_z \rangle)$ against t will not in principle be linear. However, in a large number of cases, the plot is very nearly linear, and 'T_1' can be extracted from the slope (see e.g. **inversion recovery sequence**). But what is the relationship between this measured 'T_1' and ρ and σ?. Consider two limiting cases. First, if $\rho_I \sim \rho_S = \rho$, then $\sigma_{IS} \gg |\rho_I - \rho_S|$, and (S72) becomes

S73 $$(I_0 - \langle I_z \rangle)/I_0 = 3 \exp\{-(\rho - \sigma)t\} - \exp\{-(\rho + \sigma)t\}.$$

Now ρ is always larger than σ, and thus the right-hand side of (S73) will approximate to a single exponential with

S74 $$\frac{1}{T_1} \approx \rho_I.$$

A second example considers the case when $\rho_I \neq \rho_S$, and $|\rho_I - \rho_S| \gg \sigma_{IS}$. Thus we can make the approximation

S75 $$[1 + (\sigma^2/(\rho_I - \rho_S)^2)]^{\frac{1}{2}} \approx 1 + \tfrac{1}{2}(\sigma^2/(\rho_I - \rho_S)^2)$$

and λ_1 and λ_2 become

S76
$$\lambda_1 \approx \rho_I + [\sigma^2/(\rho_I - \rho_S)] + \ldots$$
$$\lambda_2 \approx \rho_I - [\sigma^2/(\rho_I - \rho_S)] + \ldots$$

and

S77
$$[I_0 - \langle I_z \rangle]/I_0 \approx 2\exp\{-\rho_I t\}$$

which is again a single exponential with

S78
$$\frac{1}{T_1} \approx \rho_I.$$

In the absence of cross-relaxation, (S78) is exact. Equations (S74) and (S78) thus differ from (S69) only in the sense of what is being measured; in the case that $\omega_I = \omega_S$, the magnetizations of the individual spins cannot be measured independently.

The above has assumed that a dipole–dipole relaxation mechanism exists between spins. Other mechanisms exist which contribute to the spin–lattice relaxation. In the absence of **chemical exchange**, all of these (with the exception of modulated scalar coupling) contribute to ρ but not σ. When several such mechanisms contribute, the total direct relaxation rate is equal to the sum of the relaxation rates over all mechanisms.

See also **quadrupole relaxation**, **spin–rotation relaxation**, **scalar coupling relaxation**, **anisotropic chemical shift relaxation**, **anisotropic motion**, **rotating frame spin–lattice relaxation**.

FURTHER READING

See the classic paper:

Solomon, I. (1955). *Phys. Rev.* **99,** 559

Spin-locking Consider a simple pulse-and-collect NMR experiment (Fig. S22) described in terms of the **classical formalism**. A 90° pulse along the x' axis in the rotating frame generates transverse magnetization along the y' axis. If a second pulse is now applied along the y' axis, the magnetization

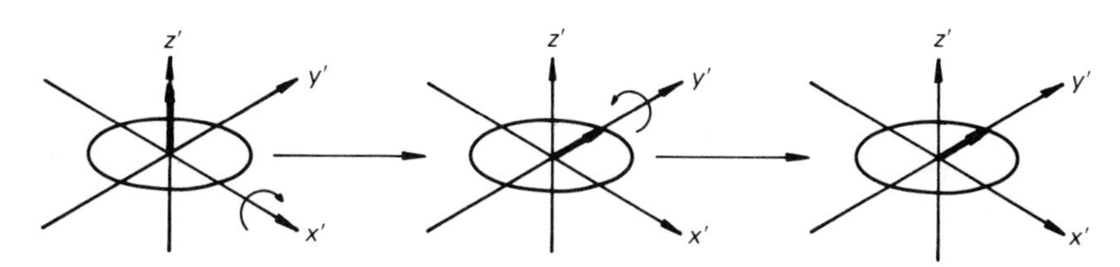

Fig. S22. Diagrammatic representation of spin locking. See text for details.

will effectively be locked along this axis by the r.f. field. This phenomenon, which is known as spin-locking, is essential for the workings of several coherence transfer experiments. In heteronuclear NMR, spin-locking can be described in terms of the doubly rotating frame. When the **Hartmann–Hahn condition** is satisfied, coherence transfer between heteronuclei becomes efficient since they are effectively 'energy matched'. A similar strategy can be employed in homonuclear NMR, giving rise to **total correlation spectroscopy** (TOCSY) and **homonuclear Hartmann–Hahn spectroscopy** (HOHAHA). Efficient spin-locking requires that off-resonance effects are compensated, such that all nuclei experience the same effective field. This is usually achieved by phase modulation of the spin-lock field, using cyclic **composite pulses**.

A second class of experiment which makes use of spin-locking is **rotating frame Overhauser effect spectroscopy** (ROESY). This is effectively a transverse **nuclear Overhauser effect** experiment which depends upon **spin–lattice relaxation** in the rotating frame (see **rotating frame spin–lattice relaxation**) rather than conventional T_1 relaxation.

Spinning sidebands In order to average the effects of inhomogeneity in the transverse components of the static magnetic field B_0, it is common practice to spin the NMR sample about its long axis at a rate which is fast compared with the linewidth of the static sample. In this manner the transverse field experienced by the sample is averaged, resulting in a higher effective resolution. Unfortunately, this procedure carries with it a class of artefacts known as spinning sidebands. Since the field experienced by any given microscopic volume element changes with time due to the rotation, then the effective field experienced by spins in this volume element will also change. The rate of precession will therefore experience **frequency modulation**, resulting in a family of sidebands spaced either side of the resonance line, at distances which are multiples of the spinner speed. Since the modulation index is low, generally only the first-order sidebands are visible, unless the transverse homogeneity is particularly poor. Correspondingly, spinning sidebands are often only visible on strong solvent resonance lines.

Apart from B_0 inhomogeneity, other effects contribute to the generation of spinning sidebands. Important amongst these is B_1 inhomogeneity. This can be understood simply in terms of an **amplitude modulation** of the free induction decay as the various microscopic volume elements rotate in the receiver coil during the detection period. The spins contained within these volume elements will induce an e.m.f. which is dependent upon the coupling of the spins to the receiver coil. However, combinations of B_1 inhomogeneity and other factors such as sample tube asymmetry can influence the magnitude of spinning sidebands, and it is difficult to optimize all of these factors for minimum spinning sideband intensity.

Spin order See **longitudinal spin order**.

Spin–rotation relaxation The spin–rotation interaction results from magnetic fields generated at a nucleus by the **magnetic moment** of the molecule (rather than another nucleus). The molecular magnetic moment derives in turn from the electron distribution in the molecule. The **Hamiltonian** for this interaction is given by

S79 $$\mathcal{H}_{SR} = \sum_m \sum_i \mathbf{I}_i \mathbf{C}_{i,m} \mathbf{J}_m$$

where $\mathbf{C}$ is the spin–rotation interaction **tensor** and $\mathbf{J}_m$ is the molecular angular momentum. Fluctuations in the local field at the resonant nuclei in the molecule arise from changes in the direction or both direction and magnitude in the angular momentum. For molecules undergoing isotropic molecular reorientation in liquids, the relaxation rate is given by

S80 $$\frac{1}{T_1} = \left[\frac{2\pi IkT}{h^2}\right] C_{\text{eff}}^2 \tau_J$$

where I is the moment of inertia of the molecule, k is the Boltzmann constant, and T is the absolute temperature. The parameter τ_J represents the angular momentum correlation time, and $C_{\text{eff}}^2 = 1/3(2C_\perp^2 + C_\parallel^2)$, where $C_\parallel$ and $C_\perp$ refer to the interaction along and perpendicular to the symmetry axis. The value of τ_J is related to the molecular reorientational correlation time by

S81 $$\tau_c \tau_J = I/6kT.$$

An important distinction between this relaxation mechanism and all others is that τ_J becomes larger with increasing temperature, whereas τ_c becomes shorter. Therefore T_1 becomes longer as the temperature decreases, which is the opposite to that observed for liquid samples in the extreme narrowing limit with regard to other relaxation mechanisms.

Spin space The **classical formalism** attempts a pictorial representation of NMR experiments in terms of the motion of classical vectors with respect to three orthogonal axes. These axes are functionally identical to the cartesian coordinate system used in simple geometry. On the other hand, the quantum mechanical treatment of NMR depends upon the commutation properties of the **angular momentum** operators. Just as the classical formalism describes manipulations in cartesian space, the quantum mechanical formalism can, by analogy, be thought of as manipulations in spin space, i.e. a vector space spanned by the relevant **operators**. Now the **density matrix** of states corresponding with a given state of the **spin system** can be expanded into a suitable basis set (see **basis state**) of operators. By judicious choice of such operators, the spin space can be functionally equated with cartesian space, as described under **product operator formalism**. In other circumstances, no such simplification exists, and it is difficult to visualize quantum mechanical manipulations classically.

The distinction between cartesian space and spin space is important when considering the effects of **averaging**.

Spin–spin relaxation, T_2 In contrast to **spin–lattice relaxation** (T_1), the phenomenon of spin–spin relaxation (T_2) is not intuitively obvious. Indeed, it is less easy to understand in simple physical terms. Just as T_1 relaxation describes relaxation processes responsible for the decay of longitudinal magnetization (see **classical formalism**), T_2 relaxation describes relaxation processes responsible for the decay of transverse magnetization, and hence is sometimes called the transverse relaxation time. However, T_2 relaxation does not involve the exchange of spin energy with the lattice, but is concerned with the exchange of energy between spins, via a flip-flop type mechanism. For this reason T_2 is usually known as the spin–spin relaxation time. According to the classical formalism the application of an r.f. field at the **Larmor precession** frequency generates a state of **phase coherence** between spins, which results in net transverse magnetization. In simple physical terms, T_2 relaxation can be understood as a process which causes a loss in phase coherence, due to the mutual exchange of spin energies. Consequently, the net transverse magnetization decays with time.

The processes responsible for spin-lattice relaxation also contribute to spin–spin relaxation (see **relaxation**), but T_2 contains an additional 'zero frequency' term, represented by the spectral density function $J(0)$, i.e.

$$\frac{1}{T_1} = J(\omega) + J(2\omega)$$

S82

$$\frac{1}{T_2} = J(0) + J(\omega) + J(2\omega).$$

In similar fashion to the measurement of T_1, T_2 can be measured by plotting the time dependence of the transverse magnetization created following a 90° pulse. This is of course identical to the time constant for the **free induction decay** (FID). However, unlike T_1 the measured value of T_2 is severely affected by instrumental imperfections. In fact the decay rate of the FID is always greater than $1/T_2$, since magnetic field inhomogeneity is an important contributor. This is because each nucleus in a given sample experiences a slightly different value of B_0, and thus precesses at a slightly different frequency from other nuclei. The result is a 'fanning out' of each individual magnetization vector, with a loss in phase coherence similar to that induced by 'authentic' T_2 processes. Sometimes the term T_2^* is introduced when the measured value of T_2 contains contributions from magnetic field inhomogeneity. Nevertheless it is possible to measure T_2 in the absence of inhomogeneous contributions by using the **Carr–Purcell–Meiboom–Gill** pulse sequence. This sequence creates a spin echo in the transverse plane, where effects due to magnetic field inhomogeneity are refocused. The decay of transverse magnetization is simply plotted as a function of the length of the spin echo sequence determined by the repetition number n:

$$90°_{+x} - \tau - [180°_y - 2\tau]_n - 180°_y - \tau - Acq$$

Since magnetic field inhomogeneity directly affects linewidth in NMR spectra, it might be anticipated that T_2 is also related to the linewidth. This is indeed the case, since the dephasing of the phase coherence leads to a 'spreading' in the frequency domain. The linewidth at half height of a resonance line is given by

S83 $$\Delta\nu_{\frac{1}{2}} = \frac{1}{\pi T_2^*}.$$

Another means by which the relationship of T_2 to linewidth may be understood is in terms of the **uncertainty principle**. As T_2 becomes smaller, the decay rate of the FID becomes larger, and we can observe the detected signal for a shorter period of time. This leads to an 'uncertainty' in the frequency components of the time-domain signal, which results in line broadening. In order to examine the relevance of T_2 measurements, it is necessary to consider the relaxation mechanism in more detail. In analogy to spin–lattice relaxation, Solomon (1955) has derived a series of equations to describe T_2 for the case of two dipolar coupled spins IS. These may conveniently be described in terms of the transition probabilities per unit time between eigenstates of the transverse components of spin operators (Fig. S23). Using a procedure identical to that described under **spin–lattice relaxation**, the following

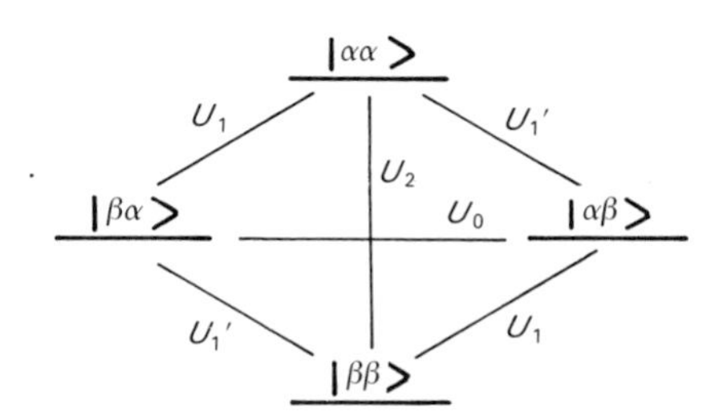

Fig. S23. Transition probabilities per unit time between eigenstates of transverse components of spin operators.

equations are obtained for the decay of transverse magnetization:

S84
$$\frac{d\langle I_x \rangle}{dt} = -(U_0 + 2U_1 + U_2)I_x - (U_2 - U_0)S_x$$
$$\frac{d\langle S_x \rangle}{dt} = -(U_0 + 2U_1' + U_2)S_x - (U_2 - U_0)I_x.$$

Unlike longitudinal magnetization components, (S84) cannot be compared directly with the macroscopic **Bloch equations** since the spin operators are time independent, and thus describe the motion of I_x and S_x in the **rotating frame**. However, it is possible to represent the motion of I_x and S_x by a set of modified Bloch equations in the rotating frame. These are given by

S85
$$\frac{dI^+}{dt} = -\nu I^+ - \mu \exp\{-i(\omega_S - \omega_I)t\}S^+$$
$$\frac{dS^+}{dt} = -\nu' S^+ - \mu \exp\{-i(\omega_I - \omega_S)t\}I^+$$

with Larmor frequencies for spins I and S equal to ω_I and ω_S respectively, with the **shift operators**

S86
$$I^+ = I_x + iI_y, \qquad S^+ = S_x + iS_y$$

and with

$$\nu = U_0 + 2U_1 + U_2$$
$$\nu' = U_0 + 2U_1' + U_2$$

and

$$\mu = U_2 - U_0.$$

Equations (S85) have a particularly simple interpretation in two limiting cases. Firstly, in the case of 'like' spins, $\omega_S = \omega_I$ and (S85) give,

S87
$$\frac{d}{dt}(I^+ + S^+) = -(\nu + \mu)(I^+ + S^+).$$

Secondly, in the case of 'unlike' spins, where the shift difference is large compared to the linewidths, the terms $\exp\{-i(\omega_S - \omega_I)\}$ and $\exp\{-i(\omega_I - \omega_S)\}$ represent rapid **phase modulation** and the last terms will average out so that

S88
$$\frac{dI^+}{dt} = -\nu I^+, \qquad \frac{dS^+}{dt} = -\nu' S^+.$$

So in these limiting cases, transverse relaxation occurs with a simple exponential decay, and the behaviour of I_x and S_x can be described by a single relaxation time:

S89 $$\frac{\mathrm{d}I_x}{\mathrm{d}t} = -\frac{1}{T_2} \cdot I_x$$

For cases where the spins are neither 'like' nor 'unlike', (i.e. partially overlapping lines), intermediate values of T_2 are expected, and the behaviour of the transverse relaxation may be non exponential. Explicit expressions for U_0, U_1, U_1', and U_2 can be obtained in an analogous manner to ω_0, ω_1, ω_2 in spin–lattice relaxation. These depend upon whether the spins are 'like' or 'unlike'. In the case of like spins, $\omega_I = \omega_S = \omega$, and

S90
$$U_0 = \frac{\gamma^4 \hbar^2 \tau_c}{8r^6}\left[\frac{1}{5} + \frac{3}{5} \cdot \frac{1}{1 + 4\omega^2 \tau_c^2}\right]$$
$$U_1 = U_1' = \frac{\gamma^4 \hbar^2 \tau_c}{8r^6}\left[\frac{3}{5} \cdot \frac{1}{1 + \omega^2 \tau_c^2} + \frac{3}{5} \cdot \frac{1}{1 + 4\omega^2 \tau_c^2}\right]$$
$$U_2 = \frac{\gamma^4 \hbar^2 \tau_c}{8r^6}\left[\frac{9}{5} + \frac{12}{5} \cdot \frac{1}{1 + \omega^2 \tau_c^2} + \frac{3}{5} \cdot \frac{1}{1 + 4\omega^2 \tau_c^2}\right],$$

and using (S87) we find

S91 $$\frac{1}{T_2} = (\nu + \mu) = 2(U_1 + U_2)$$

S92 $$= \frac{1}{20} \cdot \frac{\gamma^4 \hbar^2}{r^6}\left[9\tau_c + \frac{15\tau_c}{(1 + \omega^2 \tau_c^2)} + \frac{6\tau_c}{(1 + 4\omega^2 \tau_c^2)}\right].$$

In the case of 'unlike' spins, the transition probabilities are

S93
$$U_0 = U_2 = \frac{\gamma_I^2 \gamma_S^2 \hbar^2 \tau_c}{8r^6}\left[\frac{4}{5}\left(1 + \frac{1}{8} \cdot \frac{1}{1 + (\omega_I - \omega_S)^2 \tau_c^2}\right) + \frac{3}{10} \times \left(\frac{2}{1 + \omega_I^2 \tau_c^2} + \frac{2}{1 + \omega_S^2 \tau_c^2}\right) + \frac{3}{5}\left(\frac{1}{1 + (\omega_I + \omega_S)^2 \tau_c^2}\right)\right]$$
$$U_1 = \frac{\gamma_I^2 \gamma_S^2 \hbar^2 \tau_c}{8r^6}\left[\frac{1}{10}\left(\frac{1}{1 + (\omega_I - \omega_S)^2 \tau_c^2}\right) + \frac{3}{5}\left(\frac{1}{1 + \omega^2 \tau_c^2}\right) + \frac{3}{5}\left(\frac{1}{1 + (\omega_I + \omega_S)^2 \tau_c^2}\right)\right]$$
$$U_1' = \frac{\gamma_I^2 \gamma_S^2 \hbar^2 \tau_c}{8r^6}\left[\frac{1}{10}\left(\frac{1}{1 + (\omega_I - \omega_S)^2 \tau_c^2}\right) + \frac{3}{5}\left(\frac{1}{1 + \omega_I^2 \tau_c^2}\right) + \frac{3}{5}\left(\frac{1}{1 + (\omega_I + \omega_S)^2 \tau_c^2}\right)\right].$$

Note that these are quite different from the probabilities for 'like' spins. In contrast, the probabilities for T_1 relaxation in the case of 'like' spins are simple generalizations for those in the case of 'unlike' spins. Using (S88), the expression for T_2 in the case of unlike spins is for spin I

$$\frac{1}{T_2} = \nu = U_0 + 2U_1 + U_2$$

S94
$$= \frac{1}{20}\frac{\gamma_I^2\gamma_S^2\hbar^2}{r^6}\left[4\tau_c + \frac{\tau_c}{1+(\omega_I-\omega_S)^2\tau_c^2} + \frac{3\tau_c}{1+\omega_I^2\tau_c^2} + \frac{6\tau_c}{1+\omega_S^2\tau_c^2} + \frac{6\tau_c}{1+(\omega_I+\omega_S)^2\tau_c^2}\right],$$

where the expression for spin S is obtained by interchanging I spin and S spin labels.

In the case of like spins, in the **extreme narrowing** limit, $\omega^2\tau_c^2 \ll 1$, the expression for the transverse relaxation rate reduces to

S95
$$\frac{1}{T_2} = \frac{3}{2}\frac{\gamma^4\hbar^2}{r^6}\cdot\tau_c$$

which is exactly that for the longitudinal relaxation rate under the same conditions.

From (S92) or (S94) we can see that the transverse relaxation rate corresponds to terms in zero frequency, ω, and 2ω, which is consistent with the second of (S82). In contrast, T_1 contains no zero-frequency terms. The implication of this is that in the presence of slow molecular motion T_2 becomes very small since the zero-frequency term dominates (and, incidentally, T_1 becomes large by the reverse argument). Thus, from (S83), narrow lines are indicative of fast motions. This is a useful rule of thumb, which can be applied in macromolecular NMR to distinguish 'mobile' and 'rigid' regions of the molecule. However, it must be used with care since the term r^{-6} also contributes to T_2, and broad lines may result from a particularly efficient relaxation pathway (e.g. several nuclei at a short distance).

FURTHER READING

See the classic paper:

Solomon, I. (1955). *Phys. Rev.* **99**, 559.

Spin system In NMR, we are concerned exclusively with nuclei which possess the property of spin. A collection of such nuclei between which spin–spin interactions exist is known as a spin system. In NMR of liquids, a notation is in general use for the description of certain types of spin system. Consider the case of a loosely coupled two-spin system. We may

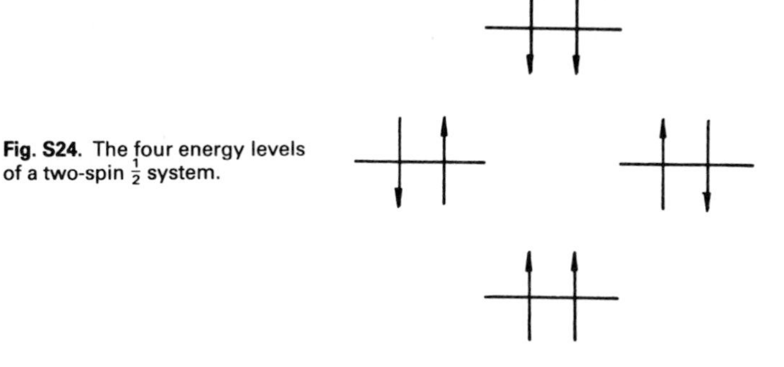

Fig. S24. The four energy levels of a two-spin $\frac{1}{2}$ system.

conveniently represent each spin by labelling it with a letter of the alphabet. We choose these letters to be well spaced in the alphabet to indicate that the spin system is loosely coupled (a large difference in Larmor frequencies). A two-spin system is thus often referred to as an *AX* or *IS* system. It is composed of four interconnecting energy levels (Fig. S24). A second type of two-spin system can be distinguished if the two nuclei are strongly coupled (see **strong coupling**). This situation arises if the difference in Larmor frequencies of the spins is of the order of the magnitude of the spin coupling constant. This system is often referred to as an *AB* system. The letters are chosen to be close in the alphabet to indicate that the system of interest is strongly coupled. The energy-level diagram is indistinguishable from Fig. S24, but the **eigenvalues** are different.

In the case of three spins, we can describe an *AMX* spin system which represents three loosely coupled spins, which has an energy-level diagram as shown in Fig. S25. Similarly we can define an *ABX* spin system to

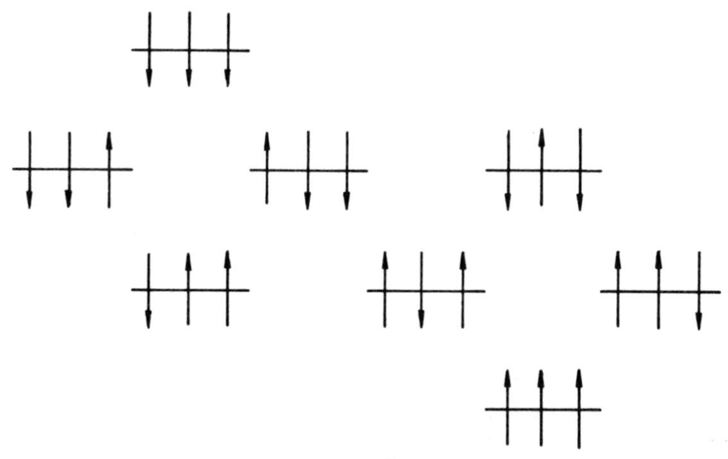

Fig. S25. The eight energy levels of a three-spin $\frac{1}{2}$ system.

indicate that protons A and B weakly coupled to X. This notation is used freely throughout this volume. Generalization to larger spin systems is obviously quite straightforward.

The concept of a spin system can in many cases considerably simplify calculations in macromolecules in the liquid state. For example, if relaxation is ignored, important features of many two-dimensional NMR experiments can be calculated by considering only those spins which are scalar coupled. In the case of proteins, each amino acid residue is essentially an isolated spin system. Likewise, the bases in nucleic acids and monosaccharide residues of oligosaccharides can often be considered in isolation. It is therefore possible, for example, to optimize a particular aspect of a given experiment in terms of the residue in question. This approach forms the basis for spin filtration (see **multiple-quantum filters**).

Spin temperature In many respects it is useful to consider a spin system as a thermodynamic system. In this way spin systems can be considered to behave in an analogous manner as those systems usually considered in thermodynamics, for which the concept of temperature has been proven experimentally.

The concept of spin temperature may be understood by reference to a spin system isolated from the lattice and subjected to spin–spin interactions. This system will proceed towards a state of internal equilibrium such that the probabilities of finding the system in any of its energy levels are given by a Boltzmann distribution $\exp\{-E/kT_s\}$, where k is the Boltzmann constant, E is the energy difference between states and T_s is the spin temperature. In most cases, the 'energy per spin' is much smaller than kT_s. Under these conditions the **density matrix** can be expanded to first order:

$$\sigma \approx 1 - \frac{\hbar \mathcal{H}}{kT_s} \tag{S96}$$

where we ignore a constant of proportionality, and $\mathcal{H}$ is a **Hamiltonian**. Equation S96 is valid in the 'high-temperature approximation' i.e. at temperatures above a few Kelvin.

FURTHER READING

Goldman, M. (1970). *Spin temperature and NMR in solids.* Oxford University Press, London.

Spin-tickling Spin-tickling refers to the selective perturbation of a single resonance line. The r.f. field is weak compared to the scalar coupling but strong compared to the linewidth such that splittings of the lines remain observable. The purpose of this procedure is to elucidate the connectivity of transitions in coupled spin systems. Each transition connected to the irradiated transition is split into a 'tickling doublet'. Transitions that are not connected to the irradiated transition remain unaffected, while the irradiated transition itself splits into a triplet.

In addition, the linewidths of the tickling doublets allow for the determination of whether the connectivity is progressive or regressive (see **connectivity networks**). For progressive connectivity, the linewidths of the tickling doublets are larger than for an unconnected transition, while for regressive connectivity the linewidths are smaller.

FURTHER READING

A comprehensive explanation of spin tickling is given by

Freeman, R., and Anderson, W. A. (1962). *J. Chem. Phys.* **37,** 2053.

See also

Ernst, R. R., Bodenhausen, G., and Wokaun, A. (1987). *Principles of NMR in one and two dimensions.* Clarendon Press, Oxford, pp. 230–233.

Spin-warp imaging See **imaging**.

Splitting See **spin coupling**.

SPT See **selective population transfer**.

Stationary state See **variational method**.

Steady state nuclear Overhauser effect See **nuclear Overhauser effect**.

Stokes–Einstein relation A major difficulty in **relaxation** studies is the determination of the correlation time τ_c characterizing the motion of the molecule. In macromolecules, the value of τ_c is unlikely to be longer than the rotational diffusion time of the molecule. This places an upper limit on the value of τ_c. The rotational diffusion time can be calculated for a globular macromolecule by use of the Stokes–Einstein relation. From Stokes' law, the rotational diffusion time for the whole molecule is given by

S97
$$\tau_R = \frac{4\pi\eta a^3}{3kT}$$

where η is the solvent viscosity, a is the radius of the macromolecule, k is the Boltzmann constant, and T the absolute temperature. Equation (S97) can be rewritten as

S98
$$\tau_R = M\bar{V}\eta/RT$$

where M is the molecular weight of the complex, $\bar{V}$ is the partial specific volume, and R is the gas constant.

Strong coupling In many situations of practical interest, a group of spins can be described as weakly coupled (see **weak coupling**). In fact, the assumption that, say, two protons are weakly coupled is an approximation, known as the weak coupling approximation or **high-field approximation**. For this approximation to be valid, the magnitude of the scalar spin coupling constant (J) between the spins must be much less than the chemical shift difference (in Hz) between them. In cases where this is not true, the two protons (or indeed any arbitrary spin system) must be considered as a strongly coupled system. The presence of strong coupling distorts the simple 'doublet of doublets' nature of the NMR spectrum of two coupled protons, until in the limit the chemical shifts of the two protons are identical, resulting in a single resonance line (see Fig. S16). A practical manifestation of strong coupling is that it is not possible to refer to a given resonance line as belonging to spin A or B. In the case of weak coupling, the flipping of one spin does not result in a tendency of any other spins to flip, and discrete resonance lines can be assigned to A spin or B spin transitions. However, in the case of strong coupling, the flipping of one spin results in a probability that its J-coupled neighbour(s) will also flip. Thus, in experiments involving phenomena such as the **nuclear Overhauser effect**, the NOE will in general be dispersed over all resonance lines of the strongly coupled system.

From this simple physical interpretation, it is clear that a theoretical analysis of strong coupling differs from the weak coupling case. In fact we need to include the finite probability that the flipping of a given spin is not independent of al the others. In quantum mechanical terms, we need to allow for mixing of the eigenstates. It was explained under **density matrix** and **matrix representation** that it is necessary to work in the **eigenbasis** of the **Hamiltonian** when calculating the result of a given NMR experiment upon a **spin system**. In the case of weak coupling the eigenbase is simply the **product basis** (Fig. S26). In this basis the weak coupling Hamiltonian is diagonal (see **weak coupling**). In the case of strong coupling, since the eigenstates mix, the simple product base of Fig. S26 is no longer appropriate, and it is necessary to work in the eigenbase of the strongly coupled system. To see why this is necessary, we must consider the form of the Hamiltonian appropriate for a strongly coupled system. This includes the Zeeman term, and the full isotropic coupling Hamiltonian. In the case of two strongly coupled protons, this is

$$\begin{aligned}\mathcal{H} &= \mathcal{H}_Z + \mathcal{H}_J = \omega_I I_z + \omega_S S_z + J\mathbf{I}\,.\,\mathbf{S} \\ &= \omega_I I_z + \omega_S S_z + J(I_x S_x + I_y S_y + I_z S_z)\end{aligned} \quad \text{S99}$$

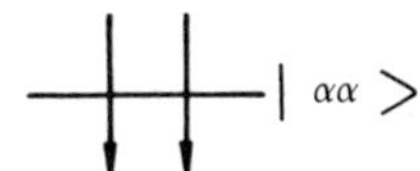

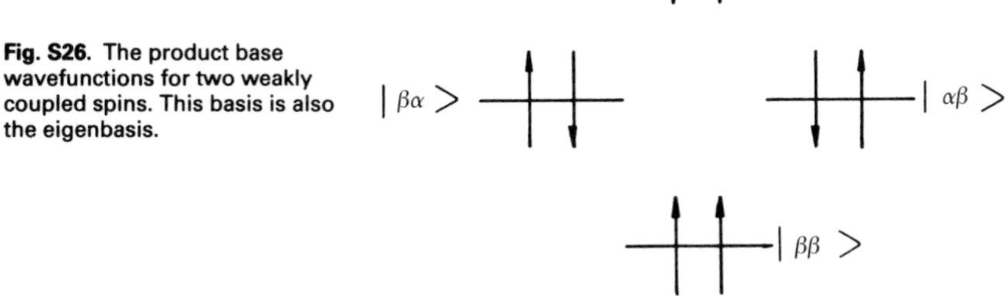

Fig. S26. The product base wavefunctions for two weakly coupled spins. This basis is also the eigenbasis.

where J is measured in Hz.

We can generate a matrix for this Hamiltonian by using the following relation (see **matrix representation**):

S100 $$\mathscr{H}_{m,n} = \langle \psi_m | \mathscr{H} | \psi_n \rangle .$$

If we use the product base wavefunctions for the ψ's, we find

S101 $$\mathscr{H} = \begin{bmatrix} \frac{1}{2}(\omega_I + \omega_S) + \frac{1}{4}J & 0 & 0 & 0 \\ 0 & \frac{1}{2}(\omega_I - \omega_S) - \frac{1}{4}J & \frac{1}{2}J & 0 \\ 0 & \frac{1}{2}J & \frac{1}{2}(-\omega_I + \omega_S) - \frac{1}{4}J & 0 \\ 0 & 0 & 0 & \frac{1}{2}(-\omega_I - \omega_S) + \frac{1}{4}J \end{bmatrix}$$

and thus the product base is not the eigenbase of the isotropic Hamiltonian since the matrix representation is not diagonal. However, if $\delta \gg J$, then the off-diagonal elements are negligible, and the product base becomes the eigenbase. This is the theoretical basis of the weak coupling approximation. It is equivalent to defining a 'truncated' Hamiltonian

S102 $$\mathscr{H} = \omega_I I_z + \omega_S S_z + J I_z S_z$$

which can be proven by recalculating (S101) using (S100) and (S102). If $\delta \approx J$, then we cannot make this approximation, and we need to find a basis set (see **basis state**) of wavefunctions, one for each energy level of the strongly coupled system, which when inserted into (S100) gives a diagonal matrix representation for $\mathscr{H}$. A suitable basis set (**eigenbasis**) can be computed using the **variational method** and is shown in Fig. S27. The angle θ is known as the strong coupling parameter, the magnitude of which is a measure of the 'degree' of strong coupling. Note that only states 2 and 3 mix. Also, when $J \ll \delta$, then θ becomes zero, and we arrive at the simple product base, as of course we should. The manner in which we perform density matrix calculations upon a system such as that shown in Fig. S27 is by generating **rotation operators** and **propagators** in a precisely analogous manner to that described for weakly coupled

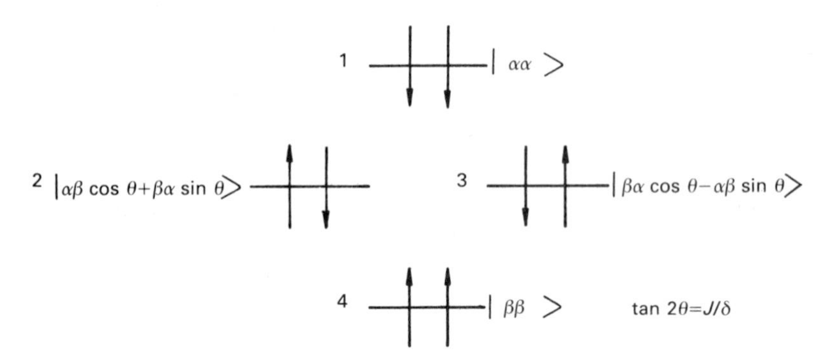

Fig. S27. The eigenbase wavefunctions for two strongly coupled nuclei.

systems (see **density matrix**, **matrix representation**). However, instead of using the product base wavefunction, we use the eigenbase functions of Fig. S27 in the calculation of matrix elements. This leads to the matrices for rotation operators as given in Appendix 4. As an example, consider the case of a strongly coupled two-spin $\frac{1}{2}$ system AB. The rotation operator for an r.f. pulse of flip-angle α along the x axis is given by

$$R_x = \exp\{-\mathrm{i}F_x\alpha\} \tag{S103}$$

which can be rewritten as (see **matrix representation**);

$$R_x = c^2\mathbf{1}_A\mathbf{1}_B - 4s^2I_xS_x - 2isc(\mathbf{1}_A I_{xB} + I_{xA}\mathbf{1}_B) \tag{S104}$$

where $c = \cos(\alpha/2)$ and $s = \sin(\alpha/2)$.

In order to compute the matrix elements $R_{x_{m,n}}$ we use the relation

$$R_{x_{m,n}} = \langle \psi_m | \, R_x \, | \psi_n \rangle \tag{S105}$$

so the matrix element $R_{x_{1,2}}$ is given by

$$\begin{aligned} R_{x_{1,2}} = \langle \alpha\alpha | \, c^2\mathbf{1}_A\mathbf{1}_B - 4s^2I_xS_x - 2isc(\mathbf{1}_A I_{xB} + I_{xA}\mathbf{1}_B) \\ \times |\alpha\beta\cos\theta + \beta\alpha\sin\theta\rangle = isc(\cos\theta + \sin\theta), \end{aligned} \tag{S106}$$

where we have applied analogous operations to those described under matrix representation. Using the notation $u = \cos\theta + \sin\theta$, $v = \cos\theta - \sin\theta$, $u^2 = 1 + \sin 2\theta$, $v^2 = 1 - \sin 2\theta$, $uv = \cos 2\theta$, the complete matrix for R_x is given by

$$R_x(\alpha) = \begin{bmatrix} c^2 & -iucs & -ivcs & -s^2 \\ -iucs & 1 - u^2s^2 & -uvs^2 & -iucs \\ -ivcs & -uvs^2 & 1 - v^2s^2 & -ivcs \\ -s^2 & -iucs & -ivcs & c^2 \end{bmatrix} \tag{S107}$$

which is identical in form to that given in Appendix 4. Free precession is given by a propagator corresponding to the **Hamiltonian** under which the spin system evolves. Since we are working in the eigenbase of the Hamiltonian this propagator is by definition a diagonal matrix:

S108 $$\exp\{-\mathrm{i}\mathscr{H}t\} = \begin{bmatrix} \exp\{-\mathrm{i}E_1 t\} & & & \\ & \exp\{-\mathrm{i}E_2 t\} & & \\ & & \exp\{-\mathrm{i}E_3 t\} & \\ & & & \exp\{-\mathrm{i}E_4 t\} \end{bmatrix}$$

in exact analogy to that formulated in the weak coupling case, except that the E's are now the energies of the states of the strongly coupled system. These can be found from the **eigenvalues** of the Hamiltonian i.e. the diagonal elements of the diagonalized matrix of this Hamiltonian. In standard notation these are

S109 $$\begin{aligned} E_1 &= \tfrac{1}{2}(\omega_A + \omega_B) + \tfrac{1}{4}J \\ E_2 &= \cos^2\theta(\tfrac{1}{2}(\omega_A - \omega_B) - \tfrac{1}{4}J) - \sin^2\theta(-\tfrac{1}{2}(\omega_A - \omega_B) - \tfrac{1}{4}J) = -\tfrac{1}{4}J + C \\ E_3 &= -\sin^2\theta(\tfrac{1}{2}(\omega_A - \omega_B) - \tfrac{1}{4}J) + \cos^2\theta(-\tfrac{1}{2}(\omega_A - \omega_B) - \tfrac{1}{4}J) = -\tfrac{1}{4}J - C \\ E_4 &= -\tfrac{1}{2}(\omega_A + \omega_B) + \tfrac{1}{4}J \end{aligned}$$

where

$$C = \tfrac{1}{2}[(\omega_A - \omega_B)^2 + J^2]^{\frac{1}{2}}, \quad (\omega_A - \omega_B)/2C = \cos 2\theta, \quad J/2C = \sin 2\theta.$$

Thus, in order to calculate the results of pulsed NMR experiments in strongly coupled spin systems, we proceed exactly as for the weak coupling case using the density matrix formalism, but we use the matrices formulated above and listed in Appendix 4. For example, in the case of a simple pulse-and-collect experiment, we would derive $\sigma(t)$ from $\sigma(0)$ using the following transformations:

S110 $$\sigma_{(\mathrm{e})}(t) = \exp\{-\mathrm{i}\mathscr{H}_{(\mathrm{e})}t\} R^{-1}_{x(\mathrm{e})} \sigma_{(\mathrm{e})}(0) R_{x(\mathrm{e})} \exp\{\mathrm{i}\mathscr{H}_{(\mathrm{e})}t\}$$

and the observable (x) magnetization is given by

S111 $$M_x = \mathrm{Tr}\{\sigma(t) F_{x(\mathrm{e})}\}$$

where the subscript (e) represents the eigenbase matrix representations.

The somewhat circuitous route described above has been chosen to describe the inner workings of strongly coupled systems. However, it is not the fastest route to the computation of the results of experiments in strongly coupled systems. A second method which is actually entirely equivalent to the first depends upon the introduction of a matrix U which transforms the matrix of the Hamiltonian computed in the product base (S101) into that in the eigenbase:

S112 $$H_{(\mathrm{e})} = U H_{(\mathrm{p})} U^{-1}$$

where U is given in the case of two strongly coupled protons by

S113 $$U = \begin{bmatrix} 1 & 0 & 0 & 0 \\ 0 & \cos\theta & \sin\theta & 0 \\ 0 & -\sin\theta & \cos\theta & 0 \\ 0 & 0 & 0 & 1 \end{bmatrix}.$$

The reader may care to prove that a diagonal matrix with elements given by (S109) is obtained upon insertion of (S113) (and its inverse) and (S101) into (S112). The value of the matrix U is that in analogy to (S112), we can transform an arbitrary operator from the product base to the eigenbase. For example, (S110) can be rewritten

S114 $$\sigma_{(e)}(t) = \exp\{-i\mathcal{H}_{(e)}t\}UR^{-1}_{x(p)}U^{-1}U\sigma_{(p)}(0)U^{-1}UR_{x(p)}U^{-1}\exp\{i\mathcal{H}_{(e)}t\}$$

and since the product of any matrix and its inverse equals unity, (S114) becomes

S115 $$\sigma_{(e)}t = \exp\{-i\mathcal{H}_{(e)}t\}UR^{-1}_{x(p)}\sigma_{(p)}(0)R_{x(p)}U^{-1}\exp\{i\mathcal{H}_{(e)}t\}$$

which shows that the calculation can be performed in the product base, and then converted to the eigenbasis with U, before considering the evolution. In some cases this is simpler than computation of all matrices in the eigenbasis.

Superoperator In many instances, it is desirable to expand the density operator (**density matrix**) into a suitable set of base operators $\{B_n\}$:

S116 $$\sigma(t) = \sum_{n=1}^{k^2} b_n(t)B_n.$$

A well-known example is the expansion of the density operator into a complete set of cartesian product operators (see **product operator formalism**). The meaning of (S116) can be understood by examining a simple example. In the case of, for example, a two-spin system, the four independent functions associated with each of the four spin states ($\alpha\alpha$, $\alpha\beta$, $\beta\alpha$, $\beta\beta$) span a **Hilbert space** of dimension 4. In the general case a k-spin system has k independent functions associated with it, and these span a Hilbert space of dimension k. When we expand the density matrix according to (S116), we therefore find k^2 independent operators, and these span an operator space of dimension k^2, called Liouville space. In the case of a two-spin system (weakly coupled) the k^2 independent operators are the so called cartesian product operators (see **product operator formalism**).

Since we can define operator relations (such as commutation relations, see **angular momentum**) in Hilbert space, it is obvious to ask whether similar relations exist in Liouville space. Such relations do exist, and they are defined by superoperators and superoperator algebra. Of particular interest in the context of pulsed NMR spectroscopy are commutation superoperators and **unitary transformation** superoperators. In their general representation, superoperators take the form

S117 $$\hat{\hat{S}}A = \sum_{jk} s_{jk} B_j A B_k.$$

As with operators in Hilbert space, we are often interested in the **matrix representation**. The supermatrix elements of the superoperator of (S117) are given by

S118 $$S_{pq,lm} = \sum_{jk} s_{jk} B_{j,pl} B_{k,mq}$$

which may be expressed in terms of direct products:

S119 $$S_{pq,lm} = \sum_{jk} s_{jk} (B_j \otimes \tilde{B}_k)_{pq,lm}$$

where $\tilde{B}_k$ is the transpose of B_k. Appendix 3 explains matrix transposition and direct products. As an example of the use of (S119), we may define the commutator superoperator

S120 $$\hat{\hat{C}}A = CAE - EAC$$

where E is the unitary operator, **1**. The matrix representation of $\hat{\hat{C}}$ is, according to (S119),

S121 $$(\hat{\hat{C}}) = (C) \otimes (\tilde{E}) - (E) \otimes (\tilde{C})$$

where C might be an angular momentum operator, I_x, I_y, or I_z.

The matrix representation of a unitary transformation superoperator

$$\hat{\hat{R}}A = RAR^{-1}$$

is given by

S122 $$(\hat{\hat{R}}) = (R) \otimes (R^*)$$

where * stands for complex conjugate (see **complex number**).

FURTHER READING

Ernst, R. R., Bodenhausen, G., and Wokaun, A. (1987) *Principles of NMR in one and two dimensions*. Clarendon Press, Oxford.

Sweep-width The sweep-width of a spectrometer determines the range of offsets (see **offset**) which may be faithfully recorded during the NMR experiment. This in turn is determined primarily by the sampling rate of the **analogue-to-digital converter** (ADC). The sampling theorem states that in order to reproduce faithfully a signal of frequency f, the sampling rate must be at least $2f$. In practice, if the sampling rate is $2f$, signals of frequency greater than f will still be detected due to **aliasing**. To prevent aliasing of noise components, an **audio-filter** is normally inserted prior to the ADC which has a bandwidth just greater than the sweep-width defined by the ADC.

T

t_1 See **two-dimensional NMR**.

T_1 See **spin–lattice relaxation**.

T_{1_ρ} See **rotating frame spin–lattice relaxation**.

T_2 See **spin–spin relaxation**.

Tensor The tensor notation is of great value in NMR since it allows the transition from one set of axes to another with comparative ease. A vector I has three components I_x, I_y, I_z when referred to a set of orthogonal cartesian axes i, j, k:

$$I = I_x i + I_y j + I_z k. \tag{T1}$$

This is also true of a tensor. However, a cartesian tensor is composed of nine components, which may conveniently be expressed in the form of a 3×3 matrix:

$$T = \begin{bmatrix} T_{xx} & T_{xy} & T_{xz} \\ T_{yx} & T_{yy} & T_{yz} \\ T_{zx} & T_{zy} & T_{zz} \end{bmatrix}. \tag{T2}$$

If T is multiplied from the left by a row vector A (using the normal matrix manipulation, see Appendix 3), the result is a second-row vector $A\,.\,T$. Multiplication from the right by a column vector B gives a new column vector $T\,.\,B$. Thus multiplication from the left by A and the right by B gives a scalar quantity $A\,.\,T\,.\,B$.

As an example of the application of tensor notation, consider the **Hamiltonian** corresponding to the dipolar interaction between two protons:

$$\mathcal{H}_{\mathrm{D}} = \gamma^2\hbar^2\left\{\frac{\mathbf{I}_1 \cdot \mathbf{I}_2}{r^3} - \frac{3(\mathbf{I}_1\,.\,r)(\mathbf{I}_2\,.\,r)}{r^5}\right\} \tag{T3}$$

where the various terms are described under **Hamiltonian**. Firstly, it is necessary to compute the various vector products in (T3). Noting that $\mathbf{I}_1$ is a row vector (I_{1x}, I_{1y}, I_{1z}) and I_2 is the equivalent column vector, and r

is the column vector (x, y, z), we find

$$\mathbf{I}_1 \cdot \mathbf{I}_2 = I_{1x}I_{2x} + I_{1y}I_{2y} + I_{1z}I_{2z}$$

$$I_1 r = I_{1x}x + I_{1y}y + I_{1z}z \qquad \text{T4}$$

$$I_2 r = I_{2x}x + I_{2y}y + I_{2z}z$$

Thus (T3) may be expanded to give

$$H_{\mathrm{D}} = \frac{\gamma^2\hbar^2}{r^5}\{I_{1x}I_{2x}(r^2 - 3x^2) + I_{1y}I_{2y}(r^2 - 3y^2) + I_{1z}I_{2z}(r^2 - 3z^2) - (I_{1x}I_{2y} + I_{1y}I_{2x})3xy - (I_{1y}I_{2z} + I_{1z}I_{2y})3yz - (I_{1z}I_{2x} + I_{1x}I_{2z})3zx\}. \qquad \text{T5}$$

Now (T5) can be written in matrix form as

$$H_{\mathrm{D}} = \gamma^2\hbar^2 \left\{ [I_{1x}, I_{1y}, I_{1z}] \begin{bmatrix} (r^2 - 3x^2)/r^5 & -3xy/r^5 & -3xz/r^5 \\ -3xy/r^5 & (r^2 - 3y^2)/r^5 & -3yz/r^5 \\ -3xz/r^5 & -3yz/r^5 & (r^2 - 3z^2)/r^5 \end{bmatrix} \begin{bmatrix} I_{2x} \\ I_{2y} \\ I_{2z} \end{bmatrix} \right\} \qquad \text{T6}$$

which is equivalent to

$$\mathcal{H}_{\mathrm{D}} = \gamma^2\hbar^2 \mathbf{I}_1 \cdot \mathbf{D} \cdot \mathbf{I}_2 \qquad \text{T7}$$

where **D** is the dipolar coupling tensor.

The presence of off-diagonal elements of **D** indicates that r is not colinear with any of the axes x, y, z (Fig. T1). However, **D** becomes diagonal if $xy = yz = zx = 0$.This condition is realized if r lies along the z axis. We may thus state that **D** is diagonal in terms of a new coordinate system in which the direction of the internuclear vector is the z axis. Under these conditions, the diagonal elements $D_{xx} = 1/r^3$, $D_{yy} = 1/r^3$, $D_{zz} = -2/r^3$ are called the principal values of the tensor. Note that the sum of these values (the trace of the tensor) is equal to zero. In NMR of liquids, D_{xx}, D_{yy}, D_{zz} will fluctuate randomly due to rapid reorientational motion. The time average of such motion is given by $\frac{1}{3}(D_{xx} + D_{yy} + D_{zz}) = 0$. Thus, on the average, the dipolar coupling between spins is zero in solution.

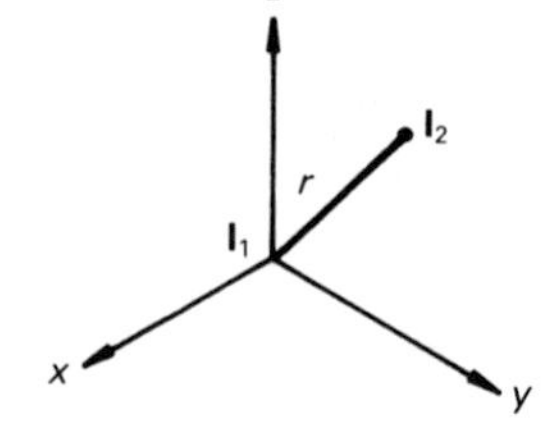

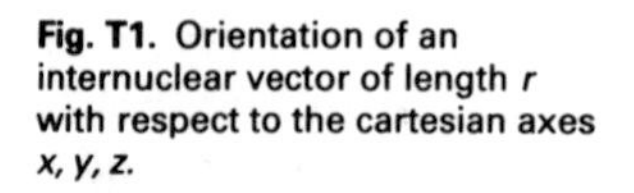
Fig. T1. Orientation of an internuclear vector of length r with respect to the cartesian axes x, y, z.

Fig. T2. Connectivities observed in the three-dimensional HCACO experiment for ^{15}N- and ^{13}C-labelled proteins.

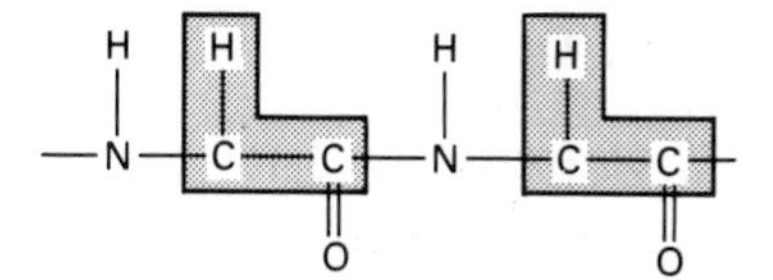

Three-dimensional HCACO experiment The HCACO experiment is a technique devised for ^{15}N- and ^{13}C-labelled proteins which correlates intraresidue Hα, Cα and C′ chemical shifts (Fig. T2). The pulse scheme for this experiment is shown in Fig. T3. An INEPT (see **Insensitive nuclei enhanced by polarization transfer**) sequence is utilized to transfer magnetization originating on Hα protons to the directly-coupled Cα neighbour. During the evolution period t_1, Cα magnetization evolves under the influence of chemical shift as well as the Cα–C′ and Cα–Cβ J couplings. Hα–Cα J coupling is removed by the 180° ^{1}H pulse at the midpoint of t_1. Simultaneous Cα and C′ 90° pulses applied at the end of t_1 result in a COSY-like transfer of magnetization from Cα to C′ and Cβ. Carbonyl evolution proceeds during t_2, while the net effects of ^{1}H–C′ and Cα–C′ couplings are removed by the ^{1}H and Cα 180° pulses applied at

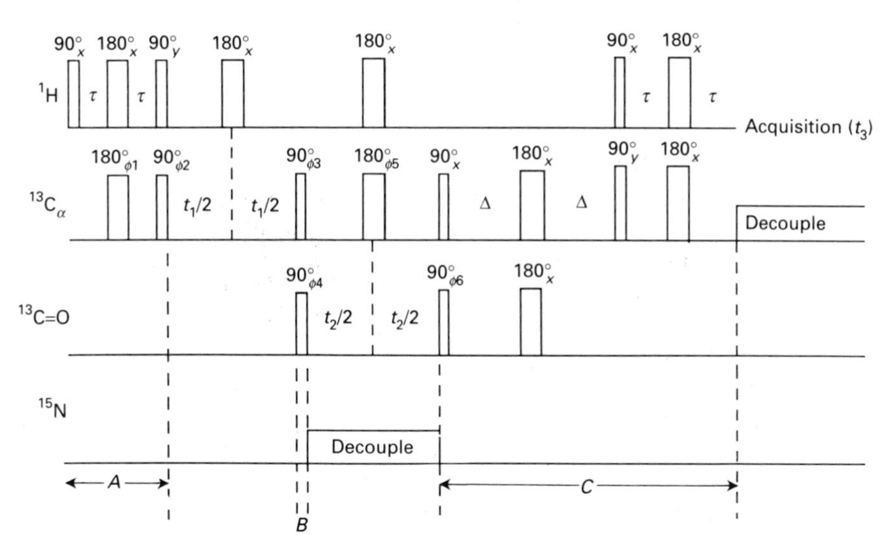

Fig. T3. Pulse scheme for acquisition of three-dimensional HCACO spectra. Typical delay durations are $\tau = 1.5$ ms and $\Delta = 3$ ms. The power levels of the Cα and C′ pulses are adjusted such that during application of a Cα pulse minimal excitation of C′ occurs, and vice versa. In order to minimize the effects of homonuclear J modulation (see ***J* spectroscopy**) by the passive Cα–Cβ couplings during the intervals Δ, a semiselective 180°_x (Cα) pulse may be used. The phase cycling employed is as follows: $\varphi_1 = x, -x$; $\varphi_2 = x$; $\varphi_3 = y, -y$; $\varphi_4 = 2(x), 2(-x)$; $\varphi_5 = 4(x), 4(-x)$; $\varphi_6 = 8(x), 8(-x)$; receiver $= 2(x, -x, -x, x), 2(-x, x, x, -x)$. The phases φ_2 and φ_4 are independently incremented by 90° with appropriate data routing for the acquisition of pure phase spectra (see **phase-sensitive experiments**).

the midpoint of t_2. Decoupling of ^{15}N during t_2 is accomplished by ^{15}N irradiation with a WALTZ (see **broadband decoupling**) modulated r.f. field. At the end of the t_2 period, C′ magnetization is transferred back to the Cα spin, and the Cα magnetization is at this point antiphase with respect to the C′ spin-state. This antiphase magnetization refocusses during the following interval 2Δ, which is set to $\sim 1/3(J_{C'C}\alpha)$ in order to minimize loss of magnetization due to relaxation and dephasing by coupling to the Cβ spin. The dephasing arising from the Cα–Cβ coupling is also reduced by application of a *semiselective* 180° Cα pulse, which results in good inversion of the Cα spins, but poor inversion of most Cβ resonances. At the end of the interval 2Δ, magnetization is transferred back from Cα to Hα via a reverse-INEPT sequence. Since the HCACO experiment detects Hα resonances during t_3 and does not require the presence of amide protons, it is most easily conducted in D_2O solution.

The above magnetization transfer steps can be described more formally by use of the **product operator formalism**. For simplicity, it is convenient to describe only those terms that contribute to the final spectrum, and the effects of certain groups of pulses can be combined into operators $\boldsymbol{A}$, $\boldsymbol{B}$, and $\boldsymbol{C}$, as shown in Fig. T3. Denoting the Hα, Cα and C′ spins by I, A, and S respectively, the salient features of the HCACO pulse sequence can be described as follows

$$I_z \xrightarrow{\boldsymbol{A}} -2I_zA_y \xrightarrow{t_1} -4A_xI_zS_z \cos\omega_A t_1 \sin\pi J_{AS}t_1 \cos\pi J_{AB}t_1 \xrightarrow{\boldsymbol{B}}$$

$$-4S_yI_zA_z \cos\omega_A t_1 \sin\pi J_{AS}t_1 \cos\pi J_{AB}t_1 \xrightarrow{t_2} \qquad \text{T8}$$

$$-4S_yI_zA_z \cos\omega_A t_1 \sin\pi J_{AS}t_1 \cos\pi J_{AB}t_1 \cos\omega_S t_2 \xrightarrow{\boldsymbol{C}}$$

$$I_x \cos\omega_A t_1 \sin\pi J_{AS}t_1 \cos\pi J_{AB}t_1 \cos\omega_S t_2$$

where pulse phases corresponding to the first step of the phase cycle have been assumed, J_{AS} is the Cα–C′ coupling constant, J_{AB} is the Cα–Cβ coupling constant, and ω_A and ω_S are the Cα and C′ chemical shifts. Also, for simplicity the effect of the ^{15}N–Cα coupling during t_1 has been neglected.

Equation T8 indicates that both the active coupling, J_{AS} and the passive coupling, J_{AB} are present during t_1. Phasing the F_1 dimension of the spectrum to pure absorption would result in multiplet components of opposite phase. In practice, it is preferable to phase signals in F_1 to the dispersive mode. If the t_1 acquisition time is set to about $1/(2J_{AB})$ the $\sin\pi J_{AS}t_1 \cos\pi J_{AB}t_1$ time dependence results in an envelope similar to that of a sine bell (see **convolution**). Fourier transformation followed by phasing to the dispersive mode then yields a non-Lorentzian **lineshape** that resembles a singlet which has been convoluted with a sine-bell function. As equation T8 indicates, the lineshapes in both the F_2 and F_3 dimensions are purely absorptive.

FURTHER READING

Theoretical details of the HNCO experiment are described in
Kay, L. E., Ikura, M., Tschudin, M., and Bax, A. (1990). *J. Magn. Reson.* **89,** 496.

For an application of this technique to proteins, see
Ikura, M., Kay, L. E., and Bax, A. (1990). *Biochemistry* **29,** 4659

Three-dimensional HCA(CO)N experiment The HCA(CO)N experiment is a technique devised for ^{15}N- and ^{13}C-labelled proteins which correlates Hα and Cα chemical shifts of one amino acid residue with the ^{15}N shift of the succeeding residue (Fig. T4). The pulse scheme for this experiment is shown in Fig. T5. The magnetization-transfer pathway for this experiment is very similar to that described for the **three-dimensional HCACO experiment**, except that in the present experiment magnetization transferred to the carbonyl carbon (C′) spin is subsequently transferred further to the ^{15}N spin of the next residue. This is accomplished by inclusion of a period $\delta \sim 0.3/J_{NC'}$ during which time the C′ magnetization becomes antiphase with respect to the directly attached ^{15}N spin. The subsequent $90^\circ_{\varphi 5}$ pulse generates two-spin ^{15}N–C′ coherence which evolves during t_2. The C′ $180^\circ_{\varphi 6}$ pulse refocusses the effects of both C′ chemical shifts and the effects of the C′–Cα J coupling so that the signal is only modulated by the ^{15}N shift in t_2. The C′–^{15}N correlation part of the pulse sequence is in fact completely analogous to a conventional **heteronuclear multiple-quantum correlation (HMQC) experiment**. At the end of t_2, magnetization is transferred back to Hα by reverse transfer. The experiment is usually performed with samples in D_2O solution, since NH protons are not required.

The above magnetization transfer steps can be described more formally by use of the **product operator formalism**. For simplicity, it is convenient to describe only those terms that contribute to the final spectrum, and the effects of certain groups of pulses can be combined into operators ***A***, ***B***, and ***C***, as shown in figure T5. Denoting the Hα, Cα and C′ spins by *I, A,* and *S* respectively, and the ^{15}N nucleus of the succeeding residue by N, the salient features of the HCA(CO)N pulse sequence can be described

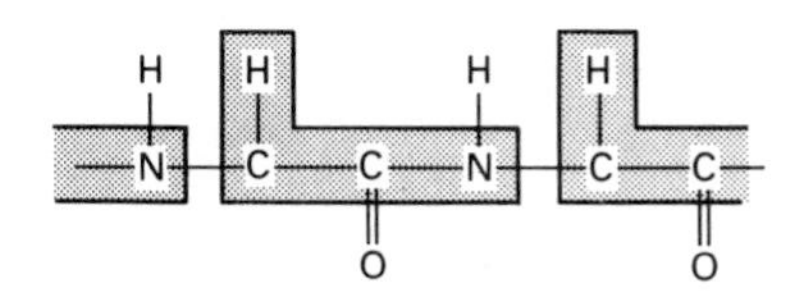

Fig. T4. Connectivities observed in the three-dimensional HCA(CO)N experiment for ^{15}N- and ^{13}C-labelled proteins.

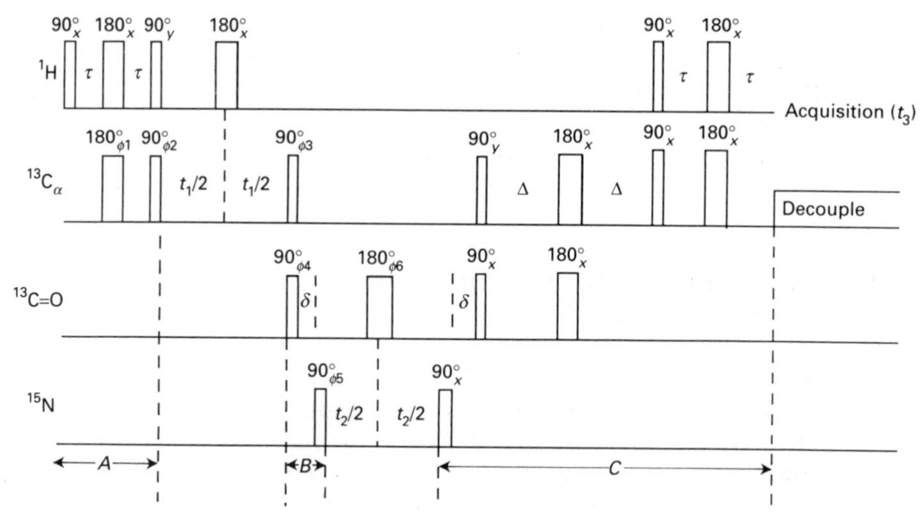

Fig. T5. Pulse scheme for acquisition of three-dimensional HCA(CO)N spectra. Typical delay durations are $\tau = 1.5$ ms, $\Delta = 3$ ms and $\delta = 18$–20 ms. The power levels of the Cα and C′ pulses are adjusted such that during application of a Cα pulse minimal excitation of C′ occurs, and vice versa. In order to minimize the effects of homonuclear J modulation (see ***J* spectroscopy**) by the passive Cα–Cβ couplings during the intervals Δ, a semiselective 180°_x (Cα) pulse may be used. The phase cycling employed is as follows; $\varphi_1 = x, -x$; $\varphi_2 = x$; $\varphi_3 = y, -y$; $\varphi_4 = 2(x), 2(-x)$; $\varphi_5 = 4(x), 4(-x)$; $\varphi_6 = 8(x), 8(y), 8(-x), 8(-y)$; receiver $= x, 2(-x), x, -x, 2(x), 2(-x), 2(x), x, -x, 2(-x), x$. The phases φ_2 and φ_4 are independently incremented by 90° with appropriate data routing for the acquisition of pure phase spectra (see **phase-sensitive experiments**).

as follows:

$$
\begin{aligned}
& I_z \xrightarrow{A} -2I_zA_y \xrightarrow{t_1} -4A_xI_zS_z \cos\omega_A t_1 \sin\pi J_{AS}t_1 \cos\pi J_{AB}t_1 \xrightarrow{B} \\
& -8S_xN_yI_zA_z \cos\omega_A t_1 \sin\pi J_{AS}t_1 \cos\pi J_{AB}t_1 \xrightarrow{t_2} \\
& -8S_xN_yI_zA_z \cos\omega_A t_1 \sin\pi J_{AS}t_1 \cos\pi J_{AB}t_1 \cos\omega_N t_2 \xrightarrow{C} \\
& I_x \cos\omega_A t_1 \sin\pi J_{AS}t_1 \cos\pi J_{AB}t_1 \cos\omega_N t_2
\end{aligned} \tag{T9}
$$

where pulse phases corresponding to the first step of the phase cycle have been assumed, J_{AS} is the Cα–C′ coupling constant, J_{AB} is the Cα–Cβ coupling constant, and ω_A, ω_S, and ω_{N} are the Cα, C′, and ^{15}N chemical shifts respectively. Also, for simplicity the effect of the ^{15}N–Cα coupling during t_1 has been neglected. Because $1/(2J_{NC\alpha})$ is smaller than either the t_1 or t_2 acquisition period, the presence of this coupling results in a small nonresolvable broadening in F_1 and F_2. Equation T9 indicates that both the active coupling, J_{AS} and the passive coupling, J_{AB} are present during t_1. Phasing the F_1 dimension of the spectrum to pure absorption would result in multiplet components of opposite phase. In practice, it is preferable to phase signals in F_1 to the dispersive mode. If the t_1 acquistion time is set to about $1/(2J_{AB})$ the $\sin \pi J_{AS} t_1 \cos \pi J_{AB} t_1$ time dependence results in an envelope similar to that of a sine-bell (see **convolution**). Fourier transformation followed by phasing to the dispersive mode then yields a non-Lorentzian **lineshape** that resembles a singlet which has been convoluted with a sine-bell function. As equation T9 indicates, the lineshapes in both the F_2 and F_3 dimensions are purely absorptive.

FURTHER READING

Theoretical details of the HNCO experiment are described in

Kay, L. E., Ikura, M., Tschudin, M., and Bax, A. (1990). *J. Magn. Reson.* **89,** 496.

For an application of this technique to proteins, see

Ikura, M., Kay, L. E., and Bax, A. (1990). *Biochemistry* **29,** 4659.

Three-dimensional HNCA experiment The HNCA experiment is a technique devised for ^{15}N- and ^{13}C-labelled proteins which correlates NH and ^{15}N chemical shifts with the intraresidue Cα shift. For a large number of residues, a connectivity is also observed from the ^{15}N shift of one residue to the Cα of the preceding residue (Fig. T6). The pulse scheme for this experiment is shown in Fig. T7. An INEPT (see **insensitive nuclei enhanced by polarization transfer**) sequence is utilized to transfer magnetization originating on NH protons to the directly coupled ^{15}N spin. During the evolution period t_1, the ^{15}N magnetization evolves under the influence of ^{15}N chemical shifts, with ^{1}H and Cα decoupling which is achieved by application of 180° pulses at the midpoint of t_1. During the following delay δ, ^{15}N magnetization precesses to become antiphase with respect to the Cα spin(s). This delay δ is tuned to an integral multiple of $1/(J_{NH})$, so that ^{15}N magnetization remains antiphase with respect to the coupled proton. In order to minimize relaxation losses and optimize transfer for those cases where a significant two-bond ^{15}N–Cα coupling is also present, the value of δ is set to approximately $1/(3J_{NC\alpha})$. Subsequent application of 90° pulses to both ^{1}H and Cα spins establishes three-spin NH–^{15}N–Cα coherence (see **multiple-quantum coherence**). The ^{1}H and ^{15}N chemical shifts are refocussed during t_2 by application of 180° ^{1}H and ^{15}N pulses at the midpoint of this interval, so that the total chemical-shift

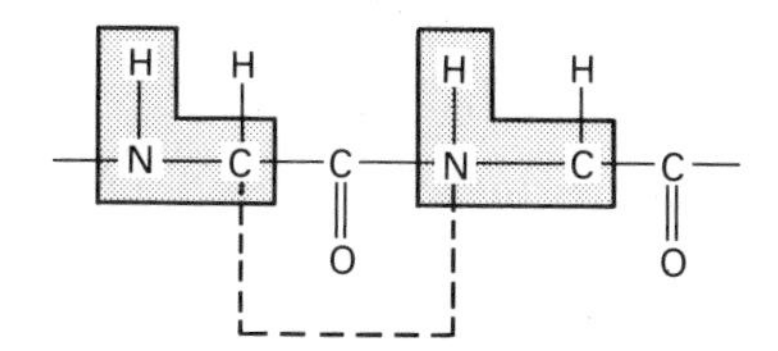

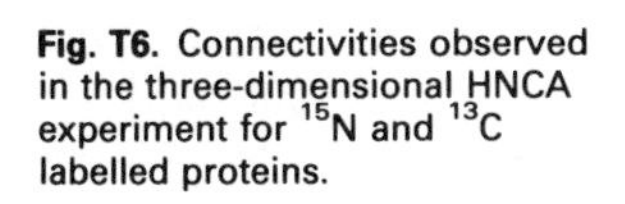

Fig. T6. Connectivities observed in the three-dimensional HNCA experiment for ^{15}N and ^{13}C labelled proteins.

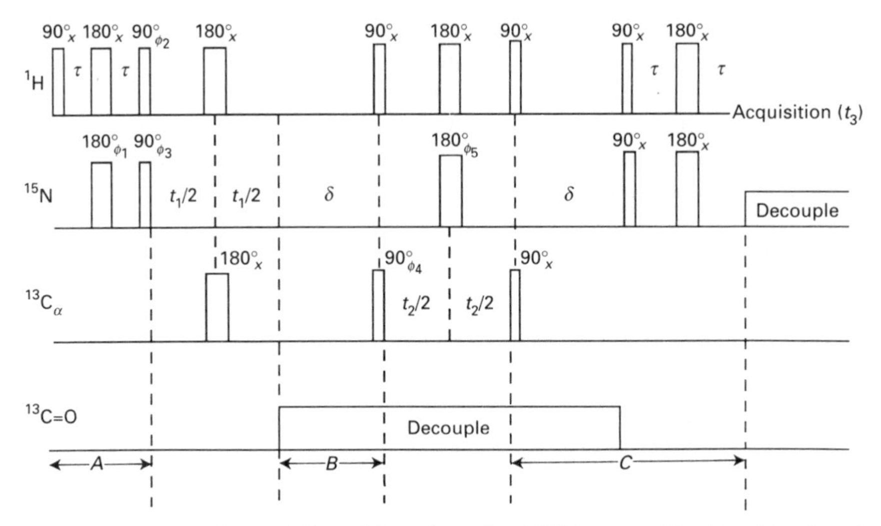

Fig. T7. Pulse scheme for acquisition of three-dimensional HNCA spectra. The delay δ is adjusted to be an integral multiple of $1/J_{NH}$ and to allow maximal magnetisation transfer between the ^{15}N and $C\alpha$ spins. The phase cycling employed is as follows; $\varphi_1 = x, -x$; $\varphi_2 = y, -y$; $\varphi_3 = x$; $\varphi_4 = 2(x), 2(-x)$; $\varphi_5 = 4(x), 4(y), 4(-x), 4(-y)$; receiver $= x, 2(-x), x, -(x), 2(x), -x$. The phases φ_3 and φ_4 are independently incremented by 90° with appropriate data routing for the acquisition of pure phase spectra (see **phase-sensitive experiments**).

evolution of the three-spin coherence depends only on the $C\alpha$ chemical shift. After the t_2 period, magnetization is transferred back to the NH protons by the reverse of the process described above.

The above magnetization transfer steps can be described more formally by use of the **product opertor formalism**. For simplicity, it is convenient to describe only those terms that contribute to the final spectrum, and the effects of certain groups of pulses can be combined into operators $\boldsymbol{A}$, $\boldsymbol{B}$, and $\boldsymbol{C}$, as shown in Fig. T7. Denoting the NH, ^{15}N, and intraresidue $C\alpha$ spins by I, N, and A respectively, and the carbonyl spin of the preceding residue by C', the salient features of the HNCA pulse sequence can be described as follows:

$$
\begin{aligned}
&I_z \xrightarrow{\boldsymbol{A}} -2I_zN_y \xrightarrow{t_1} 2I_zN_y \cos\omega_N t_1 \cos\pi J_{NC'} t_1 \xrightarrow{\boldsymbol{B}} \\
&-4I_yN_xA_y \cos\omega_N t_1 \cos\pi J_{NC'} t_1 \xrightarrow{t_2} \\
&-4I_yN_xA_y \cos\omega_N t_1 \cos\pi J_{NC'} t_1 \cos\omega_A t_2 \xrightarrow{\boldsymbol{C}} \\
&I_x \cos\omega_N t_1 \cos\pi J_{NC'} t_1 \cos\omega_A t_2.
\end{aligned}
\qquad \text{T10}
$$

where pulse phases corresponding to the first step of the phase cycle have been assumed, $J_{NC'}$ is the interresidue ^{15}N–C' coupling constant, and the J coupling and chemical shift effects removed by 180° pulses have been omitted. Also, for simplicity it has been assumed that $\delta = 1/(2J_{NA})$, where J_{NA} is the one-bond ^{15}N–Cα J coupling, and that the two-bond coupling $J_{NA'}$ between ^{15}N and the preceding Cα spin, A', is zero. In cases where a significant $J_{NA'}$ exists, the signal immediately prior to detection is given by

$$I_x \cos \omega_N t_1 \cos \pi J_{NC'} t_1 \{\cos \omega_A t_2 [\sin \pi J_{NA} \delta \cos \pi J_{NA'} \delta]^2 + \cos \omega_{A'} t_2 [\sin \pi J_{NA'} \delta \cos \pi J_{NA} \delta]^2\} \quad \text{T11}$$

Equations T10 and T11 indicate that the detected signal is amplitude modulated (see **amplitude modulation**) in both t_1 and t_2 leading to pure absorption lineshapes after three-dimensional **Fourier transformation**. The three-dimensional spectrum will comprise a series of F_3–F_2 slices containing intraresidue NH–Cα correlations together with weaker correlations between the NH of one residue and the Cα of its preceding residue. These slices are separated in F_1 by virtue of the ^{15}N chemical shift. The undesirable $J_{NC'}$ coupling present during t_1 does not greatly affect the signal since the acquisition time in this dimension is typically chosen shorter thatn $1/(2J_{NC'})$. Finally, it should be noted that the effects of J-coupling evolution during t_2 arising from NH–Hα and long-range ^{15}N–^{1}H J couplings have been omitted in the above analysis. For proteins, these couplings are typically much smaller than the 'natural linewidth' of the three-spin coherence which is dominated by the short Cα **spin–spin relaxation time, T_2**, and they may therefore be neglected.

FURTHER READING

Theoretical details of the HNCA experiment are described in

Kay, L. E., Ikura, M., Tschudin, M., and Bax, A. (1990). *J. Magn. Reson.* **89,** 496.

For an application of this technique to proteins, see

Ikura, M., Kay, L. E., and Bax, A. (1990). *Biochemistry* **29,** 4659.

Three-dimensional HNCO experiment The HNCO experiment is a technique devised for ^{15}N- and ^{13}C-labelled proteins which correlates NH and ^{15}N chemical shifts of one amino acid with the C′ (carbonyl) shift of the preceding residue, and thus provides important sequential connectivity information (Fig. T8). The pulse scheme for this experiment is shown in

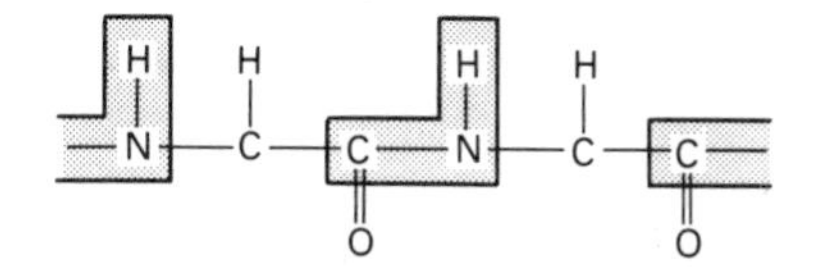

Fig. T8. Connectivities observed in the three-dimensional HNCO experiment for ^{15}N- and ^{13}C-labelled proteins.

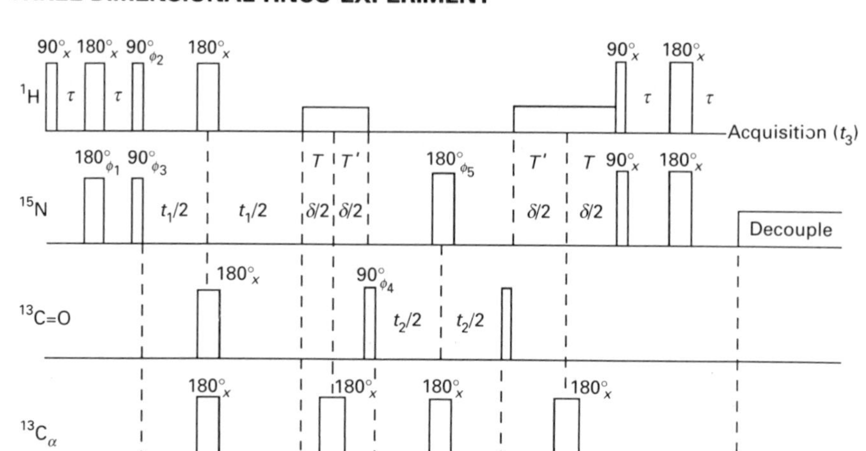

Fig. T9. Pulse scheme for acquisition of three-dimensional HNCO spectra. Presaturation of the water resonance is required during the recovery period and during both δ periods. The phase cycling employed is as follows: $\varphi_1 = x, -x$; $\varphi_2 = 2(y), 2(-y)$; $\varphi_3 = x$; $\varphi_4 = 4(x), 4(-x)$, $\varphi_5 = 8(x), 8(y), 8(-x), 8(-y)$; receiver $= 2(x), 4(-x), 2(x), 2(-x), 4(x), 2(-x)$. The phases φ_3 and φ_4 are independently incremented by 90° with appropriate data routing for the acquisition of pure phase spectra (see **phase-sensitive experiments**).

Fig. T9. An INEPT (see **insensitive nuclei enhanced by polarization transfer**) sequence is utilized to transfer magnetisation originating on NH protons to the directly-coupled ^{15}N spin. During the evolution period t_1, the ^{15}N magnetization evolves exclusively under the influence of ^{15}N chemical shifts, since ^{1}H, C′ and Cα decoupling is achieved by application of 180° pulses at the midpoint of t_1. During the following delay δ, ^{15}N magnetization precesses to become antiphase with respect to the polarization of the carbonyl spin of the preceding residue, via the one-bond coupling $^{1}J_{NC'}$, which is on the order of 15 Hz. The first 90° C′ pulse converts the antiphase ^{15}N magnetization into ^{15}N–C′ zero- and double-quantum coherence (see **multiple-quantum coherence**). The effects of the ^{15}N chemical shift and ^{1}H–^{15}N J coupling are removed during the t_2 period by the application of the $180^{\circ}_{\varphi 5}$ ^{15}N pulse. Furthermore, Cα–C′ decoupling is achieved by application of a 180° Cα pulse at the midpoint of t_2. At the end of the C′ evolution period, t_2, magnetization is transferred back to NH protons by reversing the above transfer steps.

The above magnetisation transfer steps can be described more formally by use of the **product operator formalism**. For simplicity, it is convenient to describe only those terms that contribute to the final spectrum, and the effects of certain groups of pulses can be combined into operators $\boldsymbol{A}$, $\boldsymbol{B}$, and $\boldsymbol{C}$, as shown in Fig. T9. Denoting the NH, ^{15}N and C′ spins by I, N, and S respectively, the salient features of the HNCO pulse sequence can be described as follows:

T12

$$I_z \xrightarrow{A} -2I_zN_y \xrightarrow{t_1} 2I_zN_y \cos \omega_N t_1 \xrightarrow{B} 4N_xS_yI_z \cos \omega_N t_1 \xrightarrow{t_2}$$
$$4N_xS_yI_z \cos \omega_N t_1 \cos \omega_S t_2 \cos \pi J_{\mathrm{NC}\alpha} t_2 \left\{ \prod_k \cos \pi J_{kS} t_2 \right\} \xrightarrow{C}$$
$$I_x \cos \omega_N t_1 \cos \omega_S t_2 \cos \pi J_{\mathrm{NC}\alpha} t_2 \left\{ \prod_k \cos \pi J_{kS} t_2 \right\}$$

where pulse phases corresponding to the first step of the phase cycle have been assumed, $J_{\mathrm{NC}\alpha}$ is the intraresidue ^{15}N–Cα J coupling, and J_{kS} refers to long-range coupling between the carbonyl carbon and other protons, k. For simplicity, the assumption $T' = T$ has been made and the J-coupling and chemical-shift effects removed by 180° pulses have been omitted. The two-bond interresidue ^{15}N–Cα coupling is usually small in proteins and has been neglected. Equation T12 shows that the detected signal is in-phase (I_x), and is amplitude modulated (see **amplitude modulation**) by ω_N and ω_S in the t_1 and t_2 dimensions, respectively, which gives rise to a purely absorptive **three-dimensional NMR** (3D NMR) signal after three-dimensional **Fourier transformation**. The three-dimensional NMR spectrum will comprise a series of F_3–F_2 slices which correlate the NH shifts of the nth residue with the C′ shifts of the $(n-1)$th residue, and these slices will be separated in F_1 by virtue of the ^{15}N shift of the nth residue. Equation T12 illustrates the case where $T = T' = \delta/2$, whereas the experiment can be conducted more efficiently with T set to a somewhat larger value than T'. The magnetization immediately before t_3 is then described by

T13

$$I_x \cos \omega_N t_1 \cos \omega_S t_2 \cos\{\pi J_{\mathrm{NC}\alpha}[t_2 - 2(T - T')]\} \left\{ \prod_k \cos \pi J_{kS} t_2 \right\}.$$

The effect of $T > T'$ is that the magnetization envelope in t_2 no longer begins at a maximum value at $t_2 = 0$, but reaches a maximum at $t_2 = 2(T - T')$, which is functionally equivalent to resolution enhancement in T_2 by application of a shifted sine-bell weighting function (see **convolution**). By arranging for resolution enhancement in this manner, the concomitant loss in signal-to-noise ratio associated with conventional resolution enhancement is minimized. Typically, T is about 10 ms longer than T', which yields a signal envelope in t_2 that is similar to a sine bell shifted by ~50°.

FURTHER READING

Theoretical details of the HNCO experiment are described in

Kay, L. E., Ikura, M., Tschudin, M., and Bax, A. (1990). *J. Magn. Reson.* **89,** 496.

For an application of this technique to proteins, see
Ikura, M., Kay, L. E., and Bax, A. (1990). *Biochemistry* **29,** 4659.

Three-dimensional NMR The enormous increase in resolution afforded by **two-dimensional NMR** permits the analysis of molecular systems which are otherwise too complex to be analysed by conventional one-dimensional NMR, by virtue of extreme overlap of resonances. Once the concept of an NMR spectrum in two dimensions is understood, one can envisage multi-dimensional NMR without further difficulty. Indeed, three-dimensional NMR is now utilized routinely for the structural analysis of large proteins.

A three-dimensional NMR experiment can be conceived by combining two-dimensional NMR experiments, omitting the detection period of the first experiment and the preparation period of the second. For example, a three-dimensional COSY–COSY (see **correlated spectroscopy**) pulse sequence can be devised by combining two COSY experiments as shown in Fig. T10. In exact analogy with two-dimensional NMR, time-domain data are acquired sequentially during the 'normal' detection period t_3, and are acquired point-by-point by independent incrementation of both t_1 and t_2. A convenient way to understand this procedure is to imagine a three-dimensional NMR experiment as a combination of separate two-dimensional NMR experiments. A two-dimensional NMR experiment is acquired in the normal fashion by sequential acquisition in t_3, and with incrementation of t_2 (i.e. the t_2 period can be thought of as analogous to t_1 in conventional two-dimensional NMR). The value of t_1 is then incremented and a second two-dimensional NMR experiment is acquired. This process is repeated until the desired number of datapoints has been acquired in the t_1 dimension. If quadrature detection is required in the t_1 dimension, then it is necessary to shift the phase of *all* pulses prior to t_1 by 90° in a manner analogous to conventional **phase-sensitive experiments**. Similarly, it is necessary independently to shift the phases of *all* pulses prior to t_2 to achieve quadrature detection in that dimension.

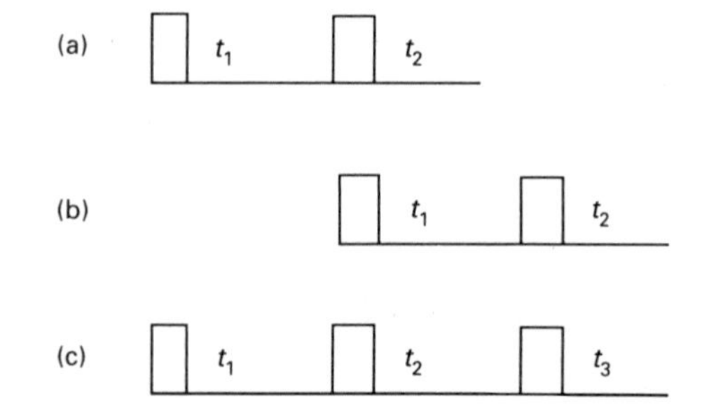

Fig. T10. A three-dimensional COSY–COSY NMR experiment (c) can be generated by a combination of two COSY experiments (a and b).

Since there are three independent time periods in a three-dimensional NMR experiment, it follows that the three-dimensional NMR spectrum is obtained by use of a three-dimensional **Fourier transform**. The analogy with two-dimensional NMR is again helpful in understanding how this may be achieved. Essentially, the time domain data will be comprised of a cube whose axes are the three orthogonal time periods t_1, t_2, t_3, as shown in Fig. T11. If the data are convoluted, Fourier transformed, and phased along the t_1 dimension, the resulting f_1, t_2, t_3 datamatrix can be thought of as a series of two-dimensional NMR spectra which, when processed as such, will consist of a series of slices through the three-dimensional NMR spectrum. Conveniently, a three-dimensional NMR spectrum can easily be processed in t_1 by use of simple fast Fourier transform routines, and processing in t_2 and t_3 can then be achieved with conventional software for two-dimensional NMR.

Various three-dimensional NMR experiments have been devised, each with particularly useful properties in certian circumstances. These are all described under the relevant heading, but here it is useful to consider briefly the general properties of three-dimensional NMR spectra. The homonuclear COSY–COSY spectrum provides a convenient example. In the simple case of three weakly-coupled spins AMX, we find three classes of peak in the three-dimensional spectrum. Diagonal peaks are found along the body diagonal from the lower left-hand to upper right-hand

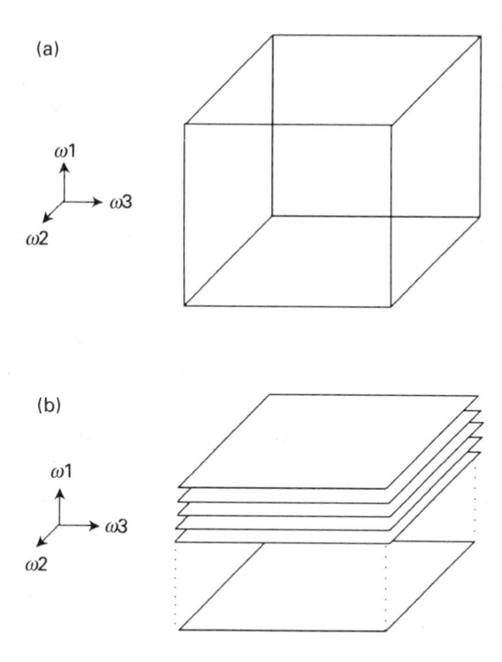

Fig. T11. A three-dimensional NMR experiment can be thought of as a cube (a) which comprises a series of two-dimensional spectra (b).

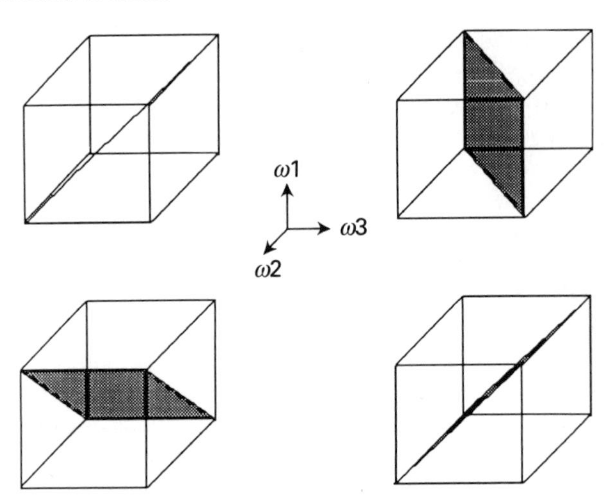

Fig. T12. Illustration of (a) the body diagonal, (b, c) cross-diagonal planes, and (d) the back transfer plane found in three-dimensional NMR spectra.

corner of the cube, corresponding to precession frequencies such as $\omega_A(t_1)$, $\omega_A(t_2)$, $\omega_A(t_3)$ (Fig. T12). These represent magnetization which has failed to migrate from one spin to another, and are analogous to diagonal peaks in two-dimensional NMR. Cross-diagonal peaks correspond to precession frequencies such as $\omega_A(t_1)$, $\omega_A(t_2)$, $\omega_M(t_3)$, and these represent magnetization associated with a given spin throughout t_1 and t_2, which is then transferred to a second coupled spin by **coherence transfer** via the third pulse. These peaks are analogous to crosspeaks in two-dimensional NMR spectra, and are found on one of two cross-diagonal planes $\omega_2 = \omega_3$ or $\omega_1 = \omega_2$ depending whether coherence was transferred by the first mixing step (second pulse) or the second mixing step (third pulse) respectively. These cross-diagonal planes contain information equivalent to the corresponding two-dimensional spectra from which the three-dimensional pulse sequence is derived. Cross-diagonal peaks can also derive from magnetization which is transferred from A to M by the second pulse, and from M back to A by the third pulse, corresponding to precession frequencies such as $\omega_A(t_1)$, $\omega_M(t_2)$, $\omega_A(t_3)$. These are found on the back-transfer plane $\omega_1 = \omega_3$. A third type of peak which has no direct analogue in two-dimensional NMR is the crosspeak, which corresponds to precession frequencies such as $\omega_A(t_1)$, $\omega_M(t_2)$, $\omega_X(t_3)$, where coherence is transferred by the second pulse, and is relayed by the third pulse. These peaks do not lie on any of the above planes.

The value of three-dimensional NMR lies primarily in the increased resolution in comparison with two-dimensional NMR. However, this must be offset against a number of practical problems. The most obvious of these is the long acquisition time required in order to achieve good digital resolution. If a three-dimensional spectrum is recorded with the digital resolution to which we are accustomed in two-dimensional NMR, the experiment would be prohibitively long. Hence in general three-dimensional spectra are recorded with rather poorer digital resolution. This can be improved by post-acquisition zero-filling. While the resulting resolution is still often worse than that in a conventional two-dimensional NMR experiment, it should be remembered that each two-dimensional slice within the three-dimensional spectrum will have a much smaller number of resonances than in the corresponding two-dimensional experiment, so the reduced digital resolution often presents a cosmetic, rather than practical problem. Ironically, this is not the case for the COSY–COSY experiment: crosspeak intensities in this experiment depend upon the creation of antiphase magnetization in an analogous manner to those two-dimensional NMR, and the resulting antiphase nature of crosspeak multiplets results in severe cancellation of intensity if the digital resolution is poor. For this reason homonuclear three-dimensional COSY–COSY is not a particularly useful experiment, and most homonuclear three-dimensional experiments utilize mixing processes which generate in-phase magnetization such as **three-dimensional NOESY–HOHAHA**.

Three-dimensional NOESY–HMQC (3D NOESY–HMQC) The three-dimensional NOESY–HMQC experiment was originally devised to achieve a simplification of conventional two-dimensional NOESY (see **nuclear Overhauser effect spectroscopy**) spectra of ^{15}N-labelled proteins. The final **three-dimensional NMR** spectrum obtained from this experiment displays NOE information between amide protons (F_3) and other protons in the protein (F_1) that are in spatial proximity to the amide protons. The three-dimensional spectrum is a collection of two-dimensional (F_1–F_3) NOE maps separated in the F_2 dimension according to the ^{15}N chemical shift of the corresponding amide nitrogen. In addition to providing information necessary for sequential assignment of the backbone resonances (NH, CαH), the spectrum provides many of the distance constraints necessary for a structure determination.

A typical pulse sequence for the NOESY–HMQC experiment is shown in Fig. T13. The variables t_1 and t_3 represent the conventional time variables in the NOESY experiment, whereas t_2 and t_3 represent the conventional time variables in the HMQC experiment (see **heteronuclear multiple-quantum correlation**). As in the NOESY experiment, proton magnetization which is excited by application of the ^{1}H 90° pulse of phase φ is chemical shift labelled during t_1 and is transferred during τ_m to all proximal spins by the NOE. Heteronuclear scalar couplings are removed

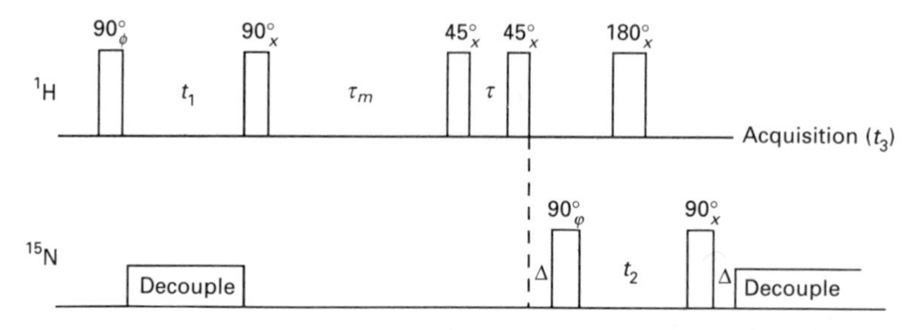

Fig. T13. Typical pulse scheme for the acquisition of three-dimensional NOESY–HMQC spectra. The phase cycling used is as follows: $\varphi = x, y, -x, -y$; $\psi = 4(x), 4(-x)$; acquisition = 2(x), 4(−x), 2(x), with appropriate data routing depending on the method by which quadrature detection is achieved in t_1 (see **phase-sensitive experiments**). The entire sequence is repeated with ψ incremented by 90° to obtain quadrature detection during t_2, together with the appropriate data routing.

during t_1 by application of ^{15}N decoupling, and a homospoil pulse may be applied in the middle of τ_m to minimize multiple–quantum interference effects between coupled spins. After τ_m, the application of an off-resonance jump-and-return read pulse (see **solvent suppression**) 45°_x–τ–45°_x, generates transverse ^{1}H magnetization. The delay τ is adjusted to minimize excitation of water magnetization ($\tau \sim 1/(2\delta_{H_2O})$). The sequence that follows the NOE mixing period is similar to the conventional HMQC shift correlation scheme, and with **phase cycling** of the first 90° ^{15}N pulse, only signals from protons directly attached to ^{15}N remain during the detection period t_3. For every t_2 value, a two-dimensional dataset is obtained which contains only amide proton resonances in the detected (F_3) dimension and all protons in spatial proximity to the amide protons in the F_1 dimension. The intensities of H–NH crosspeaks in this dataset are modulated as a function of t_2 by the ^{15}N chemical shift, and **Fourier transformation** of the three-dimensional dataset (F_1, t_2, F_3) with respect to t_2 results in the final three-dimensional spectrum. In common with most three-dimensional experiments, time considerations dictate that only a limited number of scans can be acquired for each (t_1, t_2) value. Therefore, only a short phase cycle can be utilized. It has been suggested by Kay *et al.* (1989) that a 16–step phase cycle is sufficient: the phase φ is incremented in 90° steps to obtain complex data in F_1 (see **phase-sensitive experiments**) and to suppress **axial peaks**. The phase ψ is similarly incremented in 90° steps to obtain quadrature information in F_2 and to eliminate signals during t_3 from protons not attached to ^{15}N. Finally, it should be noted that a similar three-dimensional spectrum may be obtained by permuting the NOESY–HMQC sequence to give the HMQC–NOESY experiment, whereby the NH proton shifts are recorded in F_2. However, the sensitivity of the three-dimensional experiment is essentially independent of this choice, and the NOESY–HMQC sequence is preferable for proteins since it is easier to observe the crucial NH–αH connectivities that would otherwise be buried in the wings of the intense H_2O resonance.

FURTHER READING

Additional experimental details for 3D NOESY–HMQC are described in
Kay, L. E., Marion, D., and Bax, A. (1989). *J. Magn. Reson.* **84,** 72.

The HMQC–NOESY experiment is described in
Fesik, S. W. and Zuiderweg, E. P. R. (1988). *J. Magn. Reson.* **78,** 588.

Time averaging See **average Hamiltonian theory**.

Time domain See **Fourier transform**.

Time-proportional phase incrementation (TPPI) TPPI arises from a scheme which has been used in one-dimensional Fourier transform spectroscopy to distinguish positive and negative precession frequencies without resorting to complex data acquisition (i.e. the collection of both real and imaginary **free induction decays** with a dual channel receiver). The procedure allows the transmitter **carrier** to lie in the centre of the spectrum, and yet at the same time allows the signs of the precession frequencies to be distinguished. This is achieved by shifting the apparent precession frequencies to one side of the carrier by sampling x, y, $-x$, and $-y$ components of the signal sequentially, Unlike regular **phase cycling** procedures, this sequential sampling occurs during acquisition of the FID, rather than between additions of a series of FIDs. Thus, with a sampling interval δ, a single FID is obtained which has the form

$$S(t) = \{S_x(0),\ S_y(\delta),\ -S_x(2\delta),\ -S_y(3\delta), \ldots\}. \quad \text{(T14)}$$

The **phase** increment $\pi/2$ between subsequent sampling points is equivalent to a frequency shift $\Delta\omega = \pi/2\delta$, or to half the Nyquist frequency (see **aliasing**) of the sampling process. This can be demonstrated explicitly as follows. If we consider a time-domain signal $\cos \omega_i t_1$, and add to this the phase incrementation $\pi/2\delta$, we find for the time-domain signal

$$S(t_1) = \cos(\omega_i t_1 + \pi t_1/2\delta) \quad \text{(T15)}$$

Now, if the sampling interval δ is arranged to be $1/2f_1$, where f_1 is the **sweep-width**, then (T15) can be rewritten

$$S(t_1) = \cos(\omega_i t_1 + \omega_c t_1)$$

where

$$\omega_c = \tfrac{1}{2}(2\pi f_1) \quad \text{(T16)}$$

and thus $\frac{1}{2}f_1$ has been added to the frequency of each line. The important point is that a real transform (see **Fourier transform**) with respect to t_1 can be performed with retention of relative precession frequencies.

The TPPI procedure is of use in two-dimensional NMR when spectrometers equipped for real transforms are available. In this case the use of TPPI during t_1 allows for sign discrimination despite the application of a real transform. The use of the real transform in turn allows for pure absorption-mode lineshapes to be retained (see **phase-sensitive experiments**). The experimental protocol is simply to advance t_1 in intervals of $1/(2f_1)$. Each time t_1 is incremented, the subsequent datapoint in the t_1 domain FID is being prepared, thus the phase of the desired coherence evolving during t_1 is shifted by $\pi/2$ radians. This is achieved by applying a $\pi/2$ phase shift to all pulses preceding t_1.

A similar procedure has been used to separate various orders of multiple-quantum coherence along the ω_1 dimension of two-dimensional multiple-quantum experiments. The separation lies in the fact that p-quantum coherence has a p-fold sensitivity to the sequential phase shift (see **multiple-quantum coherence**) during acquisition in t_1, and is thus shifted in frequency along the ω_1 domain after Fourier transformation.

FURTHER READING

The use of TPPI for the separation of coherence orders is described by

Drobny, G., Pines, A., Sinton, S., Weitekamp, D., and Wemmer, D. (1979). *Faraday Div. Chem. Soc. Symp.* **13,** 49.

TOCSY See **total correlation spectroscopy**.

Total correlation spectroscopy (TOCSY) In experiments such as COSY (see **correlated spectroscopy**), coherence transfer is effected by the application of a mixing pulse, following the generation of antiphase coherence during the evolution period prior to the pulse. An alternative method, total correlation spectroscopy (TOCSY), uses an extended mixing period in which a suitably tailored average **Hamiltonian** is applied, whose desired effect is to mix the various coherences. A particularly desirable Hamiltonian is the so called 'isotropic mixing' Hamiltonian

$$\bar{\mathcal{H}} = \sum_{k<1} 2\pi J_{kl}\mathbf{I}_k\mathbf{I}_l. \tag{T17}$$

A Hamiltonian such as this can be generated by suppression of the Zeeman terms of the free precession Hamiltonian appropriate for scalar coupled spins:

$$\begin{aligned}\mathcal{H} &= \mathcal{H}_Z + \mathcal{H}_J \\ &= \sum_k \omega_k I_{zk} + \sum_{k<l} 2\pi J_{kl}\mathbf{I}_k\mathbf{I}_l.\end{aligned} \tag{T18}$$

The simplest approach to suppression of $\mathscr{H}_Z$ is a string of π pulses with a repetition rate which is fast in comparison with the largest chemical shift difference. More complex spin-lock sequences (see **spin-locking**) do however give better results, in view of their rather better offset dependence (see **homonuclear Hartman–Hahn spectroscopy**). A simple physical interpretation of the effect of the isotropic mixing Hamiltonian is that the spin system becomes essentially strongly coupled under its influence. In other words, unlike weakly coupled systems (see **weak coupling**), the individual spins do not move independently under the influence of $\mathscr{H}$, but move in so-called collective spin modes. This implies that coherence transfer is possible between all pairs of nuclei, even if there is no direct coupling between them. For an extended mixing period, this is found to be the case (see Braunschweiler and Ernst, 1983).

A more formal description of the effects of $\mathscr{H}$ can be had by considering a two-spin system IS. In this case the collective spin modes are represented by the sum and difference of single spin and product spin operators:

$$\begin{aligned}
&\Sigma_\alpha = \tfrac{1}{2}\{I_\alpha + S_\alpha\},\\
&\Delta_\alpha = \tfrac{1}{2}\{I_\alpha - S_\alpha\},\\
&\Sigma_{\alpha\beta} = \{I_\alpha S_\beta + I_\beta S_\alpha\},\\
&\Delta_{\alpha\beta} = \{I_\alpha S_\beta - I_\beta S_\alpha\},\\
&\alpha, \beta = x, y, z.
\end{aligned} \tag{T19}$$

The time evolution of the difference terms is given by

$$\begin{aligned}
&\Delta_\alpha \xrightarrow{\bar{\mathscr{H}}\tau_m} \Delta_\alpha \cos(2\pi J_{IS}\tau_m) + \Delta_{\beta\gamma}\sin(2\pi J_{IS}\tau_m)\\
&\Delta_{\beta\alpha} \xrightarrow{\bar{\mathscr{H}}\tau_m} \Delta_{\beta\gamma}\cos(2\pi J_{IS}\tau_m) - \Delta_\alpha \sin(2\pi J_{IS}\tau_m)
\end{aligned} \tag{T20}$$

while the sum terms are invariant to evolution under $\bar{\mathscr{H}}$. Thus, as an example, we find explicitly for the evolution of the y component of spin I using

$$-I_y = -\tfrac{1}{2}(I_y + S_y) - \tfrac{1}{2}(I_y - S_y) = -\tfrac{1}{2}\Sigma_y - \tfrac{1}{2}\Delta_y. \tag{T21}$$

Equation (T20) gives

$$\begin{aligned}
-\tfrac{1}{2}\Sigma_y - \tfrac{1}{2}\Delta_y &\xrightarrow{\bar{\mathscr{H}}\tau_m} \{-\tfrac{1}{2}(I_y + S_y) - (\tfrac{1}{2}(I_y - S_y)\cos \pi J_{IS}\tau_m\\
&+(I_z S_x - I_x S_z)\sin \pi J_{IS}\tau_m)\}\\
&= -\tfrac{1}{2}I_y(1+\cos 2\pi J_{IS}\tau_m) - \tfrac{1}{2}S_y(1-\cos 2\pi J_{IS}\tau_m)\\
&-(I_z S_x - I_x S_z)\sin 2\pi J_{IS}\tau_m.
\end{aligned} \tag{T22}$$

An important result of this calculation is that for $\tau_m = 1/(2J_{IS})$, complete coherence transfer is expected since terms in I_y will be zero, and those in S_y will be maximal. This implies that net coherence transfer is possible, giving absorption-phase lineshapes with no antiphase components. Unfortunately, absorption-phase lineshapes are not obtained automatically, since the antiphase terms $I_zS_x - I_xS_z$ in (T22) will also be present. However, these terms can be cancelled by coaddition of signals obtained with different mixing times, τ_m. The resulting absorption mode lineshapes have been demonstrated experimentally (see Braunschweiler and Ernst, 1983).

As mentioned above, in extended coupling networks, for a sufficiently large value of τ_m, coherence transfer extends throughout the complete network, in analogy to **relayed correlation spectroscopy** with multiple relay steps. However, the TOCSY sequence is particularly useful since the efficiency of coherence transfer is essentially independent of the magnitudes of the scalar couplings in the network, which is an obvious advantage when dealing with an unknown coupling topography.

FURTHER READING

Braunschweiler, L. and Ernst, R. R. (1983). *J. Magn. Reson.* **53,** 521.

TPPI See **time proportional phase incrementation**.

TQFCOSY See **triple-quantum filtered correlated spectroscopy.**

Trace See Appendix 3.

Transfer function See **Green function**.

Transferred nuclear Overhauser effect (TRNOE, TOE) Many biological systems involve the interaction of a protein receptor with a low-molecular-weight ligand. A complete determination of the conformation of the protein with bound ligand is often not possible, due to the large size of the complex. However, for weakly binding ligands, a simpler approach termed transferred **nuclear Overhauser effect** spectroscopy is available by which the conformation of the ligand can be studied in its bound form. Provided the ligand is bound to the receptor for a sufficiently short time, NOEs between nuclei in the bound ligand are transferred to the more easily detected nuclei in excess free ligand in the same solution by virtue of **chemical exchange** of ligand molecules between the bound and free states—when a bound ligand dissociates from the receptor it carries with it a ‘memory’ of any NOEs which were generated in the bound state. The negative NOEs arising from proximal nuclei in the protein–ligand complex with a **correlation time** in the

spin-diffusion limit, are readily distinguished from the positive NOEs encountered in the ligand, which will possess a correlation time in the **extreme narrowing** limit.

It is possible to obtain quantitative distance information from TRNOEs, as the following brief theoretical discourse will show. The ^1H–^1H nuclear Overhauser effect can be expressed as $f_I(S)$, the fractional change in intensity of the resonance of proton I when that of proton S is saturated. It is given by (see **nuclear Overhauser effect**)

T23 $$f_I(S) = \sigma_{IS}/\rho_I$$

where σ_{IS} is the cross-relaxation rate between protons I and S and ρ_I is the total spin–lattice relaxation rate of proton I. Consider the case where I and S are protons on a ligand that is exchanging between a state bound to ligand (denoted by subscript B) and a second state free in solution (denoted by subscript F). If the rate of exchange of the ligand between the two states is greater than the difference in proton relaxation rates between them, protons I and S will each be characterized by relaxation rates that are the weighted mean of those in the two states. The NOE is thus

T24 $$f_I(S) = (X_{\mathrm{F}}\sigma_{IS,\mathrm{F}} + X_{\mathrm{B}}\sigma_{IS,\mathrm{B}})/(X_{\mathrm{F}}\rho_{I,\mathrm{F}} + X_B\rho_{I,\mathrm{B}})$$

where X_{B} and X_{F} are the mole fractions of the ligand in the bound and free states. Equation T24 is valid when separate resonances are observed for protons I and S in the two states, or when a single, average resonance is observed (see **chemical exchange**), provided only that the exchange rate is faster than the relaxation rates. Equation T24 can be simplified in cases where $\sigma_{IS,\mathrm{F}} = 0$, i.e. no NOEs are observed for the ligand in the absence of protein. For proteins, assuming that $\sigma_{IS,\mathrm{B}} \neq 0$ and $\rho_{I,\mathrm{B}} \gg \rho_{I,\mathrm{F}}$, equation T24 reduces to

T25 $$f_I(S) = \sigma_{IS,\mathrm{B}}/\rho_{I,\mathrm{B}}$$

If the effect on resonance I of irradiating the signal of another proton T, is measured, $f_I(T)$ will be given by

T26 $$f_I(T) = \sigma_{IT,\mathrm{B}}/\rho_{I,\mathrm{B}}.$$

Therefore

T27 $$f_I(S)/f_I(T) = \sigma_{IS,\mathrm{B}}/\sigma_{IT,\mathrm{B}} = r_{IT}^6/r_{IS}^6$$

where the r_{ij} are internuclear distances. Equation T27 holds provided that the correlation times of the I–S and I–T vectors are the same, and that indirect cross-relaxation effects are negligible. Under these conditions, the TRNOE can provide quantitative conformational information about a ligand bound to protein without direct observation of signals bound to ligand.

FURTHER READING

Clore, G. M. and Gronenborn, A. M. (1982). *J. Magn. Reson.* **48,** 402.

Clore, G. M. and Gronenborn, A. M. (1983). *J. Magn. Reson.* **53,** 423.

Two interesting applications of TRNOEs are:

Feeney, J., Birdsall, B., Roberts, G. C. K., and Burgen, A. S. V. (1983). *Biochemistry* **22,** 628.

Glaudemans, C. P. J., Lerner, L., Daves, G. D., Kovac, P., Venable, R., and Bax, A. (1990). *Biochemistry* **29,** 10906.

Transition probability See **spin–lattice relaxation**, **spin–spin relaxation**.

Transmitter See **spectrometer**.

Transverse magnetization See **classical formalism**.

Transverse nuclear Overhauser effect See **rotating frame Overhauser effect spectroscopy**.

Triple-quantum filtered correlated spectroscopy (TQFCOSY) Triple-quantum filtered COSY spectra may be recorded with the pulse sequence shown in Fig. T14. The pulse sequence is essentially identical to that used in the acquisition of double-quantum filtered COSY (DQFCOSY) spectra except that the phases ϕ of the first two pulses are cycled in steps of $\pi/3$ radians to achieve order-selective detection (see **multiple-quantum coherence**) of triple-quantum coherence. Practically, TQFCOSY is of value in the spin filtration of **spin systems** of the type

$$A-I-M-Q-S-V\begin{matrix} X \\ | \\ Z \end{matrix}$$

since only the mutually coupled spins V, X, Z will give rise to crosspeaks.

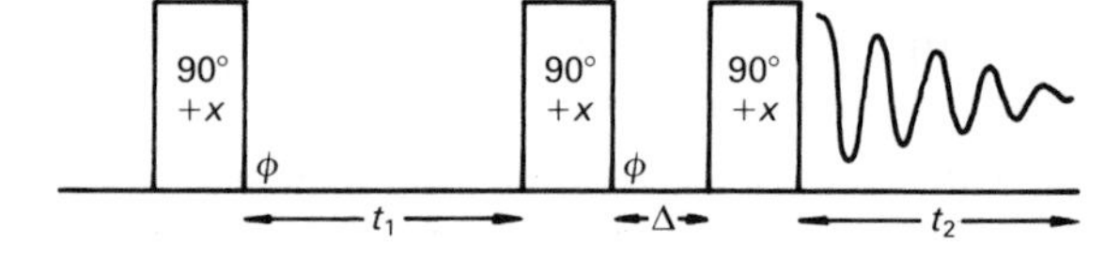

Fig. T14. Pulse sequence for the acquisition of triple-quantum filtered COSY spectra.

Such spin systems are common in carbohydrates, and TQFCOSY provides a particularly convenient method for the assignment of H5, H6 and H6′ protons. The workings of the experiment can be understood by reference to a mutually coupled three-spin system *ISM* using the **product operator formalism**. With respect to the creation of triple-quantum coherence, the relevant terms of the density operator after the second pulse are given by

$$\begin{aligned}\sigma_2 = &-4I_xM_yS_y \sin \pi J_{IS}t_1 \sin \pi J_{IM}t_1 \sin \omega_I t_1\\ &-4S_xM_yI_y \sin \pi J_{IS}t_1 \sin \pi J_{SM}t_1 \sin \omega_S t_1\\ &-4M_xI_yS_y \sin \pi J_{SM}t_1 \sin \pi J_{IM}t_1 \sin \omega_m t_1\\ &+\text{other terms}\end{aligned} \quad \text{T28}$$

where the ω's refer to the **Larmor precession** frequencies of the respective spins. Each term in (T28) consists of a superposition of pure triple-quantum coherence and single-uantum **combination lines**. For example, the first term in (T28) can be expanded in terms of **shift operators**

$$\begin{aligned}-4I_xM_yS_y = \tfrac{1}{2}(&I^+S^+M^+ - I^+S^+M^- - I^+S^-M^+ + I^+S^-M^- + I^-S^+M^+\\ &-I^-S^+M^- - I^-S^-M^+ + I^-S^-M^-).\end{aligned} \quad \text{T29}$$

During the course of the phase cycle, all terms are cancelled except those corresponding to pure triple-quantum coherence (3QC):

$$\begin{aligned}3\text{QC}_x &= \tfrac{1}{2}(I^+S^+M^+ + I^-S^-M^-) \sin \pi J_{IS}t_1 \sin \pi J_{IM}t_1 \sin \omega_I t_1\\ &= \tfrac{1}{4}(4I_xS_xM_x - 4I_xS_yM_y - 4I_yS_xM_y - 4I_yS_yM_x)\\ &\quad \times \sin \pi J_{IS}t_1 \sin \pi J_{IM}t_1 \sin \omega_I t_1.\end{aligned} \quad \text{T30}$$

The last three terms are converted into observable antiphase transverse magnetization by the final pulse:

$$\sigma_3 = (-4I_xS_zM_z - 4I_zS_xM_z - 4I_zS_zM_x) \sin \pi J_{IS}t_1 \sin \pi J_{IM}t_1 \sin \omega_I t_1. \quad \text{T31}$$

Similar expressions exist for the second and third terms of (T28). The second and third terms of (T31) give rise to crosspeaks after **two-dimensional Fourier transformation**, but only if the couplings J_{IS}, J_{SM}, and J_{IM} are non-zero. In terms of spin systems such as those described above, crosspeaks in TQFCOSY will only be seen correlating mutually coupled spins.

FURTHER READING

For the first demonstration of TQFCOSY, see

Piantini U., Sorensen, O. W., and Ernst R. R. (1982). *J. Am. Chem. Soc.* **104,** 6800.

For an application of TQFCOSY to carbohydrates, see
Homans, S. W., Dwek, R. A., Boyd, J., Mahmoudian, M., Richards, W. G., and Rademacher, T. W. (1986). *Biochemistry* **25,** 6342.

Truncation artefacts Truncation artefacts arise from the finite acquisition time in an NMR experiment. In principle, the **Fourier transform** of a decaying exponential function such as a **free induction decay** generates a Lorentzian **lineshape**. However, bearing in mind that data cannot be acquired for an infinite time in NMR, this relationship is approximate. In cases where the data have decayed to a very small value at the end of the acquisition period, the lineshape very closely approaches pure Lorentzian (Fig. T15). However, in some situations in one-dimensional NMR, or more probably in two-dimensional NMR, the signal has not decayed to zero by the end of the acquisition period. This gives rise to a peculiar lineshape after Fourier transformation (Fig. T16). This lineshape bears a

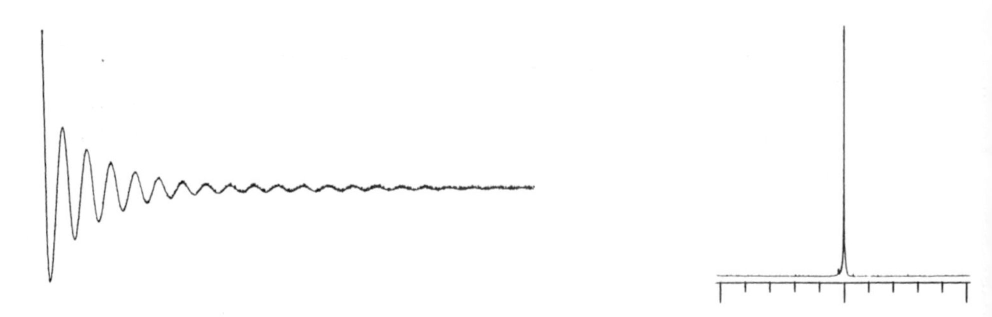

Fig. T15. Experimental free induction decay and corresponding spectrum of H_2O. The free induction decay has essentially decayed to zero at the end of the acquisition period.

Fig. T16. Experimental free induction decay and corresponding spectrum of H_2O. These data have been generated by truncating the free induction decay of Fig. T15. Note the presence of 'sinc wiggles' around the H_2O resonance.

resemblance to a 'sinc x' function (see **Fourier transform**) and is indeed related to it since the truncated free induction decay can be thought of as multiplication of the 'untruncated' free induction decay with a step function. The convolution theorem (see **convolution**) tells us that the convolution of two functions is given by the product of the Fourier transforms of each function. Thus the Lorentzian line is convoluted by the sinc function.

An analogous situation occurs if the receiver gain is set too high, resulting in overload of the **analogue-to-digital converter**. In this case the first few points of the free induction decay are truncated, which again result in lineshape distortions. Lineshape distortions such as these are known collectively as 'truncation artefacts'.

Two-dimensional Fourier transform The concept of a two-dimensional Fourier transform is central to the workings of all **two-dimensional NMR** experiments, and is a straightforward generalization of the one-dimensional **Fourier transform**.

A complex two-dimensional Fourier transform of a time-domain signal is given by

T32 $$S(\omega_1, \omega_2) = \int_{-\infty}^{\infty} \mathrm{d}t_1 \exp\{-\mathrm{i}\omega_1 t_1\} \int_{-\infty}^{\infty} \mathrm{d}t_2 \exp\{-\mathrm{i}\omega_2 t_2\} S(t_1, t_2),$$

and can be considered as two successive one-dimensional Fourier transforms. The time-domain signal may be a complex function (see **complex number**):

T33 $$S(t_1, t_2) = R_e[S(t_1, t_2)] + \mathrm{i}I_m[S(t_1, t_2)],$$

or may be composed only of the real part. In either case the two-dimensional spectrum is a complex function:

T34 $$S(\omega_1, \omega_2) = R_e[S(\omega_1, \omega_2)] + \mathrm{i}I_m[S(\omega_1, \omega_2)].$$

Two-dimensional NMR There is little doubt that the almost explosive revival of interest in high-resolution NMR techniques to study the structure and dynamics of biological macromolecules is due to the introduction of the technique known as two-dimensional NMR. Actually, this term collectively describes a large number of experiments, but nevertheless the basic principle is the same for each. Simply stated, the NMR spectrum is presented along two orthogonal frequency axes rather than one. This leads to an immediate advantage over conventional methods in the potential for a significant increase in spectral resolution. Indeed, it is probably true to say that the depressing appearance of conventional one-dimensional NMR spectra of macromolecules, in the form of a broad featureless envelope with few resolved resonances, may have led to a

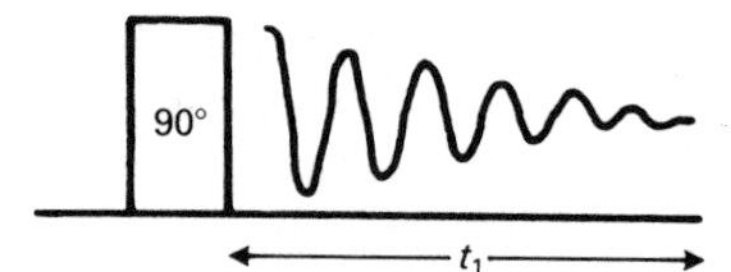

Fig. T17. The response of the spin system to an r.f. pulse is known as the free induction decay.

gradual lack of interest in the technique. The concept of two-dimensional NMR encompasses a variety of experiments, depending upon how the spin system is perturbed. Here, we will restrict the discussion to those experiments which involve exclusively the application of r.f. pulses, since these are presently the only experiments which are in general use in biological NMR. We therefore excluded perturbations involving e.g. **chemically induced dynamic nuclear polarization**. To begin, let us consider a simple pulse-and-collect NMR experiment. We apply a 90° r.f. pulse to a spin system which is initially at thermal equilibrium, and record the response, which is the **free induction decay** (Fig. T17). The free induction decay is actually time series data which are recorded as a function of the acquisition time t_1. **Fourier transformation** of the free induced decay then gives the frequency domain response or NMR spectrum (Fig. T18).

Since only one time domain is involved in this experiment, it follows that a single frequency dimension is obtained upon Fourier transformation. If we require an NMR spectrum in two frequency dimensions it therefore follows that we must record the data in two time domains. It is not intuitively obvious how we might achieve this, but consider an experiment where we simply repeat the pulse-and-collect sequence twice (Fig. T19). We now have two time domains. However, if we wait for the spin system to reach thernal equilibrium before applying the second pulse, then this is equivalent to **signal averaging** in conventional one-dimensional NMR. We therefore introduce a second requirement for two-dimensional NMR experiments: the second pulse must be applied to

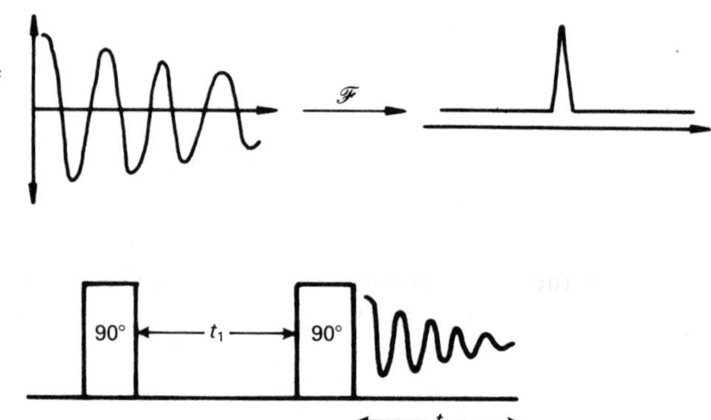

Fig. T18. Fourier transformation of the free induction decay generates the NMR spectrum.

Fig. T19. The basic two-dimensional NMR pulse sequence.

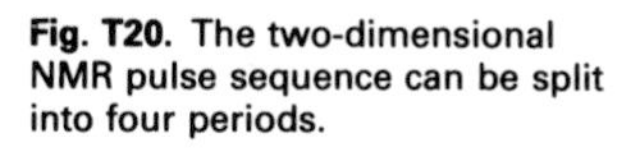

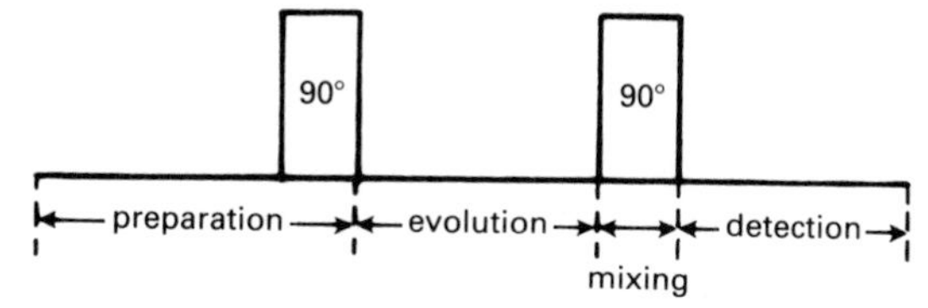

a spin system which is not at thermal equilibrium. In other words, we are probing spin systems in non-equilibrium states. This is a central concept of all two-dimensional NMR experiments. The differences between the various experiments depend precisely upon how the spin system is 'prepared' in its non-equilibrium state. To clarify this it is convenient to split the sequence of Fig. T19 into four discrete time periods (Fig. T20). During the preparation period, the system is 'prepared' in a suitable initial state. In this particular experiment, this simply consists of the creation of transverse magnetization. During the evolution period which may include additional pulses, the spin system evolves for a period t_1. During the mixing period, transfer of various coherences or polarization occurs. During the detection period, transverse magnetization created by the second pulse is observed with respect to t_2. This brings us to a tricky concept. In order to obtain a two-dimensional spectrum, we need to record data with respect to both t_1 and t_2. However, we cannot observe the evolution during t_1 and detect during t_2 simultaneously. Although we can record data in the t_2 time dimension directly, it is necessary to collect data in t_1 point by point. This is another concept which is central to a practical understanding of all two-dimensional NMR experiments. It is unfortunate that it is difficult to grasp at first. Let us try to clarify the situation with a practical example. Consider a simple pulse-and-collect experiment upon a sample of 2,5 anhydromannitol. After Fourier transformation of the free induction decay followed by **phase correction**, we obtain the conventional one-dimensional spectrum with all resonances in the absorption mode (Fig. T21). Now consider the two-pulse sequence of Fig. T19, where the two pulses of phase $+X$ are initially separated by a period t_1 which is very small, i.e. 1 μs. We can apply these pulses to the sample of 2,5 anhydromannitol and record the data during t_2 just as we would in a pulse-and-collect sequence. We can even repeat the P_1–t_1–P_2 sequence a given number of times in order to signal average the data (see **signal averaging**). After Fourier transformation with respect to t_2 we will see almost nothing since the P_1–t_1–P_2 sequence is essentially a 180° pulse. We therefore change the phase of the second pulse to $+Y$ for the purposes of this illustration without affecting its validity. We will store on disc the data corresponding to the 90_{+X}–t_1–90_{+Y} sequence for the first value of t_1. Next, suppose we increment t_1 by a fixed amount, the precise value of which will become clear shortly. The P_1–t_1–P_2 sequence can be

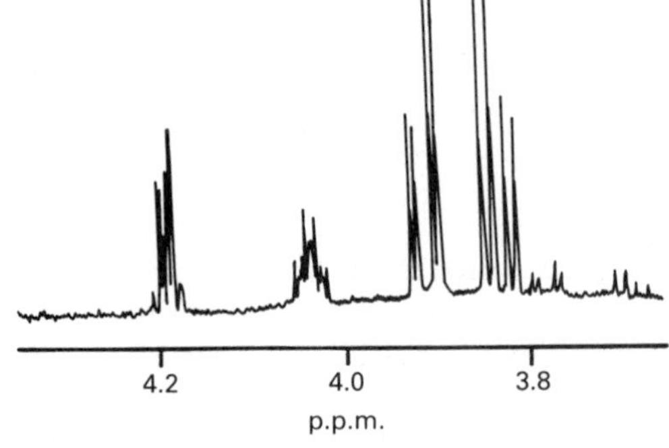

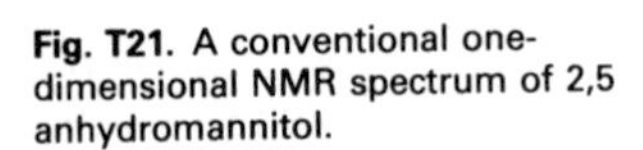

Fig. T21. A conventional one-dimensional NMR spectrum of 2,5 anhydromannitol.

repeated for this new value of t_1 and the data are again stored on disc. The value of t_1 is again incremented by the same amount, and so on until n free induction decays have been stored on disc, where n is the number of desired data points in the t_1 dimension. If, now, each free induction decay is Fourier transformed, the result is n one-dimensional spectra with respect to t_2. We must be careful to apply the same phase correction to each spectrum. The important point is that each spectrum will be different because each has been collected with a different value of t_1. In an abstract sense, each spectrum carries within it the 'memory' of events which occurred before t_2. The spectra recorded for the first four t_1 values of the two-pulse experiment of 2,5 anhydromannitol are shown in Fig. T22. If we consider a given point in each spectrum, e.g. that highlighted in Fig. T22, for all four spectra, and plot the intensity against t_1, we find that the intensity oscillates with a cosinusoidal modulation, and slowly decays due to relaxation during the increasing t_1 period. This modulation contains the frequency components with respect to t_1, of the point whose coordinate in t_2 is already defined in Fig. T22. In other words it is a free introduction decay with respect to t_1. If therefore we Fourier transform the oscillation in t_1, we will obtain a 'slice' of a two-dimensional NMR experiment with a frequency axis ω_1 (corresponding to the time period t_1) for a given value of ω_2 (corresponding to the time period t_2). A series of n such slices comprises the two-dimensional spectrum. We can thus see that the number of t_1 increments is the number of data points required in ω_1. Often n is made equal to the number of datapoints in ω_2 so that the resulting data matrix is symmetrical with respect to the data points. In addition, if the **sweep-width** in ω_1 is to be made equal to that in ω_2, it is necessary to arrange for the number of Hz per point to be the same in each dimension. This therefore determines by how much t_1 must be incremented each time we increase it. The increment must be made equal to the dwell-time between points defined by ω_2.

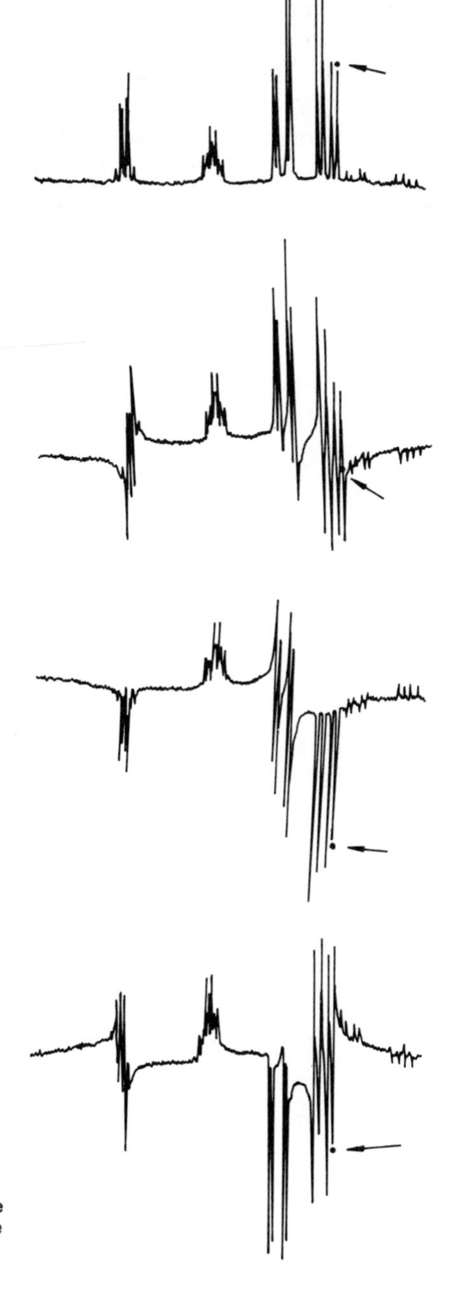

Fig. T22. Four spectra of 2,5-anhydromannitol derived from the pulse sequence of Fig. T19 Each spectrum corresponds to a sequential increment in t_1. The arrow indicates the cosinusoidal modulation of the datapoint at the peak of the lowest-field resonance line.

These are the basic principles common to all two-dimensional NMR experiments. A large variety of such experiments is now available which allow the experimenter to gain access to a variety of phenomena which can be observed with difficulty or not at all by conventional one-dimensional methods. Distributed through this volume can be found the details of the various experiments which are of value in biological NMR. In addition, the theoretical framework for an understanding of each experiment is described, and explicit reference is given to the various quantum mechanical terms where necessary.

U

Uncertainty principle There are several equivalent ways to define Heisenberg's uncertainty principle. A useful definition in terms of NMR states that the appropriate relationship between the two conjugate variables, frequency and time, is

U1 $$\Delta\nu\,\Delta t \sim 1.$$

Therefore, if we observe a phenomenon which exists in a given state for a time Δt, or we restrict observation to a time Δt, then the frequency resolution of this phenomenon is at most $\Delta\nu \sim 1/\Delta t$. This relationship recurs many times in NMR, and one manifestation is the phenomenon of uncertainty broadening of resonance lines during for example, **chemical exchange**.

Unitary transformation The equation of motion of the **density matrix** describes the time evolution of the spin system under various **Hamiltonians** corresponding to r.f. pulses and free precession periods. This equation is known as the Liouville–von Neumann equation

U2 $$\dot{\sigma} = -i\hbar^{-1}[\mathcal{H}, \sigma].$$

In order to derive an expression for the density matrix after a time t, during which $\mathcal{H}$ has been operative, it is necessary to integrate (U2). Assuming that $\mathcal{H}$ is time independent during the period t, the solution of (U2) is

U3 $$\sigma(t) = \exp\{-i\mathcal{H}t\}\sigma(0)\exp\{i\mathcal{H}t\}.$$

Since $\exp\{-i\mathcal{H}t\}$ and $\exp\{i\mathcal{H}t\}$ can be expressed in matrix form (see **matrix representation**), then (U3) is equivalent to

U4 $$\sigma(t) = U\sigma(0)U^{-1}$$

where $U = \exp\{-i\mathcal{H}t\}$. An equation such as (U4) is known as a unitary transformation of $\sigma(0)$ and can be thought of as a rotation of the density matrix. A series of such transformations is the basis by which the effects of various perturbations upon the spin system can be calculated (see **density matrix**).

Unity operator See **identity operator**.

V

Variational method Consider a system of two weakly coupled spins $\frac{1}{2}$. The **eigenfunctions** of this system consist simply of the four product functions (see **product basis**) $|\alpha\alpha\rangle$, $|\alpha\beta\rangle$, $|\beta\alpha\rangle$, $|\beta\beta\rangle$. In the case of **strong coupling** between the nuclei, these functions are no longer eigenfunctions of the **Hamiltonian** i.e. they are not stationary states. This is because the product functions $|\alpha\beta\rangle$ or $|\beta\alpha\rangle$ can no longer be assigned unequivocally to state 2 or 3, since they mix with each other. This mixing arises from the terms I_xS_x and I_yS_y in the full isotropic Hamiltonian, which cannot be neglected when the scalar coupling is of the order of the shift difference in Hz between the nuclei. It is therefore necessary to determine the type of function which should be chosen for states 2 and 3 in order for these to be eigenstates of the Hamiltonian. For this purpose the variational method is chosen. The wave function for each eigenstate is approximated by a linear combination of the form

V1 $$\psi_{2,3} = C_2\,|\alpha\beta\rangle + C_3\,|\beta\alpha\rangle.$$

We choose this form since ψ_2 and ψ_3 have certain characteristics of $|\alpha\beta\rangle$ and $|\beta\alpha\rangle$, which is intuitively what we might expect since the states mix. From this trial function we calculate the energy according to the quantum mechanical postulate

V2 $$E = \frac{\langle\psi|\,\mathcal{H}\,|\psi\rangle}{\langle\psi\,|\,\psi\rangle}.$$

The variational theorem states that the energy, E, obtained from (V2) will equal the actual value only when the trial function and the true wave function are identical. The best solution thus corresponds to a minimum in E. The best solution is obviously obtained when a variation of C_2 and C_3 no longer reduces E, i.e.

V3 $$\frac{\delta E}{\delta C_2} = \frac{\delta E}{\delta C_3} = 0.$$

We can thus proceed to calculate appropriate functions ψ_2, ψ_3 for the two-spin system by substituting (V1) into (V2):

V4 $$E = \frac{C_2^2\langle \alpha\beta|\,\mathcal{H}\,|\alpha\beta\rangle + C_2C_3\langle \alpha\beta|\,\mathcal{H}\,|\beta\alpha\rangle + C_3C_2\langle \beta\alpha|\,\mathcal{H}\,|\alpha\beta\rangle + C_3^2\langle \beta\alpha|\,\mathcal{H}\,|\beta\alpha\rangle}{C_2^2\langle \alpha\beta\,|\,\alpha\beta\rangle + C_2C_3\langle \alpha\beta\,|\,\beta\alpha\rangle + C_3C_2\langle \beta\alpha\,|\,\alpha\beta\rangle + C_3^2\langle \beta\alpha\,|\,\beta\alpha\rangle}.$$

Since each term in (V4) is a matrix element (see **bra-ket notation**, **matrix representation**), we can use the following abbreviations:

$$\mathcal{H}_{22} = \langle \alpha\beta|\,\mathcal{H}\,|\alpha\beta\rangle, \qquad \mathcal{H}_{23} = \langle \alpha\beta|\,\mathcal{H}\,|\beta\alpha\rangle$$

$$\mathcal{H}_{33} = \langle \beta\alpha|\,\mathcal{H}\,|\beta\alpha\rangle, \qquad H_{32} = \langle \beta\alpha|\,\mathcal{H}\,|\alpha\beta\rangle.$$

Using the identity $\mathcal{H}_{32} = \mathcal{H}_{23}$, and the orthonormalization conditions (see **orthonormal**), we find

V5 $$E = \frac{C_2^2\mathcal{H}_{22} + 2C_2C_3\mathcal{H}_{23} + C_3^2\mathcal{H}_{33}}{C_2^2 + C_3^2} = \frac{u}{v}.$$

According to (V3), (V5) must be partially differentiated with respect to C_2 and C_3, and the result set to zero. The rule for quotients gives

V6 $$\frac{\delta E}{\delta C_2} = \frac{1}{v}\left(\frac{\delta u}{\delta c_2} - \frac{u}{v}\cdot\frac{\delta v}{\delta c_2}\right)$$

and using (V5)

V7 $$= \frac{1}{v}\left(\frac{\delta u}{\delta c_2} - E\frac{\delta v}{\delta c_2}\right)$$

V8 $$= \frac{1}{C_2^2 + C_3^2}(2C_2\mathcal{H}_{22} + 2C_3\mathcal{H}_{23} - E2C_2).$$

Equation (V8) can only equal zero when

V9 $$(2C_2\mathcal{H}_{22} + 2C_3\mathcal{H}_{23} - E2C_2) = 0$$

i.e. when

V10 $$C_2(\mathcal{H}_{22} - E) + C_3\mathcal{H}_{23} = 0.$$

Similarly, calculation of $\delta E/\delta C_3$ gives

V11 $$C_2\mathcal{H}_{32} + C_3(\mathcal{H}_{33} - E) = 0.$$

Equations (V10), (V11) are often called secular equations. A system of homogeneous linear equations of this type has non-zero solutions for C_2, C_3 only if the secular determinant of the system is zero. In the above case this requirement is

$$\begin{vmatrix} \mathcal{H}_{22} - E & \mathcal{H}_{23} \\ \mathcal{H}_{32} & \mathcal{H}_{33} - E \end{vmatrix} = 0. \tag{V12}$$

In order to solve (V12), it is necessary to calculate explicitly $\mathcal{H}_{22}$, $\mathcal{H}_{23}$, $\mathcal{H}_{32}$, and $\mathcal{H}_{33}$ using the appropriate Hamiltonian. This procedure is explained for the strong coupling Hamiltonian under matrix representation, where the matrix elements are given explicitly (see (M36)). Inserting these values into equation (V12) we find

$$\begin{vmatrix} \{\frac{1}{2}(\omega_A - \omega_B) - \frac{1}{4}J\} - E & \frac{1}{2}J \\ \frac{1}{2}J & \{-\frac{1}{2}(\omega_A - \omega_B) - \frac{1}{4}J\} - E \end{vmatrix} = 0 \tag{V13}$$

Expanding the determinant gives the quadratic equation

$$E^2 + \tfrac{1}{2}JE - \tfrac{1}{4}(\omega_A - \omega_B)^2 - \tfrac{3}{16}J^2 = 0 \tag{V14}$$

which has solutions

$$E_{2,3} = -\tfrac{1}{4}J \pm \tfrac{1}{2}\sqrt{J^2 + (\omega_A - \omega_B)^2}. \tag{V15}$$

The coefficients in the trial function can now be calculated by substituting the solutions E_2 and E_3 into (V10) and (V11) respectively. For (V10) we find

$$C_2(\{\tfrac{1}{2}(\omega_A - \omega_B) - \tfrac{1}{2}\sqrt{J^2 + (\omega_A - \omega_B)^2}\}) + C_3 \,.\, \tfrac{1}{2}J = 0. \tag{V16}$$

The solution to (V16) can be found by defining an angle 2θ, such that

$$\cos 2\theta = \frac{(\omega_A - \omega_B)}{\sqrt{J^2 + (\omega_A - \omega_B)^2}}, \qquad \sin 2\theta = \frac{J}{\sqrt{J^2 + (\omega_A - \omega_B)^2}}. \tag{V17}$$

It follows from (V16) that

$$C_2(1 - \cos 2\theta) - C_3 \sin 2\theta = 0 \tag{V18}$$

and

$$C_2 = \frac{C_3 \sin 2\theta}{(1 - \cos 2\theta)}. \tag{V19}$$

Now since $\sin 2\theta = 2 \sin\theta \cos\theta$, $\cos 2\theta = \cos^2\theta - \sin^2\theta$, and $\cos^2\theta + \sin^2\theta = 1$, then the values for the coefficients can be obtained from (V19) together with the normalization condition $C_2^2 + C_3^2 = 1$:

$$C_2 = \cos 2\theta, \qquad C_3 = \sin 2\theta. \tag{V20}$$

An analogous calculation using E_3 gives for the coefficients

$$C_2 = -\sin 2\theta, \qquad C_3 = \cos 2\theta. \tag{V21}$$

Thus, the wavefunctions for states 2 and 3 are

V22 $$\psi_2 = \cos\theta\,|\alpha\beta\rangle + \sin\theta\,|\beta\alpha\rangle, \qquad \psi_3 = -\sin\theta\,|\alpha\beta\rangle + \cos\theta\,|\beta\alpha\rangle$$

and the states ψ_1 and ψ_4 are the same as those in the weak coupling case, since these do not mix:

V23 $$\psi_1 = |\alpha\alpha\rangle, \qquad \psi_4 = |\beta\beta\rangle.$$

The functions ψ_1, ψ_2, ψ_3, and ψ_4 are thus the eigenfunctions of the Hamiltonian for a strongly coupled two-spin system. In other words, the matrix of the strong coupling Hamiltonian will be diagonal when evaluated in this **eigenbasis**. More importantly, the **exponential operator** corresponding to this Hamiltonian will also be diagonal (see **matrix representation**).

Vector algebra See Appendix 3.

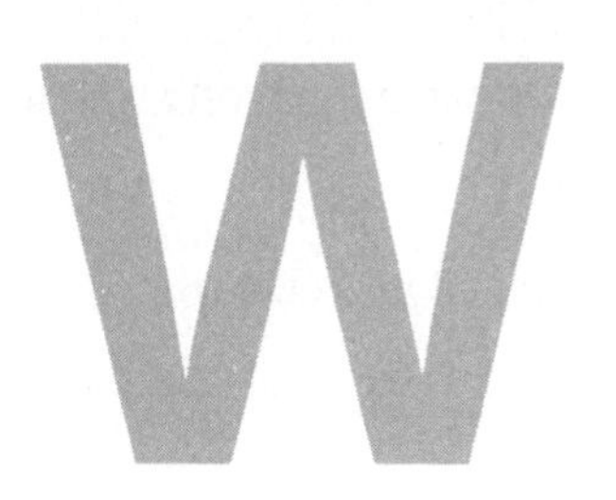

WAHUHA sequence See **average Hamiltonian theory**.

WALTZ See **broadband decoupling**.

Wavefunction See **Schrödinger equation**.

Weak coupling The **Hamiltonian** for a pair of scalar coupled spins IS is given by

W1 $$\mathcal{H} = \mathcal{H}_Z + \mathcal{H}_J = \omega_I I_z + \omega_S S_z + 2\pi J_{IS}\mathbf{I}\,.\,\mathbf{S}$$

where $\mathbf{I}\,.\,\mathbf{S} = I_x S_x + I_y S_y + I_z S_z$.

The scalar coupling Hamiltonian $\mathcal{H}_J = 2\pi J_{IS}\mathbf{I}\,.\,\mathbf{S}$ describes the interactions of the two nuclei via bonding electrons. Strictly, the Hamiltonian must be used in the form presented in (W1) in quantum mechanical calculations. However, when the magnitude of the spin coupling constant (J_{IS}) is much less than the magnitude of the difference in Larmor precession frequencies ($\omega_I - \omega_S$) of the spins, we can simplify (W1) using the weak coupling approximation. This derives from the fact that the off-diagonal elements of the matrix of $\mathcal{H}$ when evaluated in the **product basis** becomes negligible under this condition. Equation (W1) then simplifies to

W2 $$\mathcal{H} = \omega_I I_z + \omega_S S_z + 2\pi J_{IS} I_z S_z.$$

The importance of this approximation is that the **exponential operator** of $\mathcal{H}$, $\exp\{-i\mathcal{H}t\}$, is easily derived since all terms in (W2) commute (see **commutator**).

The weak coupling approximation is actually a manifestation of **averaging** in **spin space**. Clearly, the approximation is better in high magnetic field, where the chemical shift dispersion is greater. In the classical sense this means that NMR spectra can be interpreted in the first order i.e. scalar coupling is observed in terms of simple doublets, triplets, etc. This is decidedly advantageous when compared with spectra of strongly coupled systems (see **strong coupling**), where spin couplings must often be extracted by spectral simulation. Since NMR spectra of macromolecules are generally recorded at high field, weak coupling between spins is the rule rather than the exception.

Z

z-filter The z-filter is a pulse 'subsequence' which can be incorporated into several **two-dimensional NMR** experiments to obtain pure absorption-mode lineshapes. It is only of value when the procedures for the acquisition of **phase-sensitive experiments** are not applicable e.g. in **spin echo correlated spectroscopy** where lineshapes are inherently of mixed mode.

The z-filter consists of two 90° pulses separated by a variable delay τ. The first $\pi/2$ pulse converts in phase coherence components such as I_y (see **product operator formalism**) into polarization I_z (hence the term z-filter). All coherent components, which includes antiphase terms, which are present during τ are eliminated by **phase cycling** and variation of τ. The polarization terms (I_z) which are preserved during this procedure are reconverted into transverse magnetization by the second pulse. All coherences are in-phase, and pure absorption-mode spectra are obtained. Unfortunately, the procedure carries with it a sensitivity loss, together with the requirement for a longer phase cycle.

FURTHER READING

Sorensen, O. W., Rance, M., and Ernst, R. R. (1984). *J. Magn. Reson.* **56,** 527.

z-filtered correlated spectroscopy z-filtered COSY is related to both **nuclear Overhauser effect spectroscopy** (NOESY) and z–z spectroscopy. As the name suggests, the experiment consists essentially of the basic COSY experiment combined with a **z-filter**. In the basic COSY experiment, crosspeaks with simplified multiplet structure can be obtained with a mixing pulse of small flip-angle, but then diagonal peaks are found to have mixed-phase lineshapes, which are undesirable. The purpose of z-filtered COSY is to achieve absorption mode diagonal and crosspeaks with simplified multiplet structure.

The pulse sequence relevant to z-filtered COSY (z-COSY) is shown in Fig. Z1. The flip-angle β of the first pulse, although typically 90°, should be reduced if the repetition rate of the sequence is fast (compared to T_1) during **signal averaging**. The flip-angles β' must be small, typically 20°. With these conditions in mind, the workings of the experiment may be understood for a weakly coupled two-spin $\frac{1}{2}$ system *IS* (see **spin system**).

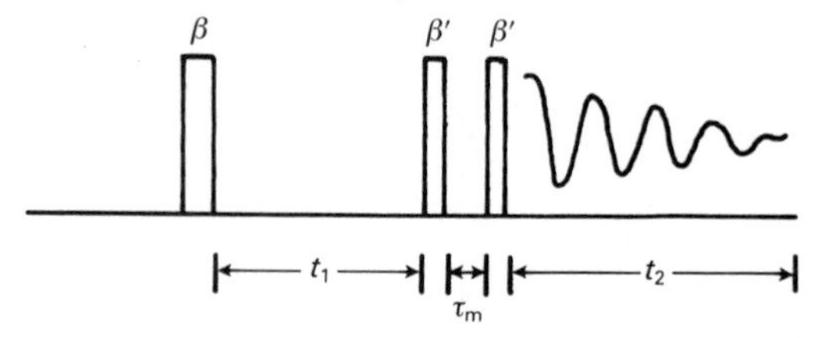

Fig. Z1. Pulse sequence for the acquisition of z-filtered COSY spectra.

As usual, it is convenient to employ the **product-operator formalism**. Assuming that the flip-angle β of the first pulse is 90°, transverse magnetization evolves during t_1 under spin couplings and chemical shifts to give at the end of the t_1 period.

Z1
$$\begin{aligned}\sigma_2 = &-I_y \cos \omega_I t_1 \cos \pi J_{IS} t_1 + 2I_x S_z \cos \omega_I t_1 \sin \pi J_{IS} t_1 \\ &+ I_x \sin \omega_I t_1 \cos \pi J_{IS} t_1 + 2I_y S_z \sin \omega_I t_1 \sin \pi J_{IS} t_1 \\ &- S_y \cos \omega_S t_1 \cos \pi J_{IS} t_1 + 2S_x I_z \cos \omega_S t_1 \sin \pi J_{IS} t_1 \\ &+ S_x \sin \omega_S t_1 \cos \pi J_{IS} t_1 + 2S_y I_z \sin \omega_S t_1 \sin \pi J_{IS} t_1.\end{aligned}$$

The second pulse of flip-angle β' then converts the various components in (Z1). For simplicity, we will consider only magnetization components corresponding to spin I without loss of generality. Thus after the second pulse, we find

Z2
$$\begin{aligned}\sigma_3 = &-I_y \cos \omega_I t_1 \cos \pi J_{IS} t_1 \cos \beta' - I_z \cos \omega_I t_1 \cos \pi J_{IS} t_1 \sin \beta' \\ &+ 2I_x S_z \cos \omega_I t_1 \sin \pi J_{IS} t_1 \cos \beta' - 2I_x S_y \cos \omega_I t_1 \sin \pi J_{IS} t_1 \sin \beta' \\ &+ I_x \sin \omega_I t_1 \cos \pi J_{IS} t_1 + 2[(I_y \cos \beta' + I_z \sin \beta') \\ &\times (S_z \cos \beta' - S_y \sin \beta')] \sin \omega_I t_1 \sin \pi J_{IS} t_1.\end{aligned}$$

During the mixing time, τ_m, which is very short such that exchange and NOE phenomena do not contribute to the final spectrum, all coherences are destroyed by phase cycling, leaving only populations just before the final pulse:

Z3
$$\sigma_4 = -I_z \cos \omega_I t_1 \cos \pi J_{IS} t_1 \sin \beta' + 2I_z S_z \sin \beta' \cos \beta' \sin \omega_I t_1 \sin \pi J_{IS} t_1.$$

After the final pulse of flip-angle β', we find

Z4
$$\begin{aligned}\sigma_5 = &-I_z \cos \omega_I t_1 \cos \pi J_{IS} t_1 \sin \beta' \cos \beta' + I_y \cos \omega_I t_1 \cos \pi J_{IS} t_1 \sin^2 \beta' \\ &+ 2[(I_z \cos \beta' - I_y \sin \beta')(S_z \cos \beta' - S_y \sin \beta')] \\ &\times \sin \beta' \cos \beta' \sin \omega_I t_1 \sin \pi J_{IS} t_1\end{aligned}$$

and the observable (see **observables**) magnetization components are given by

$$\sigma_{\text{obs}} = I_y \cos \omega_I t_1 \cos \pi J_{IS} t_1 \sin^2 \beta' - 2I_z S_y \cos^2 \beta' \sin^2 \beta' \sin \omega_I t_1 \sin \pi J_{IS} t_1 - 2I_y S_z \sin^2 \beta' \cos^2 \beta' \sin \omega_I t_1 \sin J_{IS} t_1. \quad \text{Z5}$$

After phase cycling of the final pulse we are left with the last two terms of (Z5), which evolve during t_2 to give observable antiphase magnetization. Remembering that only terms in I_x and I_y can give rise to observables, the terms in I_y are

$$\sigma'_{\text{obs}} = S_y \cos^2 \beta' \sin^2 \beta' \sin \omega_I t_1 \sin \pi J_{IS} t_1 \sin \pi J_{IS} t_2 \sin \omega_S t_2 + I_y \cos^2 \beta' \sin^2 \beta' \sin \omega_I t_1 \sin \pi J_{IS} t_1 \sin \pi J_{IS} t_2 \sin \omega_I t_2. \quad \text{Z6}$$

The first term in (Z6) is a crosspeak, and the second is a diagonal peak. Using the identity $\sin A \sin B = \frac{1}{2}(\cos(A - B) - \cos(A + B))$, we can rearrange (Z6) to give

$$\sigma'_{\text{obs}} = S_y \cos^2 \beta' \sin^2 \beta' \,.\, \tfrac{1}{2}[\cos(\omega_I - \pi J_{IS})t_1 - \cos(\omega_I + \pi J_{IS})t_1] \,.\, \tfrac{1}{2}[\cos(\omega_S - \pi J_{IS})t_2 - \cos(\omega_S + \pi J_{IS})t_2] + I_y \cos^2 \beta' \sin^2 \beta' \,.\, \tfrac{1}{2}[\cos(\omega_I - \pi J_{IS})t_1 - \cos(\omega_I + \pi J_{IS})t_1) \,.\, \tfrac{1}{2}[\cos(\omega_I - \pi J_{IS})t_2 - \cos(\omega_I + \pi J_{IS})t_2] \quad \text{Z7}$$

which describes antiphase absorption peaks in both dimensions. In contrast, diagonal peaks in **correlated spectroscopy** are in-phase dispersion. However, in z-COSY, both diagonal and crosspeaks are scaled by $\cos^2 \beta' \sin^2 \beta'$, and thus there is a loss in sensitivity compared with conventional COSY.

In order to suppress the undesirable responses described above, the phases of the first and third pulses are cycled (see **phase cycling**). To suppress axial peaks, the phase of the first pulse is alternated while the signals are alternately added and subtracted. In the τ_m period, coherences of all orders (except 0, 4, 8, etc.) are eliminated by phase cycling the last pulse and the receiver in 90° increments. Zero-quantum coherences are eliminated by stochastic variation of the duration of τ_m.

If the mixing time τ_m is deliberately lengthened, and the flip-angles β' are increased somewhat (~45°), an experiment known as z–z spectroscopy is obtained. Then the decay and diffusion of the second term in (Z3), which is known as longitudinal scalar two-spin order, can be followed during τ_m. This is the two-dimensional equivalent of a method for measuring dipolar relaxation in solids (the Jeener–Broekaert method). The $2I_zS_z$ term is not an oscillatory function of τ_m, but undergoes diffusion rather like conventional longitudinal magnetization in NOESY experiments. In the absence of any oscillatory dependence on

τ_m, lineshapes in z − z spectroscopy are obviously the same as those derived above for z-COSY.

FURTHER READING

Oschkinat, H., Pastore, A., Pfandler, P., and Bodenhausen, G. (1986). *J. Magn. Reson.* **69,** 559.

z-pulse Many important two-dimensional NMR experiments require phase shifts of the transmitter **carrier** through arbitrary angles other than 0, $\pi/2$, π, $3\pi/2$, which have been routinely used for many years. The most accurate method by which this can be achieved is by use of purpose built phase shifters. However, in the absence of such a device, a composite pulse known as the z-pulse can achieve the same effect. The composite z-pulse consists of the sequence

$$P = (\pi/2)_{\pi/2}(\beta)_0(\pi/2)_{3\pi/2}$$

where β is the flip-angle of the central pulse, which imparts a phase shift ϕ (within the x–y plane with respect to the x axis) upon the resulting magnetization. This is equivalent to a pulse β along the z axis of the rotating frame. The effect of the z-pulse may be understood geometrically (Fig. Z2). Beginning with transverse magnetization along the x axis, the first pulse creates $-z$ magnetization. The second pulse with arbitrary flip-angle β and phase $+x$ then rotates the magnetization vector through an angle β in the y–z plane. The final 90° pulse along the $-y$ axis rotates this magnetization into the xy plane with a phase β with respect to the x axis.

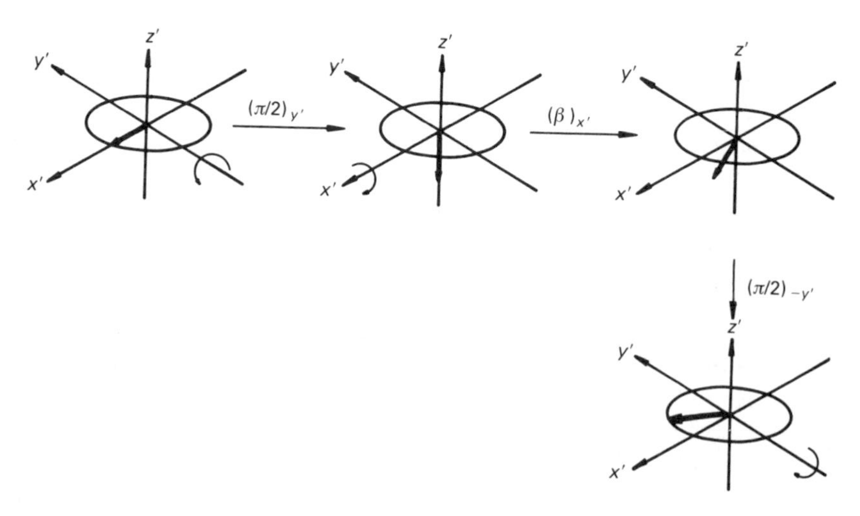

Fig. Z2. Diagram illustrating the effect of a z pulse. For details see text.

The accuracy of the z-pulse is limited by r.f. field inhomogeneity, and unless the latter is extremely good, the performance of the composite pulse will suffer. In all practical situations a purpose-built phase shifter will be found to give superior performance.

Zero-filling In general, an NMR spectrum composed of N data points is computed from a discrete **Fourier transform** of N acquired time-domain samples. However, under certain circumstances it may be desirable to compute amplitudes in the spectrum at intermediate frequencies. This can be achieved by sampling the time-domain data for a longer period. i.e. by increasing the block size of acquisition memory, or alternatively by supplementing the N time-domain samples by a string of samples with zero amplitude prior to Fourier transformation. This process is known as zero-filling. A common application of zero-filling is in **two-dimensional NMR** experiments where the number of t_1 increments is not a power of two. In these cases the **free induction decay** in t_1 is supplemented with zeroes such that the Fourier transformation algorithms can be applied in an efficient manner.

Extrapolation of time series data by a string of zeros is clearly inefficient since it is a poor representation of the 'authentic' signal. A rather more efficient procedure is the so called maximum entropy method (see **maximum entropy processing**) which nevertheless requires substantial computing time. Another useful method relies upon linear prediction, where the $N+1,\ N+2, \ldots, N+M$ absent sample points are represented in the form

$$K_{N+1} = a_0 K_N + a_1 K_{N-1} + \ldots + a_{M-1} K_{N-M+1} \quad \text{Z8}$$

which can be extrapolated iteratively to the desired number of datapoints. While both of these methods can improve the appearance of a spectrum considerably, it is difficult to overlook the zero-filling procedure in view of its simplicity.

FURTHER READING

Ernst, R. R., Bodenhausen, G., and Wokaun, A. (1987). *Principles of NMR in one and two dimensions,* p. 106. Claredon Press, Oxford.

Zero-quantum coherence Zero-quantum coherence arises when a state of **phase coherence** is created between two spin states with $\Delta M = 0$. In common with all orders of **multiple-quantum coherence**, zero-quantum coherences cannot be directly detected. The standard pulse sequence for the excitation of even-order coherences ($90°_x$–τ–$180°_y$–τ–$90°_x$) does not generate zero-quantum coherence in homonuclear weakly coupled two-spin systems. The simplest sequence $90°_x$–τ–$90°_x$ does excite zero-quantum coherence but the efficiency of excitation is not uniform since chemical shifts are not refocused. A simple modification of the first sequence, namely $90°_x-\tau-180°_x-\tau-45°_y$, does however excite zero-quantum coherence with reasonable efficiency.

The overall appearance of a two-dimensional zero-quantum correlated spectrum of a simple weakly coupled two-spin system is very similar to that of a double-quantum correlated spectrum of two weakly coupled spins. However, while double-quantum transition frequencies are composed of the sum of the **Larmor precession** frequencies of the spins, zero-quantum transition frequencies correspond with their difference. Correspondingly, since p-quantum coherences have p-fold sensitivity to shifts in r.f. phase, zero-quantum coherences are phase invariant. Although zero-quantum coherences offer attractive features such as lack of sensitivity to inhomogeneous magnetic fields, their insensitivity to r.f. phase shifts do not allow the separation of signals derived indirectly from zero-quantum coherence and from longitudinal polarization. Magnetization derived from the latter may as an example arise from relaxation during the t_1 period (see **axial peak**). The resulting peaks are very large in NMR spectra of macromolecules due to the short relaxation time, and consequently practical application of zero-quantum coherence experiments to such systems is limited.

FURTHER READING

For an application of zero-quantum correlated spectroscopy see
Müller, L. (1984). *J. Magn. Reson.* **59,** 326.

For a detailed discussion of zero-quantum correlated spectroscopy, see also
Pouzard, G., Sukumar, S., and Hall, L. D. (1981). *J. Am. Chem. Soc.* **103,** 4209.

z–z spectroscopy See **z-filtered** correlated spectroscopy.

Properties of cartesian product operators

1

The transformation properties of **angular momentum** operator products are fundamental to the workings of the **product operator formalism**. These transformations may conveniently be represented in cartesian space, resulting in the transformations illustrated in Fig. A.1.

A concept which is important in the derivation of **matrix representations** of operators is that of operator powers. For example, it is possible to operate upon a given state $|\alpha\rangle$ twice, using the same operator:

$$I_x^2\,|\alpha\rangle = I_x I_x\,|\alpha\rangle = I_x \tfrac{1}{2}\,|\beta\rangle = \tfrac{1}{4}\,|\alpha\rangle$$

and thus $I_x^2 = (\frac{1}{4})\,.\,\mathbf{1}$, where $\mathbf{1}$ is the unity operator. In a similar manner it

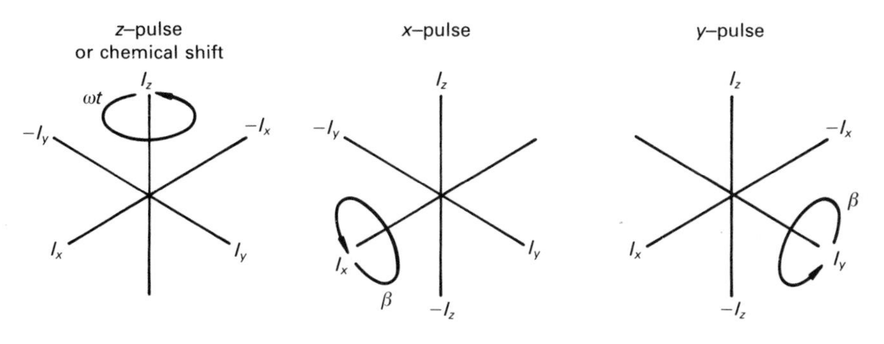

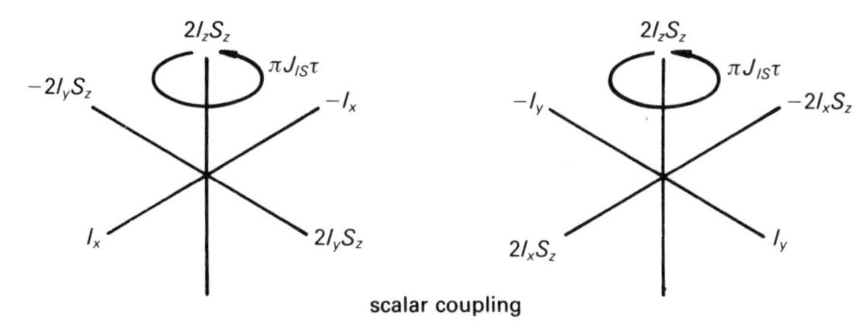

Fig. A1. Transformation properties of cartesian product operators.

can be shown that $I_y^2 = I_z^2 = (\frac{1}{4}) \, . \, \mathbf{1}$. Higher powers can be computed in the same manner, from which it will be seen that even operator powers contain the unity operator, whereas odd powers contain terms in I_x, I_y, and I_z, e.g.

$$I_y^3 = I_y I_y^2 = I_y (\tfrac{1}{4}) \, . \, \mathbf{1} = (\tfrac{1}{4}) I_y.$$

2 Trigonometric identities

The following are intended as an aid to the expansion of trigonometric terms during calculations using the **product operator formalism**:

$$\sin^2 A + \cos^2 A = 1$$

$$\sin(A \pm B) = \sin A \cos B \pm \cos A \sin B$$

$$\cos(A \pm B) = \cos A \cos B \mp \sin A \sin B$$

$$\sin A \cos B = \tfrac{1}{2}[\sin(A + B) + \sin(A - B)]$$

$$\cos A \sin B = \tfrac{1}{2}[\sin(A + B) - \sin(A - B)]$$

$$\sin A \sin B = \tfrac{1}{2}[\cos(A - B) - \cos(A + B)]$$

$$\cos A \cos B = \tfrac{1}{2}[\cos(A + B) + \cos(A - B)]$$

$$\sin 2A = 2 \sin A \cos A$$

$$\cos 2A = \cos^2 A - \sin^2 A$$

$$\sin^2 A = \tfrac{1}{2}(1 - \cos 2A)$$

$$\cos^2 A = \tfrac{1}{2}(1 + \cos 2A)$$

$$\cos A = (e^{iA} + e^{-iA})/2$$

$$\sin A = (e^{iA} - e^{-iA})/2i$$

$$e^{iA} = \cos A + i \sin A$$

$$e^{-iA} = \cos A - i \sin A$$

3 Matrix algebra

A common manipulation which is often required in the **density matrix** treatment of NMR is the product of two matrices. This is computed as follows:

3.1
$$\begin{pmatrix} a & b \\ c & d \end{pmatrix} \cdot \begin{pmatrix} e & f \\ g & h \end{pmatrix} = \begin{pmatrix} ae + bg & af + bh \\ ce + dg & cf + dh \end{pmatrix}$$

The rules for larger matrices can be derived in an obvious manner from the above.

A second manipulation which is often utilized is the direct product of two matrices. This is computed as follows:

3.2
$$\begin{pmatrix} a & b \\ c & d \end{pmatrix} \otimes \begin{pmatrix} e & f \\ g & h \end{pmatrix} = \begin{pmatrix} ae & af & be & bf \\ ag & ah & bg & bh \\ ce & cf & de & df \\ cg & ch & dg & dh \end{pmatrix}$$

and the resulting matrix has twice the number of rows and columns as the original matrices.

The trace of a matrix is defined as the sum of the diagonal elements. Thus, for the matrix on the right-hand side of equation (3.2),

3.3
$$\mathrm{Tr}[\mathbf{A}] = ae + ah + de + dh$$

where **A** represents this matrix. The bold notation indicates that **A** represents a matrix rather than a scalar variable.

The inverse of matrices commonly found in NMR theory are straightforward to compute. It is necessary simply to change the signs of the imaginary (see **complex number**) elements. Thus, if we define a matrix **A** such that

3.4
$$\mathbf{A} = \exp\{-\mathrm{i}\mathcal{H}t\} = \begin{pmatrix} \exp\{-\mathrm{i}E_1 t\} & 0 \\ 0 & \exp\{-\mathrm{i}E_2 t\} \end{pmatrix}$$

then

$$\mathbf{A}^{-1} = \exp\{\mathrm{i}\mathcal{H}t\} = \begin{pmatrix} \exp\{\mathrm{i}E_1 t\} & 0 \\ 0 & \exp\{\mathrm{i}E_2 t\} \end{pmatrix}$$

and $\mathbf{AA}^{-1} = \mathbf{1}$, the unit matrix.

4 Rotation operators

By use of the procedure described under **matrix representation**, the following rotation operators $\exp(\mathrm{i}F_x\alpha)$ may be derived for the various **spin systems** indicated. The inverses of these are obtained by changing the signs of the imaginary elements.

Abbreviations used are:

$$c = \cos(\alpha/2),\; s = \sin(\alpha/2),\; u = (\cos\theta + \sin\theta),$$
$$v = (\cos\theta - \sin\theta),\; \tan 2\theta = J_{nm}/(\omega_n - \omega_m).$$

AX SYSTEM

$$R_x = \begin{pmatrix} c^2 & ics & ics & -s^2 \\ ics & c^2 & -s^2 & ics \\ ics & -s^2 & c^2 & ics \\ -s^2 & ics & ics & c^2 \end{pmatrix}$$

AB SYSTEM

$$R_x = \begin{pmatrix} c^2 & iucs & ivcs & -s^2 \\ iucs & 1-u^2s^2 & -uvs^2 & iucs \\ ivcs & -uvs^2 & 1-v^2s^2 & ivcs \\ -s^2 & iucs & ivcs & c^2 \end{pmatrix}$$

AMX SYSTEM

$$R_x = \begin{pmatrix} c^3 & +isc^2 & +isc^2 & -s^2c & +isc^2 & -s^2c & -s^2c & -is^3 \\ +isc^2 & c^3 & -s^2c & +isc^2 & -s^2c & +isc^2 & -is^3 & -s^2c \\ +isc^2 & -s^2c & c^3 & +isc^2 & -s^2c & -is^3 & +isc^2 & -s^2c \\ -s^2c & +isc^2 & +isc^2 & c^3 & -is^3 & -s^2c & -s^2c & +isc^2 \\ +isc^2 & -s^2c & -s^2c & -is^3 & c^3 & +isc^2 & +isc^2 & -s^2 \\ -s^2c & +isc^2 & -is^3 & -s^2c & +isc^2 & c^3 & -s^2c & +isc^2 \\ -s^2c & -is^3 & +isc^2 & -s^2c & +isc^2 & -s^2c & c^3 & +isc^2 \\ -is^3 & -s^2c & -s^2c & +isc^2 & -s^2c & +isc^2 & +isc^2 & c^3 \end{pmatrix}$$

ABX SYSTEM

$$R_x = \begin{pmatrix} c^2 & isc^2u & isc^2v & -s^2c & isc^2 & -s^2cu & -s^2cv & -is^3 \\ isc^2u & c^3 - s^2c(u^2-1) & -s^2cuv & isc^2u & -s^2cu & isc^2 - is^3(u^2-1) & -is^3uv & -s^2cu \\ isc^2v & -s^2cuv & c^3 + s^2c(u^2-1) & isc^2v & -s^2cv & -is^3uv & isc^2 + is^3(u^2-1) & -s^2cv \\ -s^2c & isc^2u & isc^2v & c^3 & -is^3 & -s^2cu & -s^2cv & isc^2 \\ isc^2 & -s^2cu & -s^2cv & -is^3 & c^3 & isc^2u & isc^2v & -s^2c \\ -s^2cu & isc^2 - is^3(u^2-1) & -is^3uv & -s^2cu & isc^2u & c^3 - s^2c(u^2-1) & -s^2cuv & isc^2u \\ -s^2cv & -is^3uv & isc^2 + is^3(u^2-1) & -s^2cv & isc^2v & -s^2cuv & c^3 + s^2c(u^2-1) & isc^2v \\ -is^3 & -s^2cu & -s^2cv & isc^2 & -s^2c & isc^2u & isc^2v & c^3 \end{pmatrix}$$